PROFESSIONALISM AND ETHICS

Q & A SELF-STUDY GUIDE FOR MENTAL HEALTH PROFESSIONALS

Second Edition

D1354656

PROFESSIONALISM AND ETHICS

Q & A SELF-STUDY GUIDE FOR MENTAL HEALTH PROFESSIONALS

Second Edition

Laura Weiss Roberts, M.D., M.A.
Gabriel Termuehlen, B.A.

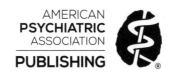

AMERICAN
PSYCHIATRIC
ASSOCIATION
PUBLISHING

American Psychiatric Association Publishing
800 Maine Avenue SW
Suite 900
Washington, DC 20024-2812
www.appi.org

Library of Congress Cataloging-in-Publication Data
Names: Roberts, Laura Weiss, 1960- author. | Termuehlen, Gabriel, author. | American Psychiatric Association Publishing, publisher.
Title: Professionalism and ethics : Q & A self-study guide for mental health professionals / Laura Weiss Roberts, Gabriel Termuehlen. \
Description: Second edition. | Washington, DC : American Psychiatric Association Publishing, [2022] | Includes bibliographical references and index.
Identifiers: LCCN 2021028088 (print) | LCCN 2021028089 (ebook) | ISBN 9781615373352 (paperback ; alk. paper) | ISBN 9781615373963 (ebook)
Subjects: MESH: Mental Health Services—ethics | Health Personnel—ethics | Professional Role
Classification: LCC RC455.2.E8 (print) | LCC RC455.2.E8 (ebook) | NLM WM 21 | DDC 174.2/9689—dc23
LC record available at https://lccn.loc.gov/2021028088
LC ebook record available at https://lccn.loc.gov/2021028089

British Library Cataloguing in Publication Data
A CIP record is available from the British Library.

Contents

CONTRIBUTORS

Paul S. Appelbaum, M.D.
Elizabeth K. Dollard Professor of Psychiatry, Medicine, and Law; Director, Center for Law, Ethics, and Psychiatry, Columbia University Vagelos College of Physicians and Surgeons, New York, New York

Glen O. Gabbard, M.D.
Clinical Professor of Psychiatry, Baylor College of Medicine, Houston, Texas

Max Kasun, B.A.
Roberts Ethics Lab, Department of Psychiatry and Behavioral Sciences, Stanford University School of Medicine, Stanford, California

Jane Paik Kim, Ph.D.
Clinical Assistant Professor, Department of Psychiatry and Behavioral Sciences, Stanford University School of Medicine, Stanford, California

Laura Weiss Roberts, M.D., M.A.
Katharine Dexter McCormick and Stanley McCormick Memorial Professor, Stanford University; Chair, Department of Psychiatry and Behavioral Sciences, Stanford University School of Medicine, Stanford, California

Gabriel Termuehlen, B.A.
Editor, Department of Psychiatry and Behavioral Sciences, Stanford University School of Medicine, Stanford, California

Thomas N. Wise, M.D., FACP
Professor of Psychiatry, Johns Hopkins University School of Medicine, Baltimore, Maryland; Professor of Psychiatry, George Washington University School of Medicine, Washington, D.C.

PREFACE

Every era of medicine has ethical challenges—some new, such as those we have experienced with the COVID-19 pandemic and effects of recent extreme weather events caused by climate change, and some not as new, such as those we face when determining how to uproot systemic barriers to equity in the workplace and in the provision of care, and how best to demonstrate respect for patients' cultural values, self-governance, and privacy. Psychiatrists, psychologists, therapists, and clinicians caring for people with mental health concerns encounter additional and specific ethical concerns, also both modern and ancient. Should a psychiatrist consider including artificial intelligence decision tools in her clinical practice, for example? How does one intervene with an exhausted, care-worn clinical colleague while maintaining appropriate boundaries? What are the best ways to support the autonomy of a patient who is living with a severe but intermittent disorder affecting mood and cognition? These are hard questions, and the answers are nuanced and dependent on multiple factors and context. For these reasons, mental health clinicians and trainees as well as practitioners in related health fields must understand the requirements of professionalism and cultivate a strong set of ethical decision-making skills.

This book is a second edition of an earlier text that sought to help clinicians and clinical trainees across the health professions to prepare for professional and ethical issues in their everyday work and education. We have structured the second edition to provide commentaries on the role of professionalism and ethics in clinical care, training, research, and leadership activities of mental health professionals. The first two chapters provide a brief overview of key elements of professionalism and ethics. These first chapters give essential guidelines, strategies, and best practices for mental health clinicians and trainees. Subsequent chapters proffer questions and answers based on terms, principles, and clinical, training, and research scenarios. The last chapter of the book provides dozens of questions that draw on content throughout the entire text.

We hope that this second edition will continue to be a resource of value to mental health professionals of different backgrounds and experiences at different points in their professional developmental paths.

This new edition includes updated references, expanded and revised introductory material on ethics and professionalism in the field of mental health, new clinical vignettes, and dozens of new questions and answers, covering timely and timeless topics, including assisted suicide, euthanasia, social media, technology, burnout, professional well-being, and belonging. The expanded bank of questions for review in Chapter 7 is intended to help readers to assess their knowledge and areas for further study.

This book would not be possible without the generous contributions of those who worked on the first edition. We wish to thank Jinger G. Hoop, M.D.; Teresa T. Anderson, M.D., M.A.; Robert A. Bailey, M.D.; Jerald Belitz, Ph.D.; Philip J. Candilis, M.D.; Carlyle H. Chan, M.D.; John H. Coverdale, M.D., M.Ed., FRANZCP; Cynthia M. A. Geppert, M.D., Ph.D., M.P.H.; Thomas W. Heinrich, M.D.; Joseph B. Layde, M.D., J.D.; Jon A. Lehrmann, M.D.; Teresita McCarty, M.D.; Joshua C. Reiher, B.A.; Ryan Spellecy, Ph.D.; Carol I. Tsao, M.D., J.D.; Paul S. Appelbaum, M.D., Laura B. Dunn, M.D.; Glen O. Gabbard, M.D.; Thomas N. Wise, M.D.; and Ann Tennier, E.L.S. for their work on the first edition. For the second edition, we also thank Jane Paik Kim, Ph.D., for her introductory comment and Max Kasun, B.A., for his diligent and thoughtful efforts in providing background literature and editing assistance.

Laura Weiss Roberts, M.D., M.A.
Gabriel Termuehlen, B.A.

INTRODUCTORY COMMENTS

Ethics can sometimes seem a bit ethereal. With its roots in philosophy and much talk of principles, virtues, and values, ethics may appear too distant from the everyday realities of clinical practice to warrant close attention by a busy mental health professional. There is, after all, so much other art and science to learn, so many skills that do not come naturally to the mind of a good person, as many imagine that ethical practice does. When it comes time to triage the hours of the day, it is understandable that time for serious ethical reflection often loses out.

But what an unfortunate result that is! Moreover, this outcome springs from a mistaken notion about the nature of ethics. Just as good people do not instinctively follow good diagnostic practices without the training required to do so, just as they cannot be expected to have an intuitive sense of interactions among medications without studying pharmacology, so good people are not necessarily able to avoid the pitfalls inherent in the ethical challenges ubiquitous in clinical work. Sound ethical practice, like good psychotherapy, requires a judicious mixture of theoretical knowledge, supervised learning, and reflective practice. And like most other aspects of the job of a clinician, learning ethics takes time and intellectual effort.

What is this body of knowledge that we call ethics? The dominant approach in mental health ethics today, which is reflected in this book, relies on a set of principles that embody actions representing moral goods. Such principles—autonomy, beneficence, justice, and fidelity among them—are part of the ordinary moral discourse of our professions and the broader society. In this view, ethical knowledge involves the ability to recognize the moral principles at play in a situation and, to the extent that different principles lead to varying courses of action, to reason through an approach to the situation that represents a justifiable prioritization of one principle or combination of principles over alternative formulations.

Consider just a sample of issues that have come across my desk recently from trainees and colleagues alike. How certain does a clinician have to be that child abuse has occurred at the hands of her patient to risk rupturing the therapeutic relationship by reporting her suspicions to the authorities? When is it appropriate, if ever, for a psychiatrist to conduct an internet search to learn more about a current or prospective patient? What information can a psychiatrist disclose to the police about a former patient, when that person is stalking the psychiatrist? How should a training program deal with a resident who has serious difficulties with supervisors and peers but whose treatment of patients seems unimpaired? To what parts of the psychiatric chart in an electronic health record should nonpsychiatric clinicians in a hospital or clinic have access to be able to provide the best care for patients? How far does a researcher have to go to protect a nonpatient participant who indicates that he is experiencing suicidal thoughts?

Far from an exhaustive list, this assortment of ethical conundrums reflects the slew of routine issues with which mental health clinicians, teachers, and researchers must cope. None would be worthy of discussion if they did not involve the opposition of principles that, taken on their own, would ordinarily point toward a clear path of action. Take the question of when to report suspected child abuse as an example. Standing alone, protecting the confidentiality of the clinical setting is ordinarily seen as a good in itself or reflective of other goods, such as fidelity to the patient's interests and respect for the patient as a person. But here in opposition to those desiderata is the well-being of a helpless child, who the clinician has reason to suspect is being endangered. Every state has codified a resolution of this ethical tension, requiring clinicians to report child abuse to the proper authorities, yet that does not fully settle the matter. How certain must the clinician be that abuse is occurring? Most states use word formulas with phrases such as "reasonable probability." Whatever such language conveys to the legal mind, it will often leave the clinician struggling to define when a probability is "reasonable" and to what extent the potential negative consequences of a report to the authorities—including the rupture of the dyadic bond on which treatment relies—can legitimately influence that conclusion. On which side are we to err, confidentiality or beneficent protection of the helpless? And on what basis can we defend our choice?

Didactic experiences of a classroom variety are in themselves unlikely to prepare clinicians to deal with challenges such as these. Whatever the benefits of extensive education in the history and theory of moral philosophy, most mental health professionals have neither the time nor the predilection for such training. Nor is it clear that even the best moral theoreticians would be well suited to confront the common dilemmas that clinicians must resolve. After all, ethical problems rarely come with clear labels attached or sort neatly into the categories beloved by authors of philosophical texts. No, this is a field in which pure theory takes one only so far.

How then to pursue the task? As clinicians, we recognize the importance of context in all aspects of our patients' lives, and the ethical dilemmas they present are no exception. The ethics of mental health practice, training, and research are best learned from situations that resemble those we face in our work, unavoidably shaped as they are by the rich details of the contexts in which they occur. We are surely not unique in that respect. Just as students of law gain most from analyzing actual legal cases and students of business focus on travails of real corporations, so clinical situations help us think through issues in ways that transfer meaningfully to our subsequent work with patients. Within the rich contexts of real life, general principles are easier to appreciate and apply and are more likely to be imprinted for future use. And the complexity of the situations that we study belies any efforts at ethical reductionism. These are inescapably complicated and difficult challenges, presenting choices that often represent significant trade-offs regardless of the course chosen.

Ideally, we might each have a tutor in ethics to accomplish this task, someone with a broad knowledge of ethical theory and an equally wide experience in dealing with the ethical dilemmas of mental health practice, training, and research. When a problem arose, we would turn to this person for guidance, learning to identify the relevant facts, clarify the principles involved, and reason to a satisfying conclusion. Few of us, however, are so blessed. Instead, we must search for more prosaic alternatives to that wise mentor.

Therein lies the value of this book and its interactive, case-oriented approach to mental health ethics. The brief case descriptions that frame each ethical question echo the real-life complexities of clinical practice. The questions test the reader's reasoning and sharpen his or her ability to engage in ethical thought. And the explanations following each question offer background information about relevant ethical concepts, related legal and clinical considerations, and suggestions for further reading. Taken as a whole, it is a most congenial and effective way for both trainees and more experienced mental health professionals to develop and polish their ethical skills.

Not even a text as useful as this one will confer on us all the knowledge and experience we need to feel confident in our ethical judgments. We must still dip into the literature of clinical ethics, consult with colleagues when tough cases come along, and inevitably make mistakes and, one hopes, learn from them. But this book is a decidedly useful vehicle to carry us down that road and to make us more accomplished professionals in the process.

Paul S. Appelbaum, M.D.
Elizabeth K. Dollard Professor of Psychiatry, Medicine, and Law; Director, Center for Law, Ethics, and Psychiatry, Columbia University Vagelos College of Physicians and Surgeons, New York, New York

When the first edition of *Professionalism and Ethics: Q & A Self-Study Guide for Mental Health Professionals* appeared in 2008, Dr. Laura Roberts' book was a highly regarded text sought out by both experienced clinicians and students from all mental health disciplines. It appeared at an auspicious time, when professionalism and ethics were gaining increasing importance in the day-to-day work of psychiatrists, psychologists, social workers, and other mental health professionals. The first edition reflected a quiet revolution that was occurring—in particular, it signaled the arrival of professionalism as deserving of a place alongside the other core competencies. Problem-based learning, didactic courses on ethical dilemmas, an emphasis on the doctor-patient relationship, and other innovations were appearing in the curricula of medical schools. Arnold and Stern (2006) have defined professionalism as follows: "Professionalism is demonstrated through a foundation of clinical competence, communication skills, and ethical and legal understanding, on which is built the aspiration to, and wise application of, the principles of professionalism: excellence, humanism, accountability, and altruism" (p. 19).

As a result of this sea change, professionalism and ethics are now universally considered essential to those in the field of mental health. There is a broad understanding that gaining the patient's confidence with respect, empathic listening, and compassion is the groundwork that must be laid to optimize the clinical encounter. There is an altruism inherent in this position—that is, practitioners must consider their own needs as secondary to those of the patient. As was true of the first edition, Dr. Roberts has provided wonderful clinical vignettes to help the reader actively think through options and their potential consequences in the clinical setting. Similarly, she takes the reader through the complexities involving conflicts of interest in research, the difficult tasks of assigning authorship, the need for disclosure, and other dilemmas that both students and experienced researchers will find of great value.

In this new, second edition, Dr. Roberts also presents new content that will be welcomed by both researchers and clinicians, not to mention educators. One of the most controversial and thorny aspects of ethics is assisted suicide and euthanasia. This area is complicated by religious views, the complexity of informed consent, and the concern that some who choose euthanasia may be clinically depressed. Another area that has presented new challenges for all practitioners emerges from the digital revolution. How does one navigate social media and the loss of anonymity, not to mention self-disclosure of all kinds? Another area that has recently been the subject of much discussion among ethicists is the increasing frequency with which clinicians may be "googling" their patients. Questions have arisen regarding the lack of concern for patient privacy, the voyeurism of the professional, and the absence of consent.

Another new area in this second edition is the unprecedented rise in problems of burnout and professional well-being. What are reasonable limits in an era of the electronic health record and increased expectations of physicians? The delicate task of reporting impaired colleagues is also addressed in this edition. In addition, neuroethics is also carefully considered. What about artificial intelligence and algorithms? What about the ethics of gene editing technology? Novel modes of prediction, evaluation, and treatment are addressed, and further information on ethical peer review is also taken up.

Throughout the book there are questions that are raised for contemplation. This new edition of *Professionalism and Ethics* is a superb text for clinicians of all mental health disciplines. Trainees will find it essential for their education. It will answer questions while also raising consciousness about dilemmas that have no easy answer. I highly recommend it for the shelves of all clinicians who must ponder the complexities of the human psyche.

Glen O. Gabbard, M.D.
Clinical Professor of Psychiatry, Baylor College of Medicine, Author of Professionalism in Psychiatry

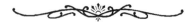

The field of psychiatry has evolved drastically since the last edition of *Professionalism and Ethics*. The BRAIN 2020 initiative has brought to the forefront the most innovative neurotechnologies, as well as machine learning and artificial intelligence, which offer great promise in realizing the goals of modern medicine. Additionally, the COVID-19 pandemic has dramatically elevated the need for and use of telehealth and digital psychiatry. No longer confined to in-person encounters, physicians can implement a myriad of digital tools, including telemedicine, smartphone applications, and wearable devices. Information technology has changed in parallel: protected health information is transferred at high volumes from patients to health providers and third-party for-profit entities, and to and from cloud servers in which machine learning and artificial intelligence algorithms are deployed. Such algorithms, enabled by increases in computing speed and power and breakthroughs in deep learning algorithm development, have the ability to improve accurate diagnoses, predict preventable health events, and make personalized treatment recommendations for individuals.

The potential for artificial intelligence applications, specifically machine learning, to prevent, predict, manage, and even cure disease sparks immense hope for the future of health care (Abràmoff et al. 2018; Esteva et al. 2017; Gulshan et al. 2019; McKinney et al. 2020; Yeung et al. 2018, 2019). And yet, we must consider the new ethical issues posed by algorithmic medicine and algorithmic psychiatry. Professionals must remain aware of the latest developments in the research landscape, including revisions to the common rule. New technological innovations will also require an understanding of data privacy and confidentiality. Professionals must consider the risks and benefits posed by data and information handling by multiple agents. Further on the horizon, and less evident at the moment, professionals will need to know how to interoperate with artificial intelligence systems, and, in particular, how to understand the origins of data and algorithms and how to follow protocols related to technology and information sharing.

Outside of medicine, algorithms are already playing a role in human decision-making in unprecedented ways, from human resources to criminal courts (Barocas and Selbst 2016). And, yet, little is known about how algorithms perform in comparison with human judgment in complex situations (Dressel and Farid 2018). Of greater concern, there is now wide recognition that algorithms may reflect, reproduce, and perpetuate bias, which has prompted an explosion of theoretical and empirical research in the field of machine learning reflecting concerns about fundamental issues of fairness, justice, and bias (Barocas and Selbst 2016; Bolukbasi et al. 2016; Buolamwini and Gebru 2018; Chouldechova 2016; Corbett-Davies et al. 2017; Dressel and Farid 2018; Flores et al. 2016; Garg et al. 2017; Jackson et al. 2019; Jiang and Nachum 2019; Nachum and Jiang 2019). These concerns foreshadow the ethically laden arguments that are certain to emerge as algorithms become increasingly common in health care. An understanding of how unconscious bias in humans can propagate through algorithmic systems will be acutely necessary in the medical professions. Psychiatrists and emergency medicine physicians will be the first adopters of machine learning systems, and thus remain at the forefront of this crucial ethical issue.

The new edition of *Professionalism and Ethics* introduces ethical concepts related to algorithmic medicine in an engaging and proactive way. Dr. Roberts and colleagues present questions and answers that will allow health professionals to navigate this new, important territory. New content speaking to professionalism and wellness is also featured. Such content is especially salient and timely, given mental health care needs and unprecedented work conditions due to a devastating combination of biological and social traumas seen in 2020, namely, the COVID-19 pandemic and racism, police brutality, and violence against Black and minority communities. This new material on wellness is timely and its importance cannot be understated.

Dr. Roberts and colleagues have compiled a collection of forward-thinking content portrayed in a challenging question-and-answer format that allows the reader to think in real time and respond—providing an opportunity for learning in and of itself, through the act of showing, before telling. Although the application of ethics in clinical care and medical research is best learned through tangible and concrete lived experiences, this book provides a critical opportunity and point of learning to prepare professionals for challenges in care and research. It also offers a concrete tool and reference that will enable many in the profession, on all stages of the career path, to work toward the goal of improving global mental health with the utmost care and respect.

Jane Paik Kim, Ph.D.
Clinical Assistant Professor, Department of Psychiatry and Behavioral Sciences, Stanford University School of Medicine, Stanford, California

Professionalism has now been identified as one of the six core competencies for residency education, and it has been defined as consisting of three domains: commitment to carrying out professional responsibilities, adherence to ethical principles, and sensitivity to diverse patient populations (Andrews and Burruss 2004). Bioethics overlaps with professional responsibility and may be considered the theoretical framework for professional behavior. The foundations of moral reasoning in patient care include respect for autonomy, nonmaleficence, beneficence, and justice (Beauchamp 1999). Only through ongoing and reinforcing discussions will trainees fully understand and incorporate the essential values and behaviors inherent in this concept of professionalism. Such teaching typically begins with a top-down outline of the basic principles of moral reasoning. This must be accompanied by a bottom-up analysis of specific cases. Volumes such as this one should therefore be introduced during the clinical clerkship and then utilized at all levels of postgraduate training.

A major training goal for nascent physicians is to understand the very clear historical and current professionally legislated contract within the physician-patient relationship. The word *patient* is used advisedly in this context. Slavney and McHugh (1987) discussed the issue of our mental health colleagues (as well as some psychiatrists) utilizing the term *client* in lieu of *patient*. Labeling individuals as clients suggests superficial understanding of psychiatric disorders and also connotes the notion of *caveat emptor* ("let the buyer beware"). This is a distortion of the medical professional relationship, and it does not reduce our fundamental fiduciary responsibility to those we treat. The ideal of *primum nocere* ("first do no harm") highlights the difference between the concepts of clients and patients and suggests professionals' true covenant with patients. This covenant has roots in the Hippocratic oath, which includes a code of duties to patients and obligations to teachers and colleagues (Andrews and Burruss 2004). This responsibility does not limit patient autonomy but is the foundation that governs physicians' behaviors and treatment approaches.

Chapter 4 of this book, "Ethics and Professionalism in Clinical Care," may be the most compelling for students who are currently immersed in clinical care. One of the more confusing moral issues for psychiatric trainees is the inequity in psychiatric care due to financial and systemic barriers. This is often an issue in our current health care system, which lacks universal access and in which managing care is often more focused on financial considerations rather than on clinically relevant evidence. Use of datasets that give quantitative guidelines for length of stay are often inaccurate and can lead to limited hospital lengths of stay or inadequate outpatient management. Alternatively, unlimited fee for service may foster financial incentives for the practitioner (Hellinger 1996). Another problematic issue arises from the competing theoretical models that psychiatry employs, which complicates trainees' ability to understand what is the best care: although the disease perspective is currently predominant, as demonstrated by advances in biological psychiatry and the importance of DSM iterations in diagnostic classification, the life-story methodology is often what attracts students to psychiatry (Slavney and McHugh 1985). However, biological and developmental explanations for a patient's problems need not be contradictory and can complement each other. Nevertheless, students can become confused when their teachers hold strong views of what constitutes the best approach. The solution is for all students to have a firm grounding in the different perspectives of psychiatry, including the strengths and weaknesses of each. Two outstanding volumes that cover these issues should be required reading for all residents: Ghaemi's *The Concepts of Psychiatry: A Pluralistic Approach to the Mind and Mental Illness* (Ghaemi 2003) and McHugh and Slavney's *The Perspectives of Psychiatry* (McHugh and Slavney 1998).

The role of psychotherapy in healing is fascinating, but unless practitioners understand transference and countertransference, dangers can arise and ethical boundary violations can occur. Thus, those teaching psychodynamic issues must focus on both the patient's and the trainee's reactions (Coburn 1997; Smith 1984; Springmann 1989). This seems to be common sense, but with the current emphasis on short-term treatments and medically oriented management, these essential elements can be minimized in curricula. One problem with the use of psychotherapy is that we have not really defined the optimal dosing of these interventions. For example, should an individual who is "medication managing" a patient see that patient every 6 months or on a more frequent basis? The answer should depend on the patient's clinical status and on the other treatment options available, but some practitioners tend to underutilize careful follow-ups in this age of managed care. A second problem occurs when individuals tend to see patients on a very frequent basis but are not fully trained to manage the transference and countertransference phenomena that arise in such intense psychotherapy relationships. Such therapeutic situations can develop into extremely dependent transferential relationships with untoward results (McHugh 1994).

It is also problematic when physicians use unorthodox tests and bio-logical treatments. (This does not refer to the common use of rational polypharmacy or off-label indications of psychotropics that have a reasonable evidence basis.) Students often see patients managed in a nonsystematic manner, with both biological and psychological interventions that make no clinical sense and do not help patients. Trainees must learn how to respond to such situations, which may result in an uncomfortable confrontation with a colleague. Similarly, when practitioners learn of individuals treated unsuccessfully for weeks to months by therapists who fail to recommend biological interventions with proven efficacy, privately complaining about the therapist is not as helpful as finding methods to educate the person or intervening in other ways. Emerging new technologies also pose ethical challenges that can be helpful adjunctive elements to care or harm when used (Torous and Roberts 2017). There are no easy answers for these and many other situations psychiatrists face, and they pose special challenges that should be considered in training (Talbott and Mallott 2006).

Psychiatrists who practice within hospital settings are easily scrutinized by peers for significant aberrations from accepted practice. Such aberrations or sentinel events as defined by the Joint Commission (formerly Joint Commission on Accreditation of Healthcare Organizations) mandate investigation into the quality and competence of the practitioner. The office-based practitioner, on the other hand, is quite independent from such attention—a fact that requires ongoing discussion during training, not just a single lecture about ethics. The isolation of full-time office-based practice should be mitigated with peer supervision groups, clinical faculty appointments, or work in community mental health settings or hospitals. Ethics curricula in psychiatric residencies may ignore "hidden" issues that are not considered but potentially arise when the trainee enters clinical practice (Gupta et al. 2016).

In the past, the practice of medicine was a more personally autonomous enterprise, regulated only by other members of the profession (Freidson 1970). Such self-determination among mental health practitioners has begun eroding, as external forces have begun to shape decisions about therapeutic options as well as professional sanctions (McHugh 1996). In Chapter 4 of this volume, "Ethics and Professionalism in Clinical Care," a vignette concerning the management of a suicidal patient whose insurer demands an early discharge cuts to the core of a dilemma facing contemporary hospital psychiatrists and should spark discussion in any hospital-based curriculum. The need to provide acute crisis management and stabilization has become the operant mode for the general hospital psychiatric program. Treatment is often limited to symptomatic change, rapidly followed by discharge. Sadly, it is all too easy to continue documentation that a patient is verbalizing self-harm when, in fact, the patient needs a few more days of stabilization but is not actively suicidal. Although one strategy is to phone the insurance reviewer and explain the need for continuing hospitalization, such feedback often falls on deaf ears and leads to further conflict. Furthermore, an increasing number of hospitals pressure physicians and psychiatric programs to reduce length of stay in an era of declining hospital benefits and increased indigent care. This points out the reality that psychiatric ethics is complex and often beset by a form of moral relativism. What is best for the patient is often not fully possible, and there are no easy answers (Beauchamp 1999).

As demonstrated by Chapter 5, "Ethics and Professionalism in Medical Research," medical research also raises many ethical questions. For example, is it ever ethical to use placebo arms in clinical trials of patients with significant psychiatric disorders? Institutional review boards struggle with such questions daily. Managing relationships with pharmaceutical companies is another challenge, particularly in academic settings (Schneider et al. 2006; Wofford and Ohl 2005), and is touched on in Chapter 6, "Ethics and Professionalism in Interactions With Colleagues and Trainees." The goal of the pharmaceutical company is to sell its products, and residents and faculty should remember that there is quite literally "no free lunch" (www.no-free-lunch.org). It may be easy to exclude pharmaceutical representatives from the training site, but residents will often see them at conferences and after work at industry-sponsored dinners. Shielding trainees from industry relationships entirely will not serve them well when they enter independent practice. One reasonable approach is to educate residents about the problems with industry-sponsored studies that often employ questionable statistics, dosing strategies, and patient selection to make a product seem better than alternatives. This kind of education will allow trainees to better assess the data they receive from industry programs and representatives.

A final topic to initiate early in training is how the resident can engage in lifelong learning, an essential aspect of professionalism. Although one of the core competencies is medical knowledge obtained and mastered during training, lifelong learning is essential given the rapidly changing advances in medical and psychiatric knowledge. It is increasingly easy to obtain and retrieve current medical knowledge through electronic journals and textbooks that allow the practitioner to have a sophisticated medical library on his or her desktop. Such resources are very often inexpensive, and it is not clear why all clinicians do not use them. The psychiatric trainee should easily incorporate knowledge acquisition as an essential part of professional practice if it is emphasized throughout their training.

In closing, this book offers a wonderful methodology for the beginning of training individuals in the basic construct of professionalism as a core competency in medicine, as well as for instilling the need for ongoing consideration of ethical behaviors and principles in the daily practice of psychiatry.

Thomas N. Wise, M.D., FACP
Professor of Psychiatry, Johns Hopkins University School of Medicine, Baltimore, Maryland; Professor of Psychiatry, George Washington University School of Medicine, Washington, D.C.

PART I

ETHICS AND PROFESSIONALISM

CHAPTER 1

ETHICS, PROFESSIONALISM, AND THE FIELD OF MENTAL HEALTH

An Overview

Laura Weiss Roberts, M.D., M.A.
Max Kasun, B.A.
Gabriel Termuehlen, B.A.

Ethics is an endeavor.
It refers to ways of understanding
what is good and right in human experience.
It is about discernment, knowledge and self-reflection,
and it is sustained through seeking, clarifying, and translating.
It is the concrete expression of moral ideals in everyday life.
Ethics is about meaning, and it is about action.

Laura Weiss Roberts (2002a)

This chapter has been adapted from Roberts LW, Hoop JG, Dunn LB: "Ethical Aspects of Psychiatry," in *The American Psychiatric Publishing Textbook of Clinical Psychiatry*, 5th Edition. Edited by Hales RE, Yudofsky SC. Washington, DC, American Psychiatric Publishing, 2002, pp. 1601–1636; and Belitz J: "On Professionalism," in *Professionalism and Ethics: Q&A Self-Study Guide for Mental Health Professionals*. Edited by Roberts LW, Hoop JG. Washington, DC, American Psychiatric Publishing, 2008. The authors would like to acknowledge Laura Bodin Dunn, M.D., Cynthia M.A. Geppert, M.D., Ph.D., M.P.H., and Jerald Belitz, Ph.D.

ETHICS AND PROFESSIONS

Ethics is a formal branch of philosophy that examines, evaluates, and seeks to more deeply understand the moral aspects (the right and wrong) of human nature and action. Within the profession of medicine, ethics has become an applied discipline, with a basis in emerging evidence as well as in historical concepts that have endured and evolved over many centuries. The fields of clinical and research ethics encompass the principles, virtues, values, decision-making approaches, accepted and expected behaviors, and rules of conduct that are fundamental to the modern profession of medicine, and the biomedical sciences, in our society.

A profession is a set of individuals who possess a distinct expertise and have been entrusted to serve a special role, with specific obligations, rights, and privileges (Roberts 2016). A central commitment of a profession is to ensure that its members possess specialized knowledge and skills and that these are used to fulfill the positive role of the profession in society. In the profession of medicine, members are concerned with activities in support of the societal aim of promoting health and diminishing disease and suffering. This is a diverse endeavor that includes engaging in the practical work of clinical care and biomedical research—generating new knowledge through inquiry; imparting expertise (both cognitive and technical skill) across the field and to the next generation of professionals; evaluating the competence of professionals and professionals in training (e.g., through specialty examinations and licensure standards); providing leadership and advocacy—and recognizing, remediating, or rooting out members who are not capable of acting or, irrespective of ability, who do not act in accordance with the expectations of the field. The vitality and legitimacy of a profession rely on cultivating a membership that reflects the broader makeup of society, appointing members of marginalized groups to positions of leadership, and detecting and reducing bias and inequity through continual, honest, and robust self-analysis.

A profession itself has moral importance because of the trust and privileges conferred on it by society as a whole. Being a member of a profession has moral standing because society requires that professionals possess certain qualities and adhere to a specific set of duties. The reasons for this are self-evident: a surgeon may cut another person with a knife so long as he possesses appropriate expertise and his intent is to help the patient or to lessen the patient's suffering. This is true even at times when consent is not possible (e.g., an unconscious trauma victim) and even if there is a poor outcome not due to negligence. Under nearly all other imaginable circumstances in everyday life, cutting another person with a knife would be considered assault. Similarly, in the course of psychotherapy, a psychologist may learn of the most deeply held private thoughts of a patient, including suicidal or homicidal fantasies or intended unlawful behavior; the psychologist in this situation is entrusted with preserving the confidentiality of the patient unless the patient expresses a specific and immediate threat to another person. A consultation-liaison psychiatrist may assess the decisional capacity of a seriously ill patient and determine that he or she is not able to decline recommended treatment. The psychiatrist, furthermore, may under certain circumstances insist that the patient undergo treatment, for example, be hospitalized or given medications against his or her preferences. These violations of the liberty of another person would not be tolerated in society under nearly all other circumstances. These violations are only tolerated because of the expectation of absolute adherence to the moral underpinnings of the profession in support of societal goals. In this case, the psychiatrist is assumed to be acting in service toward the well-being of the patient.

Medical professionals are expected to act according to an integrated set of values such as beneficence and justice and to demonstrate trustworthiness repeatedly and consistently. Distinct professional behaviors are generative of distinct types of trust, all of which are necessary in professional formation (McCullough et al. 2020). Intellectual trust, the commitment to scientific and clinical excellence, is generated by patients' confidence that clinicians are competent in diagnosing and treating their conditions, with mastery of the vocabulary and reasoning methods of their field. Intellectual trust also requires that patients actively rely on clinical competence. Moral trust is generated through the systematic privileging of the health-related interests of patients over the self-interests of organizations. Forms of organizational self-interest, such as financial incentives, may be necessary but must be kept secondary to patient interests. Moral trust also requires that patients rely on health professions' moral commitments. Both intellectual and moral trust, therefore, are sustained ultimately through their utility as perceived by patients rather than by the belief or conceptual agreement of an organization.

Clinical medical ethics refers to the integration of ethical considerations into everyday medical practice (Siegler 2017). Health professionals may apply ethical concepts in practice without being aware that they are doing so (Siegler 2017). All health professionals have professional, legal, and personal obligations to apply ethics standards in their care of patients (see Table 1–1).

TABLE 1–1. Clinical ethical standards for clinicians

Truthfulness with patients

Knowledge of how to break bad news

Ability to negotiate informed consent

Ability to assess the decisional capacity of patients

Ability to determine when to work with surrogate decision makers

Privacy and confidentiality with patients

Ability to address and relieve symptoms, including pain

Ability to discuss end-of-life care

Source. Adapted from Siegler 2017, pp. 9–16.

PROFESSIONALISM

Professionalism is notoriously difficult to define, a fact that is highlighted by the numerous and evolving ways in which it has been characterized (see Table 1–2). Standards of professionalism vary among medical specialties, and perceptions of what constitutes professional behavior are inconsistent (Dilday et al. 2018; Dubbai et al. 2019; Hendelman and Byszewski 2014; Hoonpongsimanont et al. 2018). Professionalism might be defined as the quality of being faithful to the goals of the profession, which in medicine is predicated on honoring a number of ethical obligations as well as embodying competence and exhibiting sensitivity to cultural values. A cardinal feature of professionalism is a willing acceptance of an ethical obligation to place the patient's and society's interests above one's own (Stobo and Blank 1994). Some conceptualizations of professionalism emphasize upholding the trust of patients and the public and the application of virtue to the practice of medicine (Brody and Doukas 2014). Professionalism also encompasses the socialization of emerging professionals (e.g., during training), who learn, absorb, and emulate the aims, qualities, and behaviors that characterize the profession (Koch 2019).

The traditional literature has outlined three distinct approaches to defining and understanding professionalism. The first identifies and lists specific elements and behaviors, the second delineates principles that guide behavior, and the third organizes these elements and principles into rubrics or themes (Table 1–3). Regardless of the taxonomy, all of the conceptual labors surrounding professionalism trace back to the Hippo-

TABLE 1–2.   Different conceptualizations of professionalism

Kass (1983)	Being a professional is an ethical matter, entailing devotion to a way of life in the service of others and of some higher good.
Racy (1990)	A profession is a socially sanctioned activity whose primary object is the well-being of others above the professional's personal gain.
Brandeis (1993)	A profession has three features: training that is intellectual and involves knowledge, as distinguished from skill; work that is pursued primarily for others and not for oneself; and success that is measured by more than the amount of financial return.
LaCombe (1993)	Professionalism is not a matter of trying but of being.
Reynolds (1994)	A profession is a set of values, attitudes, and behaviors that results in serving the interests of patients and society before one's own.
Stobo and Blank (1994)	Professionalism means aspiring to altruism, accountability, excellence, duty, service, honor, integrity, and respect for others.
Wynia et al. (1999)	Professionalism entails safeguarding those who are vulnerable in society—as well as "vulnerable social values."
American Board of Internal Medicine Foundation et al. (2002)	Professionalism's fundamental principles include the primacy of patient welfare, excellence in the creation and socialization of knowledge, and a commitment to be responsive to the health needs of society.
Wear and Nixon (2004)	Professionalism is a "critical educative endeavor" enacted through the sharing of "medical narratives," which foster an authentic and humanistic understanding of the profession's putative values.
Cohen (2007)	Professionalism is a way of acting. Professionalism comprises a set of observable behaviors.
Brody and Doukas (2014)	Professionalism is a trust-generating promise and an application of virtue to practice.
Koch (2019)	Professionalism describes the aims, qualities, and conduct that mark the profession. Professionalism drives the nontechnical socialization of emerging professionals.

Source.   Adapted and updated from Roberts and Dyer 2004.

TABLE 1–3.   Models for defining professionalism

Model	Key elements
Specific components of professionalism	Honesty/integrity
	Reliability/responsibility
	Respect for others
	Compassion/empathy
	Self-improvement
	Self-awareness/knowledge of limits
	Communication/collaboration
	Altruism/advocacy
Principle-based approach	Autonomy
	Beneficence
	Nonmaleficence
	Justice
	Veracity
	Fidelity
Thematic approach	Compliance to values
	Patient access
	Doctor-patient relationship
	Demeanor
	Management
	Personal awareness
	Motivation

cratic writings, particularly the convictions of beneficence and nonmaleficence: "…as to diseases make a habit of two things, to help or at least to do no harm" (cited in Siegler 2002, p. 409).

The American Academy of Pediatrics developed one early model of professionalism, which included eight components (Klein et al. 2003): honesty/integrity; reliability/responsibility; respect for others; compassion/empathy; self-improvement; self-awareness/knowledge of limits; communication/collaboration; and altruism/advocacy. Specific manifestations of these components include "is truthful with patients, peers and in professional work" and "puts best interest of the patient above self-interest."

A principle-based approach, the second model, evolves from the bioethical standards of beneficence, autonomy, nonmaleficence, and justice. The concept of justice is relatively recent and focuses attention on the distribution of and access to resources within a defined community. In 2006, the American Medical Association Council on Ethical and Judicial Affairs added a principle addressing this issue: "A physician shall support access to medical care for all patients" (p. lvii). Ethicists have added two additional principles to the bioethical model. Veracity is the principle of telling the truth, and fidelity is the principle of faithfully serving a patient or a positive objective (Beauchamp and Childress 2001; Roberts 2016). The American Psychological Association (2017) has five principles that parallel these two additional principles: beneficence and nonmaleficence; fidelity and responsibility; integrity; justice; and respect for people's rights and dignity.

Several theorists have analyzed the literature and clustered the various elements and principles into distinct themes, following the third model. Jha and colleagues (2006) differentiate seven themes that capture the concepts and behaviors of professionalism: compliance to values (e.g., maintaining confidentiality); patient access (e.g., providing continuity of care); doctor-patient relationship (e.g., treating patients with respect); demeanor (e.g., being courteous and polite); management (e.g., working in a team); personal awareness (e.g., auditing one's own practice); and motivation (e.g., protecting patients' interests).

Van de Camp et al. (2004) elegantly distilled professionalism into three rubrics: interpersonal, public, and intrapersonal. Interpersonal professionalism pertains to a health care provider's relationships and interactions with patients and other health care providers. Subsumed under this rubric are such concepts as altruism, honesty, compassion, appropriate use of power, shared decision-making with patients, and sensitivity to diverse populations. Public professionalism relates to fulfilling the demands that society places on the medical profession and involves elements including adherence to an ethical code, technical competence, and enhancing the welfare of the community. Intrapersonal professionalism concerns the responsibility of the individual to maintain the ability to function in the medical profession; specific responsibilities include lifelong learning, self-awareness, absence of impairment, and knowledge of limits.

The delineation of professionalism into the three rubrics of interpersonal, public, and intrapersonal professionalism is particularly pertinent to the interdisciplinary practice of mental health (Table 1–4). Individuals who receive psychotherapeutic services place themselves in a vulnerable situation by allowing another individual to observe and evaluate their emotions, cognitions, attitudes, values, and behaviors. Mental health clinicians are expected to facilitate the growth and development of these individuals. This responsibility requires the valuing of the patient's autonomy and integrity, respect for the patient-clinician relationship and boundaries, appreciation of power differentials, continuous focus on the needs of the patient, and sensitivity to cultural diversity and the ecological context in which patients live and function. This is especially difficult when the patient is overwhelmed by life's predicaments and is experiencing despair, has a disabling psychiatric illness, or has been ordered by a court to receive treatment.

TABLE 1–4. Variations on a theme: three concepts of professionalism

Rubric	Key concepts
Interpersonal professionalism	Relationships and interactions with patients and colleagues
	Shared decision-making
	Compassion
	Honesty
	Appropriate use of power
	Sensitivity to diverse populations
Public professionalism	Fulfilling the expectations society has for medical professionals
	Adherence to ethical codes
	Technical competency
	Enhancing the welfare of the community
Intrapersonal professionalism	Maintenance of the ability to function as a medical professional
	Self-awareness
	Knowledge of one's limits
	Lifelong learning
	Self-care

Interpersonal professionalism is also applicable to interactions with colleagues and other providers. Because patients function within an ecological environment, clinicians regularly coordinate care with an array of other providers, including other medical specialists, nurses, case managers, legal personnel, and advocates. This collaboration is critical for the delivery of optimal care to the patient. Another vital component to optimal care is a clinician's ability to recognize and address ethical lapses or professional impairment in colleagues.

Public professionalism pertains to advancing the access of care to individuals with mental health problems and to populations that are typically underserved. The New Freedom Commission on Mental Health (2003) denoted several goals that can transform mental health care: 1) to view mental health as essential to overall health; 2) to provide early mental health screening and treatment in multiple settings; 3) to eliminate disparities in services; 4) to deliver excellent care that is research based; and 5) to use information technology to improve care. Public professionalism also involves working toward the destigmatization of mental illness, creating parity in the allocation of resources between mental health and other health care, and negotiating with managed care and other social institutions to create systems of care that meet the goals of the New Freedom Commission on Mental Health.

Education is a key element of public professionalism. Senior clinicians have an obligation to teach, mentor, and act as role models of professionalism to their residents and junior colleagues. Professionals also have a responsibility to educate medical colleagues, administrators, and their communities about such issues as the relationship of mental health to physical health, lifestyle decisions (e.g., diet), and stress management.

Intrapersonal professionalism is especially relevant for mental health practitioners. Clinicians are responsible for their own self-awareness, self-care, and self-growth. Decades ago, Bugental (1965) observed that psychotherapists need to have humility, a growth orientation, fascination with psychological processes, and an evolving set of constructs related to the self, the world, therapeutic processes, and personality. Mental health professionals cannot effectively treat their patients unless they care for themselves.

Internal medicine specialists created a charter that summarizes the concept of medical professionalism in the following way:

> Professionalism is the basis of medicine's contract with society. It demands placing the interests of patients above those of the physician, setting and maintaining standards of competence and integrity, and pro-

viding expert advice on matters of health. The principles and responsibilities of medical professionalism must be clearly understood by both
the profession and society. Essential to this contract is public trust in
physicians, which depends on the integrity of both individual physicians
and the whole profession. (American Board of Internal Medicine Foundation et al. 2002, p. 244)

Professionalism is a multidimensional concept that encompasses ethics;
relationships with one's patients, colleagues, and community; public policy; and self-awareness.

Evaluating professionalism is extraordinarily challenging and has
evolved. In the mid-1980s, a holistic concept of professionalism began to
complement terms such as *clinical competence* in discourse about medical
training. Professional boards such as the American Board of Internal Medicine (ABIM) began to add new professional attributes, such as humanistic qualities, to their concepts of ideal clinical behavior. Rapid financial
and structural changes in health care resulted in an alarming increase in
novel ethical challenges that were increasingly understood to be inade-
quately addressed in medical training.

In 1990, the ABIM began Project Professionalism, a multidecade endeavor to promulgate a unified definition of medical professionalism and
"stay ahead of the wave" of its new professional challenges (American
Board of Internal Medicine 1999). The project arose from a consensus
that changes occurring both inside and outside the training environment,
such as relaxed evaluation criteria and "stress surges" caused by changes
in the health care delivery system, were eroding professional standards.
The project had three other related goals: to raise the concept of professionalism into the consciousness of all within internal medicine, to provide a way for program directors to inculcate professionalism concepts
via training programs, and to create strategies for evaluating the professionalism of medical trainees.

With the belief that professionalism entails measurable professional
qualities, Project Professionalism developed new guidelines for shaping
training programs. Furthermore, it advocated certification as a means of
ensuring integrity across the profession. The project resulted in four recommendations for curricular requirements of professional certification
programs: physician accountability, humanistic qualities, physician impairment, and professional ethics. The project brief also emphasized the
importance of vignettes in inculcating professional standards and included a section explicating the "signs and symptoms" of unprofessional
conduct to aid trainees in recognizing common patterns of unprofessional
conduct in complex everyday scenarios.

The importance of inculcating professionalism among medical trainees is underscored by the inclusion of professionalism as one of six core competencies promulgated by the Accreditation Council for Graduate Medical Education in 2002 (Educational Commission for Foreign Medical Graduates 2012). Residents in all training programs must meet a number of professionalism milestones, although these vary according to specialty.

For psychiatry, the latest iteration of professionalism competencies, effective in 2021, comprises three domains: "Professional Behavior and Ethical Principles," "Accountability/Conscientiousness," and "Well-Being" (Accreditation Council for Graduate Medical Education 2020). The inclusion of "Well-Being" attests to the growing recognition of the vital role of provider well-being in promoting professionalism and ethical behavior. This topic is explored further in the section "Professional Well-Being" later in this chapter.

THE CENTRALITY OF ETHICS IN THE CARE OF PEOPLE WITH MENTAL ILLNESS

Ethics is fundamental to the practice and identity of mental health professionals. Mental illness, by definition, affects the most basic, human aspects of ourselves—our emotions, ideas, beliefs, capacity for relationships, and abilities to engage in meaningful activities and perform diverse roles. Opportunities for people living with mental illness are frequently constrained. Living with a mental illness—whether episodic or chronic—is often associated with social isolation, alienation from family and friends, and loss of important functions. People with mental illness across the spectrum of severity and their families must muster courage and even take risks to seek help, often confronting significant barriers to care not encountered in the treatment of physical health conditions (Conner et al. 2010; Fox et al. 2018; Link and Phelan 2006). Moreover, mentally ill individuals have often struggled alone for years and are frequently misdiagnosed before receiving appropriate clinical attention. Mental illness is also often deeply stigmatizing and poorly understood, creating new sources of vulnerability (e.g., prejudicial attitudes, implicit and explicit bias) that may make some individuals more likely to experience poverty, marginalization, exploitation, neglect, and abuse (Luciano et al. 2014; Peris et al. 2008; Roberts and Roberts 1999). Individuals from certain backgrounds, moreover, may experience additional concerns about stigma related to seeking mental health care (Krill Williston et al. 2019).

Mental health professionals are expected to do what is right as healers and to regard patients as complete persons deserving of dignity and respect. Becoming worthy of the confidence and trust of people who have experienced suffering fundamentally requires that professionals develop and work to maintain a deep capacity for self-reflection and a sensitivity to the ethical nuances of their work (Roberts 2016). In this way, ethics and professionalism can be viewed as central pillars of clinical excellence (Chisolm et al. 2012). Psychiatrists, psychologists, and other mental health professionals learn patients' most sensitive thoughts, hopes, and fears; those with mental illness place great trust in their caregivers.

The mental health field is composed of professionals from a wide variety of disciplines, including, but not limited to, psychiatrists, psychiatric nurses, psychotherapists, counselors, psychiatric social workers, addiction therapists, and psychologists with diverse subspecialties. Each of these disciplines has its own ethical tradition expressed in characteristic codes of ethics that continue to be expanded and refined to meet emerging challenges. In addition, primary care practitioners have increasingly been called on to perform many mental health care functions, including routine screening for depression, anxiety, and substance use disorders (Siu et al. 2016). Mounting pressures weigh on these providers, as well as health care organizations such as accountable care organizations, to evaluate for, treat, and report on (e.g., through pay-for-performance metrics) these disorders in order to receive incentive payments, despite relatively thin evidence for the effectiveness of these incentives (Counts et al. 2019).

Given that primary care clinicians may have received relatively little education regarding the diagnosis and treatment of mental illness and are often uncoached regarding the unique ethical and legal dimensions involved in mental health care (e.g., *Tarasoff v. Regents of the University of California* [1976] rulings, involuntary commitment procedures, transference issues, manifestations of bias, and boundary crossings or transgressions), additional questions will be raised about the adequacy of the standards for such care provided within—and ethical safeguards incorporated into—these non–mental health care settings (Reynolds and Frank 2016). As integrated behavioral health models are increasingly regarded as important in cost-effective approaches to address shortages of mental health care (Woltmann et al. 2012), mental health providers may be placed in ethically challenging positions—for instance, by being asked to triage patients quickly, to parse their time differently to help manage larger panels of patients, or to provide treatment recommendations for patients whom they have not met or personally evaluated. Such scenarios involve a scarcity of individual attention and can increase clinicians' reliance on implicit and explicit individual bias in making predictive and real-time judgments and decisions (Saposnik et al. 2016). This effect can scale: by the same token, patterns of bias in the medical profession can serve to reinforce discrimination and perpetuate systemic mental health inequities (Compton and Shim 2015; Dehon et al. 2017). It is increasingly understood that many forms of bias are rooted in cognition and unconscious beliefs, and that medical professionals are just as susceptible to biased thinking as the general population (FitzGerald and Hurst 2017). Therefore, a commitment to rooting out bias is increasingly viewed as a professional value and necessary to uphold certain bioethical principles, such as nonmaleficence and justice. How to mitigate bias in mental health care, through clinician training and other means, is thus a question of immediate concern for ethics and professionalism.

In the field of mental health, clinicians must work with issues of personhood and autonomy while continuously grappling with definitions of health and illness. Ethical issues of beneficence, nonmaleficence, confidentiality, altruism, justice and nondiscrimination, professionalism, trust, and related abstract concepts are very real factors in daily work. Ethical considerations may take the form of clinical care dilemmas or conflicts—for example, in deciding whether a person should be admitted to the hospital involuntarily, in assessing whether a poststroke patient is capable of the decision to decline recommended treatment, and in determining whom to inform when a patient expresses homicidal intent. Ethically rich aspects of care also serve as the basis for some of the most gratifying work—for instance, when a clinician reaches a solution to a complex series of dilemmas.

The value of ethics to the mental health professions stems also from the unique place of mental health within the larger fields of health care and social service. Mental health professionals, as well-trained observers of behavior, have developed a broad yet nuanced understanding of human nature and are often well suited to managing complex situations that require synthesizing ethical, medical, psychological, legal, and psychosocial perspectives. Mental health clinicians are thus often called on to help clarify and resolve ethical dilemmas that arise in the care of medical patients, to join ethics committees, and to reflect publicly on ethical questions arising in society (Bourgeois et al. 2006). Mental health professionals are also frequently involved in the conduct of clinical research involving volunteers with mental illnesses. Numerous ethical challenges can arise in these studies and all deserve special attention (Dunn and Roberts 2021).

In short, the importance of ethics is rooted in the powerful and intimate role that clinicians play in the lives of their patients who experience mental illnesses. Mental illnesses cause great suffering, are complex and often misunderstood, and may give rise to significant vulnerabilities in present-day society. Ethics is critical to mental health providers because of the diverse roles, commitments, and responsibilities they assume in their professional lives.

NEUROETHICS AND NEUROSCIENCE

Over the past few decades, neuroscience has taken up a central role in medicine as the conceptual basis for understanding and treating mental illness. Mental illness, as an illness of the brain, is perceived as having a biological basis. Yet, unlike other organs, the brain gives rise to the mind, is generative of identity, and sustains the mental activity by which people develop the morals, ethics, attitudes, beliefs, and scientific facts that shape society. The study of the brain's functioning and the recursive application of advancements in our metacognitive understanding to influence the brain and mind therefore carry ethical questions that are not present elsewhere in the biological sciences. These questions belong to the emerging field of neuroethics.

Neuroethics is a capacious and interdisciplinary field implicated both in traditional ethical domains, such as human subjects research and the active question of public trust in science, as well as emerging domains, including neurotechnologies, neurolaw, and philosophy of cognition (see Figure 1–1).

The advancement of the empirical basis of neuroscience depends on the ethical participation of diverse individuals in research, including individuals with mental illness. Neuroscience research upholds the principle of beneficence by seeking to reduce the immense global disease burden represented by mental illness. Secondary interests of neuroscience research are related to concepts such as the intrinsic value of knowledge about the self and the entrusted role of basic science in making discoveries that can enable broader epistemic value for humanity. As treated by Illes (2017) in greater depth, topics in neuroethics include emerging biomedical technologies, emerging neuroimaging technologies, wearables and mobile health technology, neuromodulation, neurotechnology research, the role of technology in the lives of young people, brain death and the definition of death, ethical issues in neurodegenerative conditions, environmental neuroethics, the neurobiology of addiction, and neuroscience in the law, among other topics, which go beyond the scope of this book.

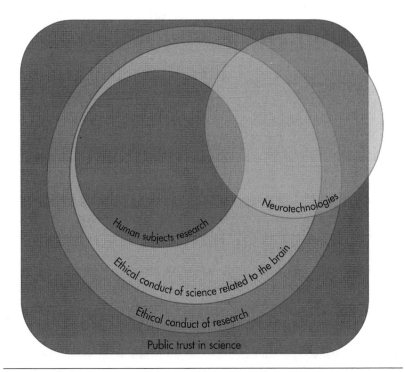

FIGURE 1–1. Overlapping ethical concerns.

Source. Copyright © 2019, Roberts Ethics Lab. Used with permission.

ETHICS EDUCATION: IMPARTING ETHICS KNOWLEDGE AND PROFESSIONAL VALUES

Ethics education, including ethics education in psychiatry and the related mental health professions, has evolved over the last four decades. Initially, ethics instruction was felt to be inappropriate, as it was believed that one's morals were learned early in life and were not necessarily teachable (Pellegrino et al. 1985). Ethics curricula have advanced from formal didactic and cognitive models of instruction to a growing recognition of the need for a developmental approach that also encompasses affective aspects of decision-making (Christakis and Feudtner 1993). Early on, ethics education emphasized rule-based codes of conduct and then the clinician-patient relationship. More recently, increasing attention is given to public health and to community obligations and responsibilities, such as those expressed in the widely adopted Professionalism Charter (American Board of Internal Medicine Foundation et al. 2002). Similarly, the need to attend to all voices—including individuals with lived experience of mental illness, consumers of mental health care services, and underrepresented populations—as full partners in clinical care represents a departure from prior, more hierarchical and paternalistic models (Institute of Medicine 2001). This shift has led mental health professionals and their teachers to encounter new ethical dilemmas, such as expanded authority and scope of practice for non-doctoral-level practitioners and the empowerment of patients in clinical decision-making expressed through novel tools like psychiatric advance directives (Murray and Wortzel 2019). To successfully negotiate this new moral territory, mental health professionals will require a different skill set from their predecessors, such as the ability to mediate disputes, negotiate power sharing, manage ever more complex legal situations, and participate in struggles for social justice and political parity, without which adequate mental health care and its funding cannot be achieved.

Cultivating an understanding of ethics is vital to providing competent and compassionate mental health care and to fulfilling mental health professionals' diverse, socially vital, yet complicated roles and obligations. Furthermore, ethical behavior is a core feature of what it means to be a health care professional. Interest in teaching, modeling, and assessing professionalism in health care includes a commitment to ensuring that professionals understand and can reason through complicated ethical issues and hold themselves to the highest ethical standards. The reinvigorated interest in ethics and professionalism derives, in part, from the perception that over the last several decades, health care providers have lost some of the moral stature historically afforded them. Another reason for the emphasis on professionalism and ethics in health care education is the rapidly changing health care environment, with numerous emerging and complex health care advances in terms of methods of care, modes of delivery, and systems of care. Concurrently, the demographic and sociocultural contexts of health care delivery demand that future clinicians be trained to attend to cultural and other dimensions of care that, although previously underappreciated and untaught, now sit squarely in the domain of professionalism.

Every professional must learn and abide by the regulations and laws governing his or her behavior; this is a fundamental commitment of a profession and a basic part of professional education. For example, regulations surrounding research involving human volunteers or participation by living human "subjects" in studies must be overseen by an appropriate institutional review board and oftentimes, in addition, by a data and safety monitoring board. These oversight bodies must be engaged prior to the initiation of research by the professional who proposes to perform the research work. The law requires that physicians and other clinicians, under nearly all circumstances, obtain a patient's informed consent prior to initiating a procedure or treatment or research participation. It is important to emphasize, however, that legal behavior is not the same as ethical behavior. The law sets parameters around choices, delimiting the acceptable options under a given set of circumstances (Roberts and Dyer 2004). In most cases, however, the law does not tell providers what to do. In other words, the law rules out certain options, providing negative imperatives; in contrast, ethical analysis helps us to construct positive imperatives, thereby "ruling in" one or more ethically defensible options. In the case of informed consent, for example, the law does not tell providers what to do when a patient refuses a recommended treatment or will not adhere to treatment recommendations. Providers must have a solid grasp of ethical aspects of care to resolve such dilemmas. These dilemmas are often evolving, dynamic situations, not easily encapsulated as a specific set of circumstances to which a single law could apply.

Professionalism expectations or standards, when interpreted as a restricted set of normative beliefs and behaviors, have come under criticism for contributing to a narrow and inflexible view of what is "acceptable" in medicine and the health professions. Professionalism has also been "weaponized" in certain situations, as noted in the literature (Frye et al. 2020; Roberts 2020), when it is used to create an unwelcome environment for individuals who identify as nonmajority. Implicit expectations of professionals defined by societal biases (e.g., around whiteness, around heteronormative identity, around hair, weight, age) also contribute to skepticism toward old-fashioned views of professionalism (Frye et al. 2020). We suggest that professionalism is intrinsically grounded in the ideals of a profession (e.g., truthfulness, respect for dignity of patients, humility), although the understanding of how such ideals are expressed at any given moment in history, society, and culture will change. A working understanding of the ideals of the profession and how they translate into professional practices and actions is crucial in informing ethical decision-making.

Ethics education, therefore, is strongly linked on conceptual grounds to the development and preservation of professionalism in trainees. For mental health providers, the special privileges and obligations accompanying their roles make ethics education a crucial component of training and lifelong learning.

Modern curricula have placed greater emphasis on both formal didactic and experiential methods—including structured ethics instruction, group discussions of real cases, and written reflections—directed at the goal of having learners acquire essential ethics-related skills as outlined above. The educational approaches used have been varied, and few data are available enabling comparison of different educational strategies. Early work conducted among medical students indicates that case-based and discussion-oriented approaches (Roberts et al. 2004b, 2005, 2007) and participant-oriented, empathy-focused approaches (Roberts et al. 2007) may be effective methods for teaching about clinical and research ethics, although much more empirical work is needed.

In addition, increasing recognition is being paid to developing ethics skills among students who are actually working with patients clinically (i.e., as opposed to those attending lectures, such as medical students in their preclinical years). Thus, ethics educators may ask students to describe cases they have encountered, given that applying ethical analytic skills to real-life situations may have more resonance for learners. Several studies have examined the content of students' reflections on ethical dilemmas they have encountered. For instance, Kelly and Nisker (2009) reported that students frequently felt that an ethical issue had arisen, but they nevertheless hesitated to bring it to their supervisors' attention, out of concern about how their performance would be evaluated. Moreover, the most commonly described dilemmas noted by students involved informed consent or inadequate care. Such findings suggest that despite trainees' attunement to ethical issues, the nature of the supervisor-trainee relationship may negatively affect students' willingness to raise these important issues.

In a survey of over 200 psychiatry residents' perspectives on ethics education, respondents affirmed the importance of ethics education, but also expressed a need for more training in core ethical concepts and issues (Jain et al. 2011a, 2011b; Lapid et al. 2009). Residents also desired educational approaches grounded in clinical practice, role modeling, and teaching by experts. Topics related to conflict of interest are also of great concern to psychiatry residents. Given that the pharmaceutical industry spends $20 billion marketing to health care professionals (Schwartz and Woloshin 2019), residents must be aware of the ethical considerations of receiving gifts from the pharmaceutical industry and how to ethically handle relationships with the pharmaceutical industry in general (Jain 2007, 2010).

Another priority for ethics-related education for mental health professionals is the goal of training clinicians who will be culturally attuned to their patients. Just as learning to identify ethical dimensions and issues in their work comprises a fundamental skill set for developing mental health professionals, gaining a working knowledge of and facility with key cultural aspects of care is also vital to upholding professional obligations. As articulated in the Accreditation Council for Graduate Medical Education (2018) competency of professionalism, residents must "demonstrate a commitment to professionalism and an adherence

---

TABLE 1–5.   Standards for professionalism in medical residency training

---

Residents must demonstrate a commitment to professionalism and an adherence to ethical principles. Residents must demonstrate competence in the following:

Compassion, integrity, and respect for others

Responsiveness to patient needs that supersedes self-interest

Respect for privacy and autonomy

Accountability to patients, society, and the profession

Respect and responsiveness to diverse patient populations, including but not limited to diversity in gender, age, culture, race, religion, disabilities, national origin, socioeconomic status, and sexual orientation

Ability to recognize and develop a plan for one's own personal and professional well-being

Capacity to appropriately disclose and address conflict or duality of interest

---

Source.   Accreditation Council for Graduate Medical Education 2018.

to ethical principles" (see Table 1–5). The National Association of Social Workers' Code of Ethics places great emphasis on cultural sensitivity, situating it solidly within the framework of social workers' set of core values as part of striving for social justice:

> Social workers pursue social change, particularly with and on behalf of vulnerable and oppressed individuals and groups of people. Social workers' social change efforts are focused primarily on issues of poverty, unemployment, discrimination, and other forms of social injustice. These activities seek to promote sensitivity to and knowledge about oppression and cultural and ethnic diversity. Social workers strive to ensure access to needed information, services, and resources; equality of opportunity; and meaningful participation in decision-making for all people. (National Association of Social Workers 2017)

PROFESSIONAL WELL-BEING: ITS FUNDAMENTAL ROLE IN ETHICS AND PROFESSIONALISM

Although, in years past, the concept of professional well-being has not frequently been encountered in the theoretical and empirical ethics literature, it is now widely acknowledged that providers' well-being is crucial to their ability to enact the virtues, knowledge, and skills that comprise ethics and professionalism. Threats to provider well-being are also threats to ethics and professionalism. As a corollary, opportunities to enhance well-being provide avenues to improving providers' capacities to practice ethically and with professionalism.

Dramatic changes over the last 30–40 years in the health care system and the practice of medicine—changes that seem to have accelerated in the last 10 years—have profoundly affected the landscape in which providers now find themselves. These changes—including significantly greater rates of clinician employment by large health care systems (vs. private practice), the proliferation of electronic health records, decreases in clinician autonomy, an emphasis on productivity, the weakening of traditional confidentiality protections, and the replacement of many licensed positions with less trained staff—are often cited as primary causes of provider "burnout" (see Figure 1–2).

Burnout, however, is not an all-or-none category (i.e., in terms of whether a provider is or is not "burned out"). Rather, it is more productive to think of burnout as residing along a continuum—from well-being and personal and professional fulfillment on one end of the spectrum, to personal and professional impairment, significant distress, and to mental illness on the other end of the spectrum (see Figure 1–3). We all have both risk and protective factors for the development of burnout. Mental health professionals may be at elevated risk, by virtue of the "secondary traumatization" that can occur by working with individuals who have experienced severe histories of mental illness, abuse, or trauma (Maslach and Leiter 2016). Additional risk factors for burnout among mental health providers are listed in Table 1–6.

Definitions of "burnout," it should be noted, continue to evolve. Although initially described as having three cardinal features—emotional exhaustion, depersonalization, and a decreased sense of personal accomplishment (Maslach and Jackson 1981)—these features have been more recently elaborated on as "dimensions" (see Figure 1–4):

> The exhaustion dimension was also described as wearing out, loss of energy, depletion, debilitation, and fatigue. The cynicism dimension was originally called depersonalization (given the nature of human services occupations), but was also described as negative or inappropriate attitudes towards clients, irritability, loss of idealism, and withdrawal. The inefficacy dimension was originally called reduced personal accomplishment, and was also described as reduced productivity or capability, low morale, and an inability to cope. (Maslach and Leiter 2016, p. 103)

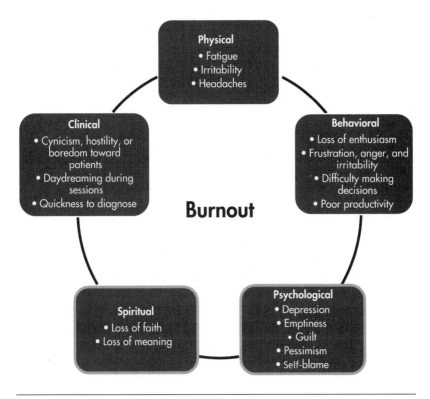

FIGURE 1–2. Symptoms of burnout.
Source. Adapted from Grosch and Olsen 1994.

In the field of mental health care, an additional and perhaps less discussed source of distress is the enormous moral pressure of feeling constantly that one or one's team is being "asked to do more with less." For example, a social worker on an inpatient psychiatric unit may be asked by a resident to find apartment housing for an individual with serious mental illness whom the social worker knows cannot survive without intensive case management, which is unavailable; or a psychologist may be told he can only provide six sessions of psychotherapy for a profoundly depressed adolescent and must submit detailed session notes if he wishes to receive payment from an insurance company.

Yet another pressure affecting professional development is the pressure to conform. Professionalism is both a set of discernible qualities and an embodied social construct that relies, in part, on images and narratives selected according to specific norms and preferences. Many images of the physician overlap in the history of medicine; the overwhelming

Negative Factors
Poor health
Lack of purpose
Excessive stress
Poor coping style
Poor mentorship and supervision
Inadequate psychosocial support
Interpersonal conflict
Excessive work demands
Adverse work environment

Positive Factors
Good health
Strong sense of purpose
Stimulation and engagement
Adaptive coping style
Mentorship and supervision
Strong psychosocial support
Harmonious relationships
Appropriate work demands
Constructive work environment

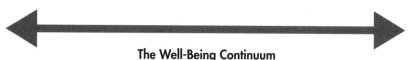

The Well-Being Continuum

Languishing   Flourishing

FIGURE 1–3. Factors influencing the well-being of professionals.

Source. Copyright © 2015, Laura Weiss Roberts, M.D., M.A. Used with permission.

majority of these images are white and male. Physicians continue to hold an implicit white preference (Sabin et al. 2009). Members of the profession must guard against normalizing privileged, racist, and arbitrarily constrained forms of professional identity and behavior. Conforming pressures can cause inequity and distress for individuals who do not see any room for themselves in their field—many of these individuals may already face compounded inequities due to race, gender identity, religion, cultural background, or other factors. For individuals whose identities remain underrepresented in medicine, professional self-discernment may be stifled by perceived "necessary behavior" (Babaria et al. 2009). Microaggressions, othering, and belittlement are examples of derivative forms of harm based in implicit and explicit bias that increase risk for burnout and prevent equity in our professional fields.

Fostering one's own well-being, as well as the well-being of one's colleagues and trainees, will remain critical to maintaining and promoting professionalism and ethics within the field of mental health care. Professionals with a greater sense of well-being will not only experience greater personal and professional fulfillment but will also be better able to practice the essential ethical skills of mental health professionals.

TABLE 1–6. Risk factors for burnout among mental health professionals

Intrapersonal or internal factors	External or systems factors
Reduced resilience	Shortage of providers
Reduced sense of belonging	Compounded inequity based on race, gender, or religious identity
Personal history of mental illness (e.g., depression or anxiety)	Productivity demands
Suboptimal social support networks/social isolation	Electronic health records
	Erosion of autonomy
Negative self-talk	Patient or family dissatisfaction
Reduced self-care (e.g., diet, exercise, sleep, substance use)	Administrative burdens (e.g., prior authorizations)
Perfectionism	Culture of shame around help seeking
Internalized stigma of help seeking	

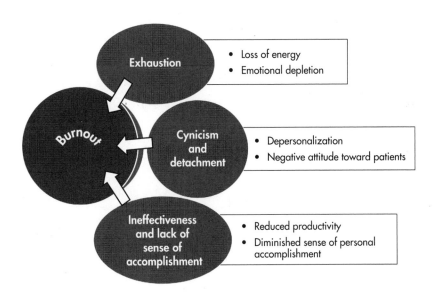

FIGURE 1–4. Dimensions of burnout.

Source. Reprinted from Gengoux G, Zack SE, Derenne JL, et al.: *Professional Well-Being: Enhancing Wellness Among Psychiatrists, Psychologists, and Mental Health Clinicians.* Washington, DC, American Psychiatric Association Publishing, 2020, p. 59.

CHAPTER 2

ETHICS IN THE MENTAL HEALTH PROFESSIONS

Laura Weiss Roberts, M.D., M.A.
Max Kasun, B.A.
Gabriel Termuehlen, B.A.

ESSENTIAL ETHICAL SKILLS OF MENTAL HEALTH PROFESSIONALS

Six Essential Skills

The clinical and interpersonal skills of the well-trained mental health professional ideally should translate into a facility with ethical problem solving, beyond a simple adherence to written guidelines, laws, and codes. Clinical training and, frequently, natural aptitude enable clinicians to attend to subtleties and nuances, to look beyond the surface for hidden motivations, and to form habits of self-reflection and self-scrutiny. These skills and habits can form the basis for sensitivity to moral issues and an ability to solve ethical dilemmas in a systematic and thoughtful way.

This chapter has been adapted from Roberts LW, Hoop JG, Dunn LB: "Ethical Aspects of Psychiatry," in *The American Psychiatric Publishing Textbook of Clinical Psychiatry*, 5th Edition. Edited by Hales RE, Yudofsky SC. Washington, DC, American Psychiatric Publishing, 2002, pp. 1601–1636; and Belitz J: "On Professionalism," in *Professionalism and Ethics: Q&A Self-Study Guide for Mental Health Professionals*. Edited by Roberts LW, Hoop JG. Washington, DC, American Psychiatric Publishing, 2008. The authors would like to acknowledge Laura Bodin Dunn, M.D., Cynthia M.A. Geppert, M.D., Ph.D., M.P.H., and Jerald Belitz, Ph.D.

TABLE 2–1.   Essential ethics skills in clinical practice

Ability to identify and describe ethical features of a patient's care and to outline various relevant dimensions of ethical dilemmas

Ability to see how one's own life experiences, attitudes, and knowledge may influence one's care of a patient (e.g., awareness of one's biases and countertransference)

Ability to identify one's areas of clinical expertise (i.e., scope of clinical competence) and to work within those boundaries

Ability to anticipate ethically risky or problematic situations (e.g., boundary crossings)

Ability to gather additional information and to seek consultation and additional expertise to clarify and, ideally, resolve ethical conflicts

Ability to build additional ethical safeguards into the patient care situation

---

Source.   Reprinted from Roberts LW, Dyer AR: *Concise Guide to Ethics in Mental Health Care.* Washington, DC, American Psychiatric Publishing, 2004. Copyright © 2004, American Psychiatric Publishing. Used with permission.

All mental health professionals whose work embodies the highest ethical standards tend to rely on a set of six core ethics skills that are learned during or before professional training and are continually practiced and refined throughout one's career (Roberts 2016). These six skills are listed in Table 2–1. Acquiring these skills in support of professional conduct unites all the mental health disciplines in a common developmental process, with certain predictable issues and milestones that occur in relation to the nature of the work and the societal roles with which mental health professionals are entrusted (Fann et al. 2003; Hoop 2004).

The first of these core skills is the ability to identify ethical issues as they arise. For some, this will be an intuitive insight (e.g., the internal sense that something is not right), and for others this will be derived more logically (e.g., the awareness that arranging for involuntary treatment of a patient, seeing patients remotely through telehealth, being asked by an administrator to limit care for certain types of patients, or handling a patient's request for exceptions to typical clinical care can all pose specific ethical problems). Tables 2–2 and 2–3 outline some common ethical issues in mental health practice and related activities.

The ability to recognize ethical issues requires some familiarity with key ethics concepts and the interdisciplinary field of bioethics. As a corollary, this ability presupposes the clinician's capacity to observe and translate complex phenomena into patterns, using the common language of the helping professions (e.g., conflicts among autonomy, beneficence,

TABLE 2–2. Ethical tensions in common clinical situations

Clinical situation	Relevant ethical principles	Conflicts and tensions
A patient refuses a medically indicated treatment.	Autonomy and beneficence	The patient's right to make his or her own decisions is in tension with the physician's duty to do good by providing medically indicated treatment.
A patient tells his psychiatrist that he plans to harm another person.	Confidentiality and beneficence	The physician's duty to guard his patient's privacy must be balanced against the obligation to protect the threatened third party.
A close friend asks a psychiatrist to write a prescription for a sleep medicine.	Nonmaleficence	The desire to oblige a friend may conflict with the psychiatrist's duty to avoid harm by prescribing without conducting a thorough medical evaluation and establishing a treatment relationship.
The parent of an adolescent patient asks the psychiatrist for information about the patient's sexual activity and drug or alcohol use.	Confidentiality and beneficence	The psychiatrist's duty to guard his patient's privacy may be in tension with the psychiatrist's desire to do good by educating the parent about the child's high-risk behaviors.
A patient asks a psychiatrist to document a less-stigmatizing diagnosis when filling out insurance forms.	Veracity and nonmaleficence	The psychiatrist's obligation to document the truth may be in tension with the desire to avoid the harm that may occur if the insurance company learns of the diagnosis.

TABLE 2–2. Ethical tensions in common clinical situations *(continued)*

Clinical situation	Relevant ethical principles	Conflicts and tensions
A psychiatrist is sexually attracted to a patient.	Fidelity and nonmaleficence	Sexual activity with a patient violates the psychiatrist's obligation to remain faithful to the goals of treatment and the duty to avoid harming the patient by sexual exploitation.
A rural patient needs a treatment the psychiatrist is not competent to provide; no other practitioner is available.	Nonmaleficence	The psychiatrist's duty to avoid harming the patient by practicing outside his scope of competencies is in conflict with the obligation to avoid harming the patient by leaving him without any treatment provider.
A medical student performs a lumbar puncture for the first time on a patient.	Nonmaleficence and beneficence	The medical student's obligation to avoid harming the patient by performing a procedure without sufficient expertise must be balanced against the student's need to learn by doing in order to help future patients.
A psychiatrist treating a physician believes the physician is too impaired to practice medicine safely; the patient/physician refuses to close his practice because he has no other source of income.	Confidentiality, nonmaleficence, and beneficence	The psychiatrist's duty to guard his patient's privacy and to avoid harming him is in tension with the obligation to protect the impaired physician's patients by reporting the impairment to the proper authorities.
A pharmaceutical company offers a psychiatrist an unusually large fee for referring patients to a research trial.	Fidelity	Financial self-interest threatens the psychiatrist's duty to remain faithful to the goals of treatment and to the role of healer.

TABLE 2–2. Ethical tensions in common clinical situations *(continued)*

Clinical situation	Relevant ethical principles	Conflicts and tensions
A psychiatrist transfers the care of a difficult patient to another provider.	Fidelity, nonmaleficence, and beneficence	The psychiatrist's obligations to remain faithful to the goals of treatment and to avoid the harm of patient abandonment must be balanced against the duty to do good by transferring care to a more competent or appropriate provider when clinically necessary.
A psychiatrist provides mental health care for medical students at their training institution.	Confidentiality, nonmaleficence	The ethical obligations of the psychiatrist's clinical role should have primacy; in general, overlapping roles introduce ethical "risks" or potential conflicts related to competing obligations of the dual or multiple roles.
A patient requests that a psychiatrist employed by a large multispecialty health system not document the patient's use of an illicit substance in the electronic medical record.	Confidentiality, truth telling, nonmaleficence	The psychiatrist's obligation to provide competent care includes documenting truthfully any relevant information that may affect the patient's overall health and medical care. Communicating with other providers is considered crucial to competent, beneficent patient care. Acquiescence to a patient's requests to not document certain aspects of their care must be carefully balanced against potential harms.

TABLE 2–2. Ethical tensions in common clinical situations *(continued)*

Clinical situation	Relevant ethical principles	Conflicts and tensions
A psychiatrist, trying to be helpful, makes an exception to her normal practice and acquiesces to giving her cellphone number to her "VIP" patient, who then begins to text her frequently, including in the evenings and on weekends, with requests for additional support in between scheduled sessions. The psychiatrist begins to feel resentful of these interruptions into her other work and her home life.	Boundaries, beneficence, nonmaleficence	The psychiatrist's exception to her usual boundaries has led to a common ethical dilemma. Although in some instances a level of flexibility is important, before making these kinds of exceptions—whether it is spending more time with a patient by extending their sessions, or providing one's cellphone number—clinicians must consider their own motivations for exceptions to boundaries (e.g., an unconscious desire to please her "special" patient). They must also consider the potential harms to the patient and to the provider-patient relationship of these exceptions.
A patient with a history of severe, treatment-resistant depression develops respiratory symptoms during a global viral pandemic. The patient presents to the emergency room for evaluation of these symptoms; several hours later her test comes back positive. During the medical evaluation, she states that she is suicidal and is actively planning to harm herself. The inpatient psychiatric unit is not equipped, however, to care safely for patients with the virus without exposing other patients and staff.	Altruism, beneficence, nonmaleficence, justice, and provider well-being	Major crises (e.g., the COVID-19 pandemic, but also natural disasters or other crises) can reveal both the strengths and fissures in health systems and practices. The vignette illustrates the tensions that may arise when the medical requirements of caring safely for patients collide with the equally urgent psychiatric care needs. Crises such as these also highlight the importance of making contingency plans ahead of time for such complex scenarios (e.g., an on-call psychiatric response team who would be activated only when circumstances require).

TABLE 2–3. Examples of ethical challenges in special clinical circumstances

Clinical circumstance	Key ethical challenges
Academic psychiatry	Conflicts between clinical and supervisory roles of faculty and between clinical and student roles of trainees
	Financial conflicts of interest related to accountable care, relationships with insurance and other payers, and relationships with industry
	Duty to provide competent care despite trainee status of resident physicians and medical students
Academic-industry partnerships	Ground rules for collaboration
	Ownership of intellectual property and profit-sharing issues
	Conflicts of interest—real or perceived
Addiction psychiatry	Confidentiality, due to potential adverse legal consequences and social implications of substance use disorders and associated behaviors
	Justice, due to the disparities in available treatment for persons with addictive disorders compared with other conditions
Child and adolescent psychiatry	Confidentiality and truth telling for patient and parents or guardians
	Informed consent for treatment, which may require the consent of parents or guardians
Consultation-liaison psychiatry	Assessment of decision-making capacity when patients refuse recommended treatment
Forensic psychiatry	Conflicts between roles as forensic expert and physician
Geriatric psychiatry	Informed consent for treatment when decisional capacity may be impaired; seeking appropriate, informed surrogate consent
	Truth telling regarding diagnosis and prognosis for patients with dementia
	Assessment of various types of capacity (e.g., financial, testamentary, treatment refusal, treatment withdrawal)

TABLE 2–3. Examples of ethical challenges in special clinical circumstances *(continued)*

Clinical circumstance	Key ethical challenges
Military psychiatry	Conflicts between roles as physician and member of the military
Psychotherapy and psychoanalysis	Confidentiality, due to the intensely private nature of patient disclosures
	Maintenance of therapeutic boundaries
Public psychiatry	Duty to provide competent care despite limited resources
	Justice, in terms of the need to distribute social resources fairly
Remotely delivered psychiatry	Confidentiality in ensuring patients can talk from a private setting
	Beneficence, in screening for patient safety when providing remote care
	Informed consent regarding limitations of remotely delivered care
Rural psychiatry	Confidentiality in a setting where everyone knows everyone
	Conflicts among multiple roles of physician and patients within community
	Duty to provide competent care in the absence of specialists
	Nonabandonment of patients in a setting in which there may be a lack of qualified clinicians to provide backup coverage
Treatment of difficult patients	Duty to provide competent care to patients with clinically challenging presentations and behaviors
	Nonabandonment despite countertransference feelings or physician burnout

Source. Adapted from Roberts and Dyer 2004.

and justice when a person with mental illness threatens the life of a specific individual and is thus involuntarily held for evaluation).

A second key ethics skill is the ability to understand how one's personal values, beliefs, and sense of self may affect one's care of patients. Just as all clinicians involved in therapeutic work must be able to recognize and therapeutically manage transference and countertransference in the doctor-patient relationship, clinicians must also be able to understand how their own personalities, identities, beliefs, experiences, and biases may influence their ethical judgment. For instance, a psychiatric nurse who places a high value on his ability to do good as a healer should recognize that this may subtly influence his judgment when evaluating the decisional capacity of patients who refuse medically necessary treatments. A psychologist with a strong commitment to personal self-care and athleticism may have difficulty accepting patients who do not share this commitment and who engage voluntarily in high-risk behaviors with both ethical and clinical consequences. Attentiveness to these interpersonal aspects of the clinician-patient relationship is a crucial safeguard for ethical decision-making by professionals in order to serve the needs and best interests of patients. In recent years, the role of implicit bias has been identified and studied vigorously, demonstrating the influence of attitudes and social stereotypes related to gender, race, cultural background, and other aspects of identity on many aspects of health care. The impact of implicit bias is felt by patients and health professionals and can adversely affect patient care practices, quality, safety outcomes, and health system policies. Amelioration of implicit bias issues is an important skill.

The third key ethics skill is an awareness of the limits of one's own medical knowledge and expertise and the willingness to practice within those limits. Providing competent care within the scope of one's expertise fulfills both the positive ethical duty of doing good and the obligation to do no harm. In some real-world situations, mental health professionals may feel compelled to perform services outside of their area of competence. Such circumstances are often encountered in geographically isolated communities. For instance, rural providers may be faced with the dilemma of being asked to provide care for which they are not adequately trained or to treat people with whom they have other relationships (e.g., neighbors or local businesspeople). Rural practitioners may also be unable to provide care for all of the patients who need help (Roberts 2016), although increasingly the use of care delivered remotely (e.g., telepsychiatry) and integrated behavioral health models hold promise in addressing these challenges (Fortney et al. 2015). In such settings, clinicians may feel ethically justified in choosing to do their best in the clinical situation, while simultaneously trying to resolve the problem (American Psychiatric Association 2001b; Roberts 2016). For example, a rural psychologist may expand his or her zone of competence by obtaining consultation by telephone or by using teleconferencing.

The fourth skill is the ability to recognize high-risk situations in which ethical problems are likely to arise. Such circumstances can occur when a mental health professional must step out of the usual treatment relationship to protect the patient or others from harm or to protect the patient's or others' best interests (even when the patient may not agree). These situations include depriving patients of autonomy (e.g., involuntary treatment or hospitalization, reporting a diagnosis of neurocognitive disorder to a public health department to prevent a patient from driving), reporting suspected child or elder abuse or neglect, and informing an identified third party of a patient's intention to inflict harm. Inhabiting multiple roles can also introduce ethical risks, as the obligations that accompany the roles may conflict (see Figure 2–1).

The fifth skill is the willingness to seek information and consultation when faced with an ethically or clinically difficult situation and the ability to make use of the guidance offered by these sources. All mental health professionals should tackle clinically difficult cases by reviewing the relevant literature and consulting with more experienced colleagues, colleagues with different expertise, or internal or external advisors who can provide guidance on tricky situations (e.g., attorneys or risk management officers). Mental health professionals should also strive to clarify and resolve ethically difficult situations by looking for data, referring to ethics codes and guidelines, discussing the circumstances with supervisors or consultants, and conferring with ethics committees when appropriate.

The sixth and final essential skill for the mental health professional is the ability to build appropriate ethical safeguards into one's work. For example, clinicians who treat children and adolescents should routinely inform new patients and their parents at the initiation of treatment about limits of confidentiality and the clinician's legal mandate to report child abuse (Johnson et al. 2019). Similarly, clinical researchers can prevent some ethical conflicts from arising in the course of their research by designing protocols that incorporate safeguards throughout the entire life of the project (see Figure 2–2), such as careful training for research staff, participant education sessions in conjunction with the informed consent process, operating procedures that protect personal information gathered from study volunteers (e.g., data encryption), and a priori exit criteria for withdrawing participants (Roberts 1999; Ross et al. 2010).

PRACTICAL ETHICAL PROBLEM-SOLVING

Many clinicians use an eclectic approach to ethical problem-solving that makes intuitive use of principles, case experiences, lessons learned from colleagues, and a combination of inductive and deductive reasoning. Such an approach typically yields not one "right" answer but, rather, an array

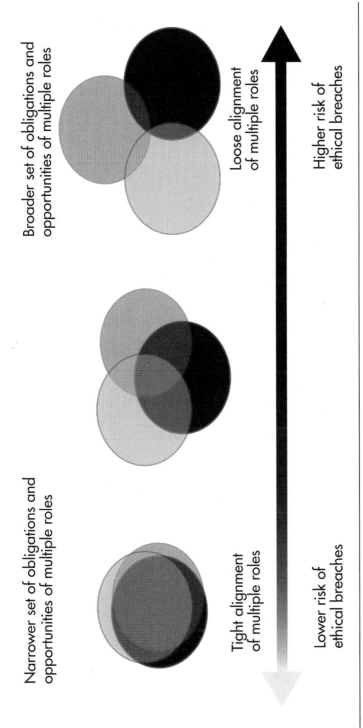

FIGURE 2–1. Ethical risks associated with multiple roles.

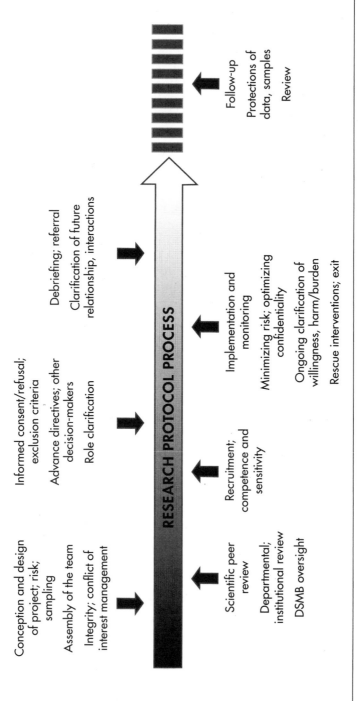

FIGURE 2–2. Multiple opportunities to safeguard research participants during the research process.

Source. Copyright © 2007, Laura Weiss Roberts, M.D., M.A. Used with permission. DSMB=data and safety monitoring board.

of possible and ethically justifiable responses that may be acceptable in the specific set of circumstances. For lower risk decisions (e.g., introducing a new medication into the care of a reluctant patient this visit vs. the next visit), this style of decision-making is often quite adequate. For higher risk decisions that must now or may later have to stand up to more rigorous scrutiny, a more systematic and explicit approach is better and often necessary.

In the clinical setting, a widely used approach to ethical problem solving is the four-topics method described by Jonsen and colleagues (2002). This method entails gathering and evaluating information about 1) clinical indications, 2) patient preferences, 3) patient quality of life, and 4) contextual or external influences on the ethical decision-making process. The model for this approach is depicted in Figure 2–3.

The four-topics methodology has the advantage of being pragmatic, offering an implicit prioritization of issues that arise in complex, real-world situations. The four-topics method has also been successfully used to analyze ethical issues in a variety of clinical settings and decision contexts. This method has been widely disseminated, and many ethics committees in hospitals use it in their evaluations and decisions regarding ethical dilemmas. In the psychiatric context, less attention has been paid to developing ethical decision-making models specifically addressing the unique characteristics of psychiatric patients, settings, and decisions (Roberts et al. 1996a). With practice, however, the four-topics method can be used to help psychiatrists and other mental health professionals think through both straightforward and complex ethical cases. Strategies for systematically evaluating ethical issues in clinical supervision of multidisciplinary colleagues and clinicians in training may also be helpful in academic and community-based patient care settings (Roberts et al. 1996b).

Many ethical dilemmas in clinical care (e.g., see Table 2–2) involve a conflict between clinical indications and patient preferences, the first two topics of the four-topics model. Consider, for instance, a severely depressed older adult, with dangerous weight loss, who is refusing recommended electroconvulsive therapy; an adolescent who is experiencing new-onset psychotic symptoms who becomes behaviorally threatening, and is brought to a hospital against his will; a psychologist attempting to form a therapeutic alliance with an individual who is angry at past providers and requests the psychologist's personal cell-phone number; or a college mental health provider who evaluates a student who is severely depressed and suicidal, but refuses hospitalization because he wants to finish his exams. In each scenario above, the patient's preferences conflict with medical, therapeutic, or ethical obligations, creating clear tensions—

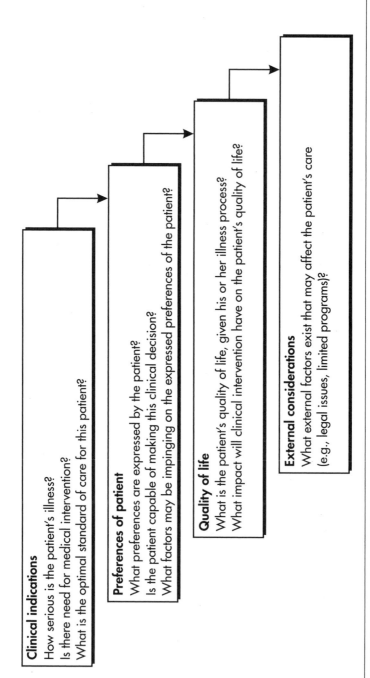

Clinical indications
How serious is the patient's illness?
Is there need for medical intervention?
What is the optimal standard of care for this patient?

Preferences of patient
What preferences are expressed by the patient?
Is the patient capable of making this clinical decision?
What factors may be impinging on the expressed preferences of the patient?

Quality of life
What is the patient's quality of life, given his or her illness process?
What impact will clinical intervention have on the patient's quality of life?

External considerations
What external factors exist that may affect the patient's care
(e.g., legal issues, limited programs)?

FIGURE 2–3.   A model for ethical decision-making.

Source.   Reprinted from Roberts LW, Dyer AR: "Health Care Ethics Committees," in *Concise Guide to Ethics in Mental Health Care.* Washington, DC, American Psychiatric Publishing, 2004, p. 307. Copyright © 2004, American Psychiatric Publishing. Used with permission.

often not quickly or easily resolved—between duties of beneficence (promoting patient welfare) and respecting patient autonomy (respecting patient wishes).

To work through dilemmas in which two vital ethical principles are at odds, one must first explore fully and thoughtfully the patient's preferences as well as the clinical indications. Why does the patient refuse treatment? Does the patient have the cognitive and emotional capacity to make this decision at this time? Are there a range of options, perhaps some that have not been previously considered, that may offer benefit? How urgent is the clinical situation, and is time available for discussion, collaboration, and perhaps compromise? If the patient does not have decision-making capacity, the dilemma is at least temporarily resolved by identifying an appropriate alternative decision-maker. If the patient does have the ability to provide informed consent—involving capacity for decision-making (Appelbaum and Grisso 1988) and capacity for voluntarism (Geppert 2007; Roberts 2002b)—then, under most foreseeable circumstances, his or her preferences must be followed. However, by engaging the patient in a meaningful dialogue in which the mental health professional describes the full range of treatment options and demonstrates sensitivity to the reasons for the patient's refusal, it may often be possible to discover a solution that the patient can willingly accept and the clinician can justify as medically beneficial.

FOUNDATIONS OF CLINICAL AND RESEARCH ETHICS

Empirical Basis

Empirical data have become increasingly important in understanding the ethical aspects of clinical practice and clinical research. Perhaps the most influential early empirical ethics work was Henry Beecher's 1966 article in *The New England Journal of Medicine* in which he provided descriptions of 22 published biomedical research projects with significant ethical violations, including studies in which individuals were injected with cancer cells or deliberately infected with hepatitis (Beecher 1966). Interestingly, none of these studies involved psychiatric research or mentally ill individuals, although some of the projects included developmentally disabled individuals (e.g., the Willowbrook Hepatitis Studies [Fletcher et al. 1997]).

Empirical studies can provide valuable support for more rigorous ethical decision-making throughout the field of biomedicine. Scientific evidence can establish the utility of medical interventions, facilitate respect for persons by surveying the perspectives and values of patients and research volunteers, and describe how the benefits and burdens of a health care policy are distributed among members of society. Empirical work can inform us about differences among different ethics guidelines developed by various professional organizations and other groups. For instance, early work by Berkman and colleagues (2004) surveyed physicians' professional organizations, group practices, and health plans to examine whether ethics policies were concordant or discordant and in what ways. They found important gaps in many of these policies in terms of the ethical concerns addressed. In particular, societal issues, such as distribution of resources and addressing the needs of and advocating for vulnerable populations, were frequently not mentioned. Finally, evidence about the views of clinicians on ethical issues has provided valuable data regarding clinicians' attitudes and perspectives regarding ethically challenging aspects of care (Sjöstrand et al. 2015) as well as perceived ethical dilemmas encountered in real-world practice (Saigle and Racine 2018).

Ethical decision-making according to the values of beneficence, nonmaleficence, and justice requires an understanding of the cognitive nature of bias and a capacity to recognize possible manifestations of bias in clinical decision-making. Empirical work on bias is necessary to detect and, ultimately, root out bias across the whole range of clinical activities, from professional training to patient diagnosis and treatment. Empirical work can inform us of the disproportionate influence bias wields over members of marginalized groups already at risk for compounded inequities (Chapman et al. 2013). Early work on implicit and explicit bias has found compelling evidence that racism and gender bias pervade clinical decision-making. In an early study of 287 physicians by Green et al. (2007), physicians were found to have an implicit preference for white patients versus Black patients, holding implicit stereotypes of Black patients as being uncooperative generally and with respect to medical treatment. More recent work by Fadus and colleagues (2020) has found that similar symptom profiles in white and nonwhite children lead to racialized diagnoses and treatments: ethnic and racial minority youth were more likely to receive diagnoses of oppositional defiant disorder and conduct disorder, whereas white youth were most likely to receive diagnosis for ADHD. These findings suggest that diagnostic categories themselves may be shaped by systemic inequities and sociocultural biases.

Social injustice has shaped the mental health system and drives mental illness and mental health inequities (Shim and Vinson 2021). Mental health professionals have an obligation to examine and research the social determinants of mental health, which are often enforced by public policy and upheld by social norms (Shim and Vinson 2021). Implicit and explicit biases held by health professionals perpetuate an unjust, inequitable system of care. Mental health professionals can mitigate biases through education, introspection, and training. Understanding a patient's clinical situation may involve an assessment of social determinants of mental health; caring for a patient may involve programs such as housing support that help to address social determinants of mental health.

In terms of the four-topics method for clinical ethical decision-making, investigators have been gathering empirical evidence relevant to understanding a patient's clinical situation for many years. These data concern disease prognosis, the relative efficacy of treatment options, and the treatments' risks and benefits. Investigators began many years ago to compile data that may be helpful in understanding patient preferences, quality-of-life issues, and contextual features.

Empirical studies have also been helpful in identifying and working through some of the complex ethical issues that arise in psychiatric research. For example, in the MacArthur Treatment Competence Study, Appelbaum and Grisso (1995) assessed the decision-making abilities of people with major depression, schizophrenia, ischemic heart disease, and a control group of nonpatient volunteers. The results of this landmark project revealed areas of decision-making capacity that were more difficult for acutely ill psychiatric patients than for the medically ill patients or members of the control group. This study demonstrated that decisional capacity was most impaired among the psychotic psychiatric patients but, very importantly, also showed that clinical treatment significantly improved the deficits in the decisional capacity of the acutely ill psychiatric patients. Subsequently, a substantial body of empirical work evaluating capacity to consent among people with severe mental illnesses (including schizophrenia, bipolar disorder, and severe depression) has supported the notion that psychiatric illness, in and of itself, does not automatically indicate lack of capacity to make treatment or research decisions (Dunn et al. 2006b; Lapid et al. 2003; Palmer et al. 2007; Stroup et al. 2005).

In addition, Roberts and colleagues have constructed a body of empirical work that provides further evidence challenging the idea of psychiatric "exceptionalism" in research—that is, the assumption that psychiatric illnesses, and people who suffer from them, are inherently "special" or more vulnerable (Roberts and Kim 2014; Roberts et al. 2002b).

Finally, empirical findings have also been helpful as a guide to monitor the ethical attitudes and behaviors of mental health trainees and to suggest, refine, or validate outcomes of educational interventions. For example, medical students and residents perceived a need for more education about the ethical and professional dilemmas that occur during medical training and the practice of medicine (Roberts et al. 2005). In addition, psychiatry residents reported a greater need than residents in other specialties for more education about specific ethical problems that occur during training, including conflicts between residents and attending physicians and performing work outside the trainee's area of competence. A recent, updated survey regarding perceptions of the ethics and professionalism curricula of child and adolescent psychiatry residency programs found that a substantial minority (22%) of respondents (program directors) believed that the amount of teaching on these topics was inadequate, whereas the majority (77%) felt that the amount of teaching was adequate (Dingle and Kolli 2020). Compared with the previous survey (conducted in 1992), the authors found that training programs had increased their use of more interactive methods of teaching. However, the authors noted that there were a number of issues related to the adequacy of training in ethics and professionalism that remained, despite increased attention to these topics overall.

Philosophical Basis

Several theories of moral behavior form the philosophical foundation of contemporary medical ethics. Each theory delineates an aspect of ethics that is relevant to particular situations or conditions in biomedical ethics. Although the theories described below are often discussed separately, the value of understanding them in practice arises from the ability to draw on them as a tool kit; that is, different tools or considerations derived from different theories may need to be combined to approach complex ethical dilemmas faced in psychiatric practice, in the development of professional guidelines, and in policy making related to mental health.

Kantianism is a philosophical theory based on the work of Immanuel Kant (1724–1804). Kantianism suggests that the morality of an action may be independent of its consequences and that some actions, such as telling the truth, are morally obligatory in almost all circumstances. To be ethical, a person must follow these moral obligations unconditionally. Kantian theory is at the core of how contemporary bioethicists think about ethical behavior in patient care—that is, serving the needs and interests of the individual patient above other goals in a clinical situation. For instance, most Western clinicians believe that it is always important to tell patients the truth, even though the truth in some circumstances may be difficult to speak or painful to hear. Kantian ideals, however, may be challenging to live out in some real-world medical situations in which there are scarce resources (e.g., allocation of organs for transplantation or of highly expensive medications). Often, these situations involve conflicting moral obligations, such as balancing the needs of others or of the community against the preferences of an individual (e.g., insisting on involuntary treatment in the care of a mentally ill person voicing a homicidal threat toward a specific person). Kantianism is complementary to another theory, deontology, which posits that decisions ought to be made based on adherence to moral norms (i.e., "doing what is right") (Alexander and Moore 2016).

Utilitarianism refers to an ethical theory supported by the writings of Jeremy Bentham (1748–1832) and John Stuart Mill (1806–1873). Utilitarian philosophy posits that the most ethical actions and rules are those that bring about the greatest good for the most people—that is, those actions that have the greatest utility. Questions of what has the greatest "good" or "utility" in complex ethical systems are questions of axiology— the study of the nature of valuation. Utilitarian philosophy emphasizes the importance of the consequences of one's actions and highlights beneficence and justice as guiding ethical principles. Whereas Kantianism is particularly relevant to the ethical treatment of individuals, utilitarianism is vital to ethical reasoning about larger systems. The principles of utility and justice are the ethical foundation of public health policies, for example. However, a rigidly utilitarian viewpoint could justify practices that most people would consider immoral—for example, coercing a small, randomly selected group of people to enroll in a risky medical research trial to derive significant benefits for the rest of the population.

Principle-based ethics, as described by contemporary theorists James Childress and Thomas Beauchamp, suggests that ethical dilemmas should be resolved through the specification and balancing of the principles of nonmaleficence, beneficence, respect for autonomy, and justice (Beauchamp and Childress 2001). By contrast, casuistry describes a bottom-up approach to ethical decision-making, in which ethicists focus first on the details of a particular case rather than overarching rules and principles. Casuistry also highlights the importance of ethical reasoning by analogy with similar cases from the past (Jonsen and Toulmin 1988).

Whereas Kantian, utilitarian, deontological, and principle-based ethics primarily ask questions that are directly amenable to paternalistic patterns of logic and reason, care ethics emphasizes modes of cognition such as empathy and compassion that have traditionally laid outside bioethical models (Gilligan 1987). The care ethics model is skeptical of naturalized concepts of "moral development" that have been elevated by empowered groups (usually, white and male) in the history of ethical thought, holding that the exclusion of historically marginalized voices and privileging of prescriptive ethical constructs amounts to arbitrary moral indifference. Care ethics is focused on pragmatic elements of care, such as attentiveness, responsiveness, and interdependence, that require epistemic openness, humility, and tolerance of ambiguity. It affirms the decision-making value of all individuals cooperating in a context of care provision according to these ideals. Care ethics can complement a deontological view when situational ambiguity or specificity exceed or are incompatible with prevailing moral rule sets, affirming the moral basis and restorative potential of local, context-sensitive, and nonnormative ethical approaches.

Other philosophical approaches to biomedical ethics include virtue ethics, which defines as ethical the actions of virtuous people; relationship ethics, emphasizing commitments and relationships to others as the basis of ethical life; and communitarian ethics, which defines morality based on social values and traditions.

ETHICAL PRINCIPLES AND VIRTUES

It is important for clinicians to be fluent in the language of ethics discourse so that they can identify and conceptualize the ethical components of their work. From a technical perspective, a principle is a basic truth, law, rule, or assumption that is inherently distinct and has enduring meaning. Examples of principles are autonomy and justice, as discussed below. A virtue is an attribute or quality that inclines an individual toward doing good acts and/or avoiding harmful acts. Historically, virtues have been linked with habits or with the habitual disposition toward positive aims and recognized excellence. Examples of virtues are compassion and self-effacement. Principles and virtues necessarily overlap because principles are terms for things that are seen as good and virtues are the qualities of an individual that lead to his or her doing good, such as fidelity (principle) and faithfulness (virtue).

Brief definitions of many principles and virtues are provided in this discussion and in Table 2–4. The key principles of moral behavior with special importance to the field of medical ethics include nonmaleficence, beneficence, autonomy, respect for persons, justice, veracity, fidelity, and the linked concepts of privacy and confidentiality (Beauchamp and Childress 2001).

Nonmaleficence is a modern term for the old, perhaps ancient, rule of *primum non nocere* ("first, do no harm"). In medical ethics, harm is defined broadly, including killing, causing physical or emotional suffering, or depriving others of beneficial things.

TABLE 2–4. Glossary of ethics terms

Altruism   The virtue of acting for the good of another rather than for oneself, at times entailing self-sacrifice.

Autonomy   Literally "self-rule." In medical ethics, autonomy is the ability to make deliberated or reasoned decisions for oneself and to act on the basis of such decisions.

Beneficence   The performance of an action done to benefit others. The principle of beneficence in medicine signifies an obligation to benefit patients and to seek their good.

Charity   Voluntary giving to provide for others in need. Charities and charitable giving have intrinsic moral and social value. Modern health care is funded more effectively from taxation or insurance than from charity (Boyd et al. 1997).

Coercion   The use of some form of pressure to persuade or compel an individual to agree to a belief or action.

Compassion   Literally, "suffering with" another person, with kindness and an active regard for his or her welfare. Compassion is more closely related to empathy than to sympathy, as sympathy connotes the more distanced experience of feeling sorry for the individual.

Confidentiality   The obligation of physicians not to disclose information obtained from patients or observed about them without their permission. In clinical care, confidentiality entails taking precautions to protect the personal information of patients. Confidentiality is a privilege linked to the legal right of privacy and may at times be overridden by exceptions stipulated in law.

Conflict of commitment   A type of conflict of interest in which a physician's or researcher's outside interests, relationships, or commitments compete for time and effort with the physician's or researcher's duties to his or her institution and prevent the physician or researcher from meeting his or her usual obligations to the institution (Marcello 2010).

Conflict of conscience   A type of conflict of interest in which one's personal beliefs interfere with one's abilities to perform one's professional duties (Marcello 2010).

Conflict of interest   In medicine, a situation in which a physician has competing roles, relationships, or interests that could potentially interfere with the ability to care for patients. Such situations may naturally occur in clinical care and research, and they are not inherently unethical. Conflicts of interest must be recognized and managed appropriately to safeguard the well-being of vulnerable individuals (e.g., patients, research participants) and to prevent exploitative practices.

TABLE 2–4.   Glossary of ethics terms *(continued)*

Duty of care   An expression used as a reminder about the key duties of the profession. Duty of care could loosely equate with the principle of beneficence. Duty of care prevents a doctor from stopping work in the middle of a clinical task, for example, and requires that a doctor keep his or her skills up to date. In terms of the law, duty of care relates to negligence and the harm of failing to avert harm. Duty of care is usually seen as being owed to patients, but could be owed to others or to oneself (Boyd et al. 1997).

Empathy   Entering into someone else's frame of reference in terms of thoughts, feelings, and experiences to have an authentic understanding of the other person's experiences imaginatively as one's own.

Equipoise   A term used in justification of randomization in clinical trials. Equipoise describes having no rational preference among treatment options being compared. A moral dilemma occurs if a clinician does not share the collective equipoise of specialists in her field and is invited to recruit and randomize patients in a trial, especially if her preferred treatment is only available to patients randomized to it in the trial (Boyd et al. 1997).

Euthanasia   A form of physician-assisted death in which the physician deliberately and with compassionate intent acts to end the life of a person with an incurable and progressive disease that will cause imminent death.

Fidelity   The virtue of promise keeping, truthfulness, and honor. In clinical care, the faithfulness with which a clinician commits to the duty of helping patients and acting in a manner that is in keeping with the ideals of the profession.

Fiduciary   An entity in a position of trust with a duty to act on behalf of another for the other's good. Physicians are fiduciaries with respect to their patients.

Futility   A term referring to medical treatment that is unlikely to achieve its desired aim. The concept of futility is used to justify the medical decision not to provide requested life prolonging treatment. Although physicians are not obligated to provide treatment that they perceive as futile, carefully reviewing the therapeutic options and reaching a joint decision together with the patient and family is preferable (Boyd et al. 1997).

Honesty   A virtue in which one conveys the truth fully, without misrepresentation through deceit, bias, or omission.

Human dignity   The belief that every person, intrinsically, is valued and worthy of respect. In medical ethics, every patient is believed to have innate and inalienable worth as a human being that requires that he or she be treated with respect and compassion and full interpersonal regard as expressed in attitudes, behaviors, and nondiscriminatory practices.

Informed consent   In the clinical setting, the legal and ethical obligation for clinicians to inform patients about their illnesses and alternatives for care and to assist them in making reasoned, authentic decisions about treatment. In the research setting, this is the similar obligation for a researcher to inform participants about the research protocol and help them make reasoned, authentic decisions about research participation.

TABLE 2–4. Glossary of ethics terms *(continued)*

Integrity   A virtue literally defined as wholeness or coherence. It connotes professional soundness and reliability of intention and action.

Justice   The ethical principle of fairness. Distributive justice refers to the fair and equitable distribution of resources and burden through society.

Medical decision-making   The intentional process associated with making a choice in clinical care. Medical decision-making pertains to a patient's capacity to make decisions related to his or her health or health care and to the clinician's process of deliberation, consultation, and data gathering that results in the development of a diagnosis and of therapeutic alternatives for a patient.

Medical negligence   The legal concept of a breach of duty of medical care. Medical negligence rests on the existence of a duty of care, failure to fulfill that duty, and the existence of harm.

Nonmaleficence   The duty to avoid doing harm.

Personhood   Having full moral status as a human being.

Quality of life   The expression of a value judgment regarding the experience of life as a whole or some aspect of it by an individual.

Respect   The virtue of fully regarding and according intrinsic value to someone or something. In clinical care, respect is reflected in treating another individual with genuine consideration and attentiveness to that person's life history, values, and goals.

Self-understanding   Awareness of one's own values and motivations. Self-understanding based on insight and careful self-scrutiny is a key ethical skill of special importance to mental health care ethics.

Therapeutic boundaries   The set of concepts, rules, and duties that structure the clinician-patient relationship to ensure psychological safety, to optimize therapeutic benefit, and to prevent potentially exploitative practices.

Trustworthiness   A virtue that pertains to a disposition that inspires confident belief in and reliance on the physician's character and ability to act beneficently and honestly.

Voluntary   The attribute in which a belief or act derives from one's own free will and is not coerced or unduly influenced by others.

Vulnerability   The capacity to be wounded or hurt physically, emotionally, spiritually, or socially and being without the means to defend or advocate for oneself fully.

Source.   Adapted from Roberts and Dyer 2004; with additional entries adapted from Boyd et al. 1997 and Marcello 2010 as noted.

Beneficence refers to the belief that individuals should try to do good and to seek benefit for others. Beneficence encompasses the notion of *utility*, the duty to act in a way that provides the greatest positive consequences and the least negative consequences.

Autonomy, which means "self-rule," suggests a moral principle based on the importance of respecting others' right to self-governance. To be autonomous, an individual must be free from coercive influences and capable of making independent decisions and actions. To respect a patient's autonomy requires one to behave in a way that allows for and enhances the ability of the patient to make voluntary decisions on his or her own behalf (Roberts 2002b).

Respect for persons is a broad concept that encompasses respect for autonomy plus a deep regard for the worth and dignity of all human beings. The protection of potentially vulnerable groups of people represents a key aspect of respect for persons and is embodied in specific ethical guidelines.

Justice is a moral principle that relates to treating people fairly and, in modern society, without prejudice. *Distributive justice* refers to equitable distribution of benefits and burdens among members of society. "Parity" legislation that seeks to ensure provision of insurance for mental illness and related conditions that is equal or equivalent to insurance for physical illness illustrates a real-life effort at distributive justice in the United States.

Veracity refers to honesty or truth telling. Upholding the moral ideal of veracity involves both a positive ethical duty—that is, being truthful in one's statements—and a negative ethical duty—that is, not telling lies and avoiding misimpressions or misrepresentation (such as misleading others by withholding the truth or some aspects of it).

Fidelity is the ideal of faithfulness. In medicine, physicians who demonstrate fidelity are steadfast in their role of healer. They do not abandon or exploit patients, and they do not place self-interest or the interest of third parties above patients' needs.

Privacy generally refers to the right to be free from the intrusions of others on one's physical body, one's mind, or one's personal information. In medicine, *confidentiality* is the privilege of having one's privacy protected by a health professional. Keeping the confidences of patients has been an acknowledged duty of physicians from at least the time of Hippocrates, more than 24 centuries ago. Confidentiality is covered in the ethical codes of every mental health discipline.

Many of the conditions under which the privilege of confidentiality is suspended touch directly or indirectly on issues subsumed under mental health, such as child and elder abuse and dangers to third parties. On the other hand, it is important to protect patient confidentiality to whatever extent it is possible, even when there are legal requirements to provide patient information. To give just one example, one should never turn over a patient's entire medical record to a police officer who is investigating the circumstances of a sexual assault; providing only the salient elements of the medical record is sufficient and appropriate according to both ethical and legal directives and prevents inadvertent disclosure of irrelevant (but perhaps very sensitive) personal material.

Although the principles of medical ethics are crucial, they are primarily cognitively based and have been, to some extent, historically limited and culturally determined. Ethical virtues, understood as qualities of character and habits of disposition, are crucial to providing compassionate care for the potentially vulnerable mental health patient. Virtues of particular importance in mental health care are *charity*, *compassion*, *integrity*, and *altruism* (see Table 2–4).

Virtues stand in contrast to cynicism and burnout and can assist clinicians to morally respond to unforeseen and rapidly changing circumstances in which ethical principles may provide general guidance but not the specificity of real-time contextualized decisions.

For example, *respect* as a virtue implies a reverence for the innate dignity of human life and reverence for the freedom of the human being even if, as often occurs in mental health care, the person exercises autonomy in directions that, from the clinician's view, are not in the person's best interests. As mentioned earlier, *fidelity*, or the fiduciary duty, is the core of the clinician-patient relationship and denotes faithfulness expressed in advocacy for the good of the patient over all other priorities. This fiduciary duty is under great pressure in modern mental health care from economic and political forces. *Compassion*, or empathy, is the most powerful counterweight to these pressures because it enables the mental health professional to feel the enormous suffering of the psychiatrically ill and to practice an active regard for their welfare manifested in kindness and mercy in the alleviation and prevention of suffering wherever possible. *Discernment*, or prudence, is the ancient Aristotelian virtue of insight into clinical situations and the ability to exercise practical moral judgment on behalf of the patient's well-being.

CODES OF ETHICAL CONDUCT

Ethical Codes for Physicians

Practical guidelines for the ethical conduct of physicians have been codified in various forms since the Hippocratic oath was documented about

2,500 years ago. Hippocratic writings describe the importance of benef-icence, confidentiality, and nonmaleficence and proscribe exploitation of patients, euthanasia, and abortion. In 1803, the English physician Thomas Percival published *Medical Ethics; or a Code of Institutes and Precepts*, and this document formed the basis of the American Medical Association's (AMA) first Code of Medical Ethics (American Medical Association, Council on Ethical and Judicial Affairs 2005). The most re-cent version of the AMA Code of Medical Ethics can be found online (www.ama-assn.org/about/publications-newsletters/ama-principles-medical-ethics).

The AMA Code of Medical Ethics was first published in 1973 in the form of annotations to the AMA Judicial Council's *Principles of Medical Ethics* (American Medical Association 1957). The AMA Council of Eth-ical and Judicial Affair's ethical guidelines are described as "not laws, but standards of conduct" (American Medical Association, Council of Ethical and Judicial Affairs 2016b, p. 1). All psychiatrists should be fa-miliar with *The Principles of Medical Ethics With Annotations Especially Applicable to Psychiatry* (selections from this brief document are found in Table 2–5; American Psychiatric Association 2010).

A cardinal feature of a profession is its ethical obligation to support and evaluate the ethical conduct of its members. Complaints of unethi-cal behavior by a member of the American Psychiatric Association are investigated by local ethics committees who conduct reviews of docu-ments and testimony, offer education-oriented supportive interventions, and, when necessary, render sanctions, sometimes as serious as expul-sion from membership of the national organization. It is important to recognize that professional codes of ethics exist for several reasons—in-cluding promoting high ethical standards, enhancing the public trust, and providing resources for professionalism education.

Ethical Codes of Other Mental Health Practitioners

Codes of ethics have been drafted by many professional groups who work with patients with mental illness, including psychologists, social workers, and nurses. The groups' different professional orientations are demonstrated by subtle variations in emphasis and philosophy among the codes. The American Psychological Association's (2017) *Ethical Prin-ciples of Psychologists and Code of Conduct* is similar in scope to the AMA guidelines. The psychologists' code outlines five aspirational ethical prin-ciples (beneficence and nonmaleficence; fidelity and responsibility; in-tegrity; justice; and respect for people's rights and dignity) and provides specific guidelines for the ethical handling of numerous professional ac-

TABLE 2–5.   Selections from *The Principles of Medical Ethics*
With Annotations Especially Applicable
to Psychiatry

Section 1   A physician shall be dedicated to providing competent medical
care with compassion and respect for human dignity and rights.

Section 1.2 A psychiatrist should not be a party to any type of policy that
excludes, segregates, or demeans the dignity of any patient
because of ethnic origin, race, sex, creed, age, socioeconomic
status, or sexual orientation.

Section 1.4 A psychiatrist should not be a participant in a legally authorized
execution.

Section 2   A physician shall uphold the standards of professionalism, be
honest in all professional interactions, and strive to report
physicians deficient in character or competence, or engaging in
fraud or deception to appropriate entities.

Section 2.1 The requirement that the physician conduct himself/herself with
propriety in his or her profession and in all the actions of his or
her life is especially important in the case of the psychiatrist
because the patient tends to model his or her behavior after that
of his or her psychiatrist by identification. Furthermore, the
necessary intensity of the treatment relationship may tend to
activate sexual and other needs and fantasies on the part of both
patient and psychiatrist, while weakening the objectivity
necessary for control. Additionally, the inherent inequality in
the doctor-patient relationship may lead to exploitation of the
patient. Sexual activity with a current or former patient is
unethical.

Section 2.3 A psychiatrist who regularly practices outside his or her area of
professional competence should be considered unethical.
Determination of professional competence should be made by
peer review boards or other appropriate bodies.

Section 2.4 Special consideration should be given to those psychiatrists who,
because of mental illness, jeopardize the welfare of their
patients and their own reputations and practices. It is ethical,
even encouraged, for another psychiatrist to intercede in such
situations.

TABLE 2–5. Selections from *The Principles of Medical Ethics With Annotations Especially Applicable to Psychiatry (continued)*

Section 4.2	A psychiatrist may release confidential information only with the authorization of the patient or under proper legal compulsion. The continuing duty of the psychiatrist to protect the patient includes fully apprising him/her of the connotations of waiving the privilege of privacy. This may become an issue when the patient is being investigated by a government agency, is applying for a position, or is involved in legal action. The same principles apply to the release of information concerning treatment to medical departments of government agencies, business organizations, labor unions, and insurance companies. Information gained in confidence about patients seen in student health services should not be released without the students' explicit permission.
Section 4.14	Sexual involvement between a faculty member or supervisor and a trainee or student, in those situations in which an abuse of power can occur, often takes advantage of inequalities in the working relationship and may be unethical because: a. Any treatment of a patient being supervised may be deleteriously affected. b. It may damage the trust relationship between teacher and student. c. Teachers are important professional role models for their trainees and affect their trainees' future professional behavior.
Section 6.2	An ethical psychiatrist may refuse to provide psychiatric treatment to a person who, in the psychiatrist's opinion, cannot be diagnosed as having a mental illness amenable to psychiatric treatment.
Section 7.3	On occasion psychiatrists are asked for an opinion about an individual who is in the light of public attention or who has disclosed information about himself/herself through public media. In such circumstances, a psychiatrist may share with the public his or her expertise about psychiatric issues in general. However, it is unethical for a psychiatrist to offer a professional opinion unless he or she has conducted an examination and has been granted proper authorization for such a statement.
Section 7.5	Psychiatrists shall not participate in torture.

Source. Reprinted from American Psychiatric Association: *The Principles of Medical Ethics With Annotations Especially Applicable to Psychiatry: 2013 Edition.* Arlington, VA, American Psychiatric Association, 2010. Available at: www.psychiatry.org/psychiatrists/practice/ethics. Accessed March 8, 2021. Copyright © 2010, American Psychiatric Association. Used with permission.

tivities. A separate code describes the ethical use of animals in psychological research (American Psychological Association 2012).

The *Code of Ethics* of the National Association of Social Workers (2017) places a high premium on the ethical ideal of justice in its description of core values central to the profession of social work. These core values include service, social justice, dignity and worth of the person, importance of human relationships, integrity, and competence. The American Nurses Association's (2015) *Code of Ethics for Nurses: With Interpretive Statements*, 2nd Edition, embraces a commitment to social justice and to the well-being of individual patients, families, and communities. Additionally, the Code includes the duties of "professional growth, maintenance of competence, preservation of wholeness of character, and personal integrity" (American Nurses Association 2015). The National Board for Certified Counselors' (2016) *Code of Ethics* provides guidelines for ethical behavior in the counseling relationship, counselor supervision, measurement and evaluation, research and publication, consulting, and private practice.

Codes of Research Ethics

Codes of ethics formulated in the last century to govern research involving human volunteers form the basis for modern-day ethical practices in the design, conduct, and oversight of biomedical research. The most famous code of ethics related to medical research is the Nuremberg Code. Developed after World War II in response to experimentation on humans conducted under the Nazis (Annas and Grodin 1992), the Nuremberg Code was a 10-point statement intended to protect human subjects in research. Its famous first sentence is "The voluntary consent of the human subject is absolutely essential" (Annas and Grodin 1992). Necessary elements of informed consent were also emphasized as part of this first point, including requirements for legal capacity to give consent, the absence of coercion, and comprehension of the "nature, duration, and purpose" of the research, the procedures involved, the reasonably foreseeable risks, and the possible effects on the participant's health. Table 2–6 describes the major principles articulated in the Nuremberg Code in 1947 (Trials of War Criminals 1946–1949) and other major ethics codes promulgated in the last century regarding biomedical experimentation.

In 1964, the World Medical Association issued the *Declaration of Helsinki* (which has undergone several revisions and clarifications since then). The *Declaration of Helsinki* substantially expanded on several areas that were either not discussed or only briefly mentioned in the Nuremberg Code, including issues of undue influence and coercion in recruit-

TABLE 2–6. Historical codes of research ethics

Code	Major principles articulated
Nuremberg Code (Katz 1972)	Voluntary participation, legal capacity for informed consent, elements of informed consent
	Results must be useful to society and unobtainable by other means
	Human research must be justified based on animal research and other knowledge informing the basis of the planned study
	Unnecessary physical and mental suffering must be avoided
	Research must not occur if there is reason to believe that death or disabling injury will occur
	Degree of risk should be justified by the importance of the research question
	Even remote possibilities of injury should be protected against
	Qualified people must conduct the experiment
	Participants must be able to voluntarily withdraw at any time
	Study must be terminated by the researcher if continuation is likely to result in injury, disability, or death
Declaration of Helsinki (World Medical Association 1964)	Physician duty to protect life, health, privacy, and dignity of the human subject
	Scientific basis and validity of methods of medical research
	Respect for environment and animals
	Independent protocol review and monitoring
	Qualified and supervised persons must conduct the research
	Assessment of risks and burdens must precede the research; risks must be managed; study must be terminated if positive and conclusive evidence of benefit
	Favorable risk-benefit ratio
	Voluntary, informed consent
	Protection of privacy, confidentiality
	Elements of informed consent

TABLE 2–6. Historical codes of research ethics *(continued)*

Code	Major principles articulated
Declaration of Helsinki *(continued)*	Safeguards for informed consent process
	Provision for informed consent from legally authorized representative for legally incompetent, physically or mentally incapable, or legally incompetent minors
	Other provisions for proxy consent: requirement of scientific necessity of enrolling the decisionally incapable population, assent from incompetent individual
	Ethical obligations of authors and publishers: accuracy, publication of negative findings, sources of funding and possible conflict of interests declared
	Provisions for the combining of research with clinical care
	New method should be tested against best currently available methods; access at end of study to best methods identified by study (placebo-controlled trial acceptable in specific circumstances [scientifically valid methodological reasons, or no additional risks from placebo])
	Inform patients which aspects of clinical care are research
	Ability, based on physician judgment, to use unproven or new methods in some situations; ideally should be focus of research
The Belmont Report (National Commission for the Protection of Human Subjects of Biomedical and Behavioral Research 1979)	Respect for persons: Treat individuals as autonomous agents; protect those with diminished autonomy
	Beneficence: Do not harm; maximize possible benefits/minimize possible harms
	Justice: Addresses principles of fairness in recruitment and in distribution of fruits of knowledge gained

ment, potential vulnerability in research subjects, and surrogate consent. It has also been a source of disagreement because of its stance (modified in a clarification in 2004) on the ethics of placebo-controlled trials in situations in which standard treatments already exist.

The Belmont Report, issued in 1979 by the National Commission for the Protection of Human Subjects of Biomedical and Behavioral Research, is another important document in the history of research ethics. It set out three core principles of research with human subjects—respect for persons, beneficence, and justice—and discussed the potential for tensions and conflict among the principles; described particular applications flowing from these principles, such as informed consent; and highlighted gaps where ethical issues remained.

The Common Rule, created in 1981 in the United States, established a set of minimal ethical guidelines for conducting research on human volunteers (see Table 2–7 for a history of the Common Rule). The Common Rule also defined a human subject as any living individual about whom a researcher obtains data (inclusive of both healthy individuals and patients). Subpart A enumerated requirements for assuring compliance by research institutions; requirements for obtaining, waiving, and documenting informed consent; and administrative and operational requirements for the institutional review board (IRB), which had already been established in 1974. In Subparts B, C, and D, the Common Rule established additional protections for "vulnerable" research subjects, including pregnant women, fetuses, and newborn children; prisoners; and children.

A significant revision to the Common Rule was added in 2018. This revision upheld the previous definition of a human subject. However, it elaborated on what is meant by "obtaining data" from volunteers, changing this language to "using, studying, or analyzing individuals' information or biospecimens or generating identifiable private information or identifiable biospecimens." The revision added a provision requiring an assessment by the Common Rule agencies of whether analytic technologies could be capable of generating identifiable private information. The revision also expanded IRB exemption more broadly to scholarly and journalistic activities, public health surveillance, criminal justice or investigative purposes, and certain national security purposes.

EXAMPLES OF KEY CLINICAL ETHICS ISSUES

Clinical ethical decision-making in mental health care can be very difficult because of the complexities of the clinician-patient relationship in the biobehavioral disciplines and the need for careful attention to ethical safeguards when working with people with disorders and treatments that affect mental processes. For instance, maintaining treatment boundaries is important for all who work therapeutically with others, but it is especially so in the intimacy of the psychotherapeutic setting. Similarly, the con-

TABLE 2–7.   History of the Common Rule

Year	Title	Summary
1974	National Research Act	Moratorium on federally funded fetal research Institutional review board (IRB) review of human research for studies funded by U.S. Department of Health, Education, and Welfare (DHEW)
1974–1978	National Commission for Protection of Human Subjects of Biomedical and Behavioral Research	Report on research involving fetuses, prisoners, children, individuals with mental infirmity, psychosurgery, IRB informed consent Belmont Report criteria and ethics of protecting subjects differentiating research and clinical practice
1978	Revised DHEW	Regulations protecting pregnant women, fetuses, prisoners, and in vitro fertilization
1980–1983	President's Commission for the Study of Ethical Problems in Medicine and Biomedical and Behavioral Research	Review of federal policies governing human research Recommendation that all federal agencies adopt the U.S. Department of Health and Human Services (DHHS; i.e., DHEW) regulations for the protection of subjects
1981	Revised DHHS	IRB responsibilities and procedures Revision of FDA regulations to correspond to those of DHHS
1982	President's Science Advisor/Office of Science and Technology	Head of interagency committee developing a common policy for protection of human research subjects
1983	DHHS Regulation	Protections governing children in research

TABLE 2–7. History of the Common Rule *(continued)*

Year	Title	Summary
1991	Final Common Federal Policy: The Common Rule	Codified 15 federal agencies' regulations, including CIA under executive order Identical to basic DHHS policy for protection of human research subjects Additional protections for pregnant women, fetuses, prisoners, children, in vitro fertilization FDA informed consent and IRB regulations changed to meet these standards

Source. Reprinted from Roberts LW, Dyer AR: *Concise Guide to Ethics in Mental Health Care.* Washington, DC, American Psychiatric Publishing, 2004, pp. 262–263. Copyright © 2004, American Psychiatric Publishing. Used with permission.

cept of confidentiality is a vital practice in all health professions, but it is particularly relevant to patients with illnesses that are socially stigmatized and for whom treatment may involve revealing deeply private, often shaming information about themselves. As another example, the process of informed consent for treatment may require more careful efforts in mental health because of the possibilities that patients with severe and persistent mental illness may suffer episodic, fluctuating, and/or progressive impairments of decisional capacity. Finally, all clinicians have an obligation to use their power ethically, but only psychiatrists (and, in some states, locales, and practice settings, psychologists) are routinely asked and authorized to appropriately use their legal power to impose involuntary treatment and hospitalization.

In this section, we provide an overview of many, although not all, of the most challenging and relevant clinical issues for mental health professionals. These include 1) maintaining therapeutic boundaries; 2) patient nonabandonment; 3) informed consent and treatment refusal; 4) alternative decision-making and advance directives; 5) ethical use of power; 6) confidentiality; 7) overlapping roles, dual agency, and conflicts of interest; 8) social stigmatization of mental illness and advocacy for better mental health care; 9) responding to colleague impairment or misconduct; 10) issues in multidisciplinary practice; 11) issues in novel modes of prediction, evaluation, and treatment (including social media, electronic footprints, and digital health); 12) caring for complex patients; and 13) caring for special populations.

Maintaining Therapeutic Boundaries

The intimate nature of the psychotherapeutic relationship requires all those who practice psychotherapy (i.e., in the United States, psychiatrists, clinical nurse specialists, psychologists, and social workers) to establish and adhere to appropriate professional boundaries. The concept of boundaries has been defined as the "edge or limit of appropriate behavior…in the clinical setting" (Gabbard 1999, p. 142).

Therapeutic boundaries are important in any type of clinical work, but they have been most thoroughly defined in the context of psychoanalysis and psychodynamic therapy (Gabbard 1999; Gabbard and Lester 1995). These boundaries include temporal and spatial limits: therapeutic encounters typically occur at the clinician's office during business hours, except in crisis situations. Limits are also observed in the nature of the relationship, which involves the professional being paid for services and acting as a fiduciary, a professional who is worthy of the patient's trust. Nontherapeutic encounters, including business arrangements, social relationships, and sexual activity, are forbidden. Within the therapeutic relationship, limits are also observed: the patient is encouraged to share intimate feelings, thoughts, and memories, whereas the therapist generally avoids self-disclosure and adopts a posture of neutrality. Physical contact other than handshakes is avoided.

Boundary violations are actions by the therapist that are outside normal professional limits and that have the potential to harm patients. The most widely studied boundary violation is sexual contact. Although sexual and romantic entanglements between psychiatrists and patients were not uncommon in the early days of psychiatry (Gabbard and Lester 1995), the damage such relationships may cause has become increasingly clear over the last several decades. Psychiatrists must never exploit patients, use interactions with patients to gratify their own impulses, or influence the patient in a manner that threatens treatment goals (American Psychiatric Association 2015). Sexual contact between patients and physicians is prohibited by the American Psychiatric Association (American Psychiatric Association 2010), the AMA, and the American Psychological Association (American Psychological Association 2017), and is illegal in many states. A review of qualitative and quantitative studies of therapists who had sexual relations with their patients suggests that risk factors for such behavior include inadequate training, isolation from colleagues, and narcissistic pathology (Epstein 1994). Gabbard classified these errant therapists into four groups based on the underlying psychodynamics: 1) psychotic individuals whose sexual transgression stems from a delusion; 2) therapists with predatory psychopathology and paraphilias, who prey on patients because they are easy to exploit; 3) lovesick therapists, whose own psychological vulnerabilities cause them to become infatuated with a particular patient; and 4) therapists who give in to a patient's demands for sex as a form of masochistic surrender (Gabbard 1999; Gabbard and Lester 1995). Although 1.6% or less of physicians are disciplined for sexual boundary violations, 7% of physician respondents of anonymous self-report surveys, on average, report a history of sexual relationships with patients (Sansone and Sansone 2009). In a recent study of 101 cases of sexual violations in medicine, 16.8% of perpetrators practiced psychiatry or neurology (DuBois et al. 2019).

Sexual contact with former patients is also understood as inherently unethical and exploitative. In the interest of beneficence and nonmaleficence, even the possibility or suggestion of a romantic relationship with a current or former patient should be avoided (American Psychiatric Association 2015). Sexual or romantic involvement with key third parties to a treatment relationship, such as the parent or spouse of a patient, threatens the therapeutic relationship and presents a conflict of interest that should be avoided (American Psychiatric Association 2020).

Nonsexual boundary violations have been less well studied than sexual violations. These transgressions include seeing patients outside of normal office hours and in nonclinical locations, engaging in social or business relationships with patients, accepting gifts from patients, and making nonsexual physical contact (American Psychiatric Association 2010, 2015; Roberts 2006). "Friending" a patient on social media or googling a patient is generally considered a boundary violation because these actions are likely to serve the interests of the therapist rather than the best interests of the patient (de Araujo Reinert and Kowacs 2019; Sabin and Harland 2017; Zilber 2014). Any of these violations carries the potential to exploit the patient or to harm the treatment relationship and should therefore be avoided.

The term *boundary crossing* has been used to describe a subtle, nonsexual transgression that is helpful to the patient because it advances the treatment (Gutheil and Gabbard 1998). As an example of a boundary crossing, Gabbard describes a guarded, paranoid patient who offers her psychiatrist a cookie. By accepting this token gift graciously, the psychiatrist helps the patient feel more relaxed in the treatment setting and more willing to discuss her symptoms. Boundary crossings such as this are common and not unethical, but differentiating crossings from actual boundary violations may be difficult in the course of treatment (American Psychiatric Association 2015; Gabbard 1999). The Exploitation Index (Epstein and Simon 1990) is most salient to analytically oriented psychotherapy performed in an urban setting, but despite this potential limitation to its generalizability and applicability, it is a useful tool to educate clinicians about potential boundary violations in their own practice. An adaptation of the Exploitation Index is summarized in Table 2–8.

A different type of boundary violation occurs when clinicians provide mental health treatment to friends or family. In this case, the established relationship is a nonprofessional one, and the boundary is crossed when the clinician provides the friend or relative with services that are more appropriately reserved for the health care setting. This most commonly occurs when a friend or family member asks a physician for a prescription medication. Although the physician may have altruistic reasons for obliging the friend, by prescribing outside of a formal treatment relationship, the physician prevents the "patient" from receiving a thorough, confidential evaluation and appropriate ongoing care. These concerns are similar to those surrounding caring for VIP patients.

Patient Nonabandonment

According to accepted ethical standards in medicine, except in emergencies, physicians are "free to choose whom to serve" (American Psychiatric Association 2010). Once an ongoing doctor-patient relationship has been established, however, the physician may not ethically abandon the patient. As a practical matter, this means that psychiatrists must arrange for clinical coverage when on vacation and must give adequate notice to patients when closing their practices. It is not considered patient abandonment to transfer a patient's care to another physician if the treating psychiatrist is not able to provide necessary care and if the situation is not an emergency. This may occur because the treating doctor is not trained in the therapeutic modality that the patient needs or because, despite diligent work, it has not been possible to form a therapeutic alliance. Nevertheless, psychiatrists must be aware that a covert, even unconscious, form of patient abandonment may occur when countertransference issues or burnout cause a psychiatrist to subtly encourage a difficult patient to leave treatment. Self-reflective clinicians who recognize this pattern benefit their patients by seeking consultation or supervision.

Informed Consent and Treatment Refusal

Informed consent is the process by which individuals make free, knowledgeable decisions about whether to accept a proposed intervention, such as clinical care or research study participation. Informed consent is thus a cornerstone of ethical practice in both treatment and research settings. Although informed consent is a legal requirement in both contexts, its phil-

TABLE 2–8.   Warning signs of problems maintaining therapeutic boundaries

Doing any of the following for your family members or social acquaintances: prescribing medication, making diagnoses, offering psychodynamic explanations for their behavior

Accepting gifts or bequests from patients

Engaging in a personal relationship with patients after treatment is terminated

Following a patient on social media

Googling a patient out of personal curiosity or to satisfy personal needs

Making exceptions for a patient, such as providing special scheduling or reducing fees, because you find the patient attractive, appealing, or impressive

Touching patients (other than shaking hands or performing appropriate medical procedures)

Using information learned from patients, such as business tips or political information, for your own financial or career gain

Asking patients to do personal favors for you (e.g., bring lunch, mail a letter)

Asking patients to attend social gatherings with you

Arranging business deals with patients

Seeking philanthropic gifts from patients directly

Accepting for treatment persons with whom you have had social involvement

Disclosing sensational aspects of a patient's life to others (even when protecting the patient's identity)

Accepting a medium of exchange other than money for professional services (e.g., work on one's office or home, trading of professional services)

Making exceptions in the conduct of treatment because you feel sorry for a patient or because you believe that the patient is in such distress or so disturbed that there is no other choice

Recommending treatment procedures or referrals that you do not believe to be necessarily in the patient's best interests but that may instead be to your own direct or indirect financial benefit

Making exceptions for a patient because you are afraid the patient will otherwise become extremely angry or self-destructive

Failing to deal with the following patient behavior(s): paying the fee late, missing appointments on short notice and refusing to pay for the time (as agreed), seeking to extend the length of sessions

Telling patients personal things about oneself

TABLE 2–8. Warning signs of problems maintaining therapeutic boundaries *(continued)*

Trying to influence patients to support political causes or positions in which you have a personal interest

Seeking social contact with patients outside of clinically scheduled visits

Joining in an activity with a patient that may serve to deceive a third party (e.g., misleading an insurance company)

Source. Adapted from Epstein and Simon 1990.

osophical roots as a medicolegal doctrine are deeply embedded in our societal and cultural respect for individual persons and in affirming individuals' freedom of self-determination. An adequate process of informed consent thus reflects and promotes the ethical principle of autonomy.

Yet autonomy without the incorporation of other key ethical principles would embody neither the spirit nor the intent of informed consent, which is to enhance meaningful, shared decision-making. The principle of beneficence is therefore also crucial in this context and entails a thorough appraisal, on the part of the clinician or investigator, of the degree to which the informed consent process has adequately met the patient's needs. These needs are not just informational. Providing individuals with meaningful, interactive opportunities to learn about their diagnosis, prognosis, and treatment options better enables them to discuss choices and arrive at a treatment plan that is most consistent with their own authentic understanding, preferences, and values (Roberts 2002b).

This model of shared, deliberate decision-making fits with a larger commitment to patient-centered care. Shared decision-making and patient-centered care are grounded in the principle of respect for persons and demonstrate deep regard for the dignity of individuals who receive clinical care. Actions that promote shared decision-making include ensuring that patients are well-informed, encouraging the patient to play a direct role by making choices and making clear the values and preferences underneath these choices, and protecting and supporting the patient's interests (Lo 2020a). Information should be provided in a clear, unbiased, and understandable form, and preferably in multiple but different formats; this information should be discussed to ensure that the facts and implications are understood. Patient goals should be explored in relation to the information provided, and special efforts should be made to address misunderstandings or hopes that may influence the decision in a manner that is not in the patient's best interests. Additional time may be needed to allow the patient to consider the decision carefully, especially if the medical facts or psychosocial implications are serious or complicated. Shared decision-making is an ideal model for the informed consent process.

Viewing informed consent as more than a medicolegal requirement also helps frame it as part of an overall therapeutic relationship and as a further opportunity for respectful dialogue and interaction. Informed consent thus represents not only an ethical obligation but also an opportunity to enhance the provider-patient relationship and patient care. When performed in a way that is attuned to the full intent of informed consent, the process consists of repeated opportunities over time to gather relevant clinical information and to discuss and clarify patients' (and often families') values, preferences, informational needs, decisional abilities, and decision-making processes.

As noted above, informed consent ideally reflects true "shared" or "participatory" decision-making. Shared decision-making represents a formal recognition of the professional's respect for the individual; awareness and incorporation of personal, familial, and sociocultural dimensions of the provider-patient relationship; and compassion for the often difficult decision-making processes that patients encounter. Patients' fuller participation in decision-making about treatment has been associated with higher levels of treatment adherence, more engagement in their own care, and better clinician-patient communication. Distinct from the paternalistic models of decision-making formerly dominant in medicine (Faden and Beauchamp 1980), the Institute of Medicine encourages shared, freely flowing knowledge and a system in which the patient is the source of control (Institute of Medicine 2001).

Elements of Consent

Informed consent has been conceptualized as consisting of three distinct yet related features: information, decision-making capacity, and voluntariness (a model of informed consent is shown in Figure 2–4; Faden et al. 1986; Roberts 2016). Each of these features is discussed in turn. Recently, the focus on these primarily cognitive aspects of informed consent has been increasingly criticized as an overly narrow focus (particularly in the research context), neglecting the importance of emotional aspects of motivation and decision-making (Glannon 2006; Roberts et al. 2000b; Roberts et al. 2002b). Thus, the construct of informed consent, although foundational to the ethical practice of psychiatry and psychiatric research, will and should remain an important topic of both conceptual and empirical work (Appelbaum 2006; Dunn et al. 2006a).

Although there is no clear index for deciding how stringent the standard for consent should be, a general rule of thumb is to use a "sliding

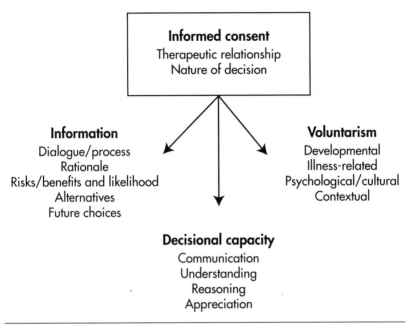

FIGURE 2–4.   Elements of informed consent.

Source.   Reprinted from Roberts LW, Dyer AR: "Informed Consent and Decisional Capacity," in *Concise Guide to Ethics in Mental Health Care.* Washington, DC, American Psychiatric Publishing, 2004, p. 52. Copyright © 2004, American Psychiatric Publishing. Used with permission.

scale" approach (Drane 1984; Roberts 2016), titrating the expectation for consent to the potential risk of the decision. Figure 2–5 depicts this concept: decisions involving higher risks or greater risk-benefit ratios generally require a more stringent standard for decisional capacity, whereas more routine, lower risk decisions generally require a less rigorous standard for decisional capacity. This sliding scale concept and the three critical elements comprising informed consent—information provision, decisional capacity, and voluntarism capacity—pertain to the informed consent process for both treatment-related decisions and for research-related decisions.

Information

Information provision, or information sharing, the first element, refers to a dialogue in which the patient or potential research participant is given all relevant information about treatment options, proposed tests, or the research protocol. Although the legal standard for how much information should be provided differs among jurisdictions, many states use

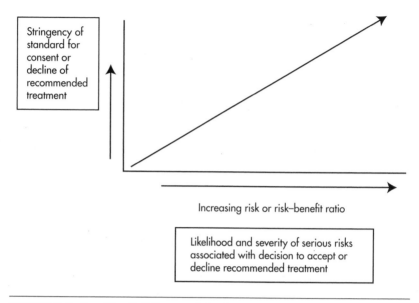

FIGURE 2–5. The "sliding scale" of consent standards.

Source. Reprinted from Roberts LW, Dyer AR: "Informed Consent and Decisional Capacity," in *Concise Guide to Ethics in Mental Health Care.* Washington, DC, American Psychiatric Publishing, 2004, p. 61. Copyright © 2004, American Psychiatric Publishing. Used with permission.

the *professional standard,* referring to the information (amount and content) that would be disclosed by most physicians. Another standard used in other states is the *reasonable person standard,* indicating the need to disclose what a reasonable person would want to know. Such information must include the purpose, the procedures involved, any foreseeable risks, and potential benefits. The issues that need to be covered include immediate issues, but potential benefits include eligibility for other forms of treatment in the future, and foreseeable risks may encompass ineligibility for future treatment as well. In many instances, particularly for some research protocols, the possibility of no benefit is a key piece of information that must be provided. In clinical trials of early experimental therapies, in fact, there may be no expectation of benefit and some clear expectation of risk or harm to the volunteer, such as in toxicity studies. In the research context, it is crucial that participants understand which procedures are experimental and which are standard and what the usual standard of care is. A thorough consent process requires that alternatives be described as part of information sharing, including the option of nonintervention (i.e., no treatment or preexisting treatment). This point is worth emphasizing, since empirical studies in which clinicians in training are observed obtaining informed consent and retrospective interviews with former study subjects suggest that alternatives are one information category more often forgotten than other content areas (see Roberts et al. 1999, 2003; U.S. Advisory Committee on Human Radiation Experiments 1996).

Increasingly, the process of the information-sharing component of informed consent is emphasized in both clinical and research settings. As described above, this has benefits for the patient/participant, the provider/investigator, and the overall relationship between them. The process provides the opportunity for patients to ask questions; to involve family, friends, or other important third parties in their decision-making process; and to become an active participant in making what may be a very complex decision. However, it is important for mental health care providers to realize that different individuals have varying levels of desire to be involved in decision-making for their own condition. In addition, the inherent power differential in the clinician-patient relationship may make many patients uneasy about asking questions during the informed consent process or stating that they do not understand health-related information. Rather than substituting the provider's own preferences for that of an indecisive or hesitant patient, the provider is ethically obligated to try to provide information in an easily understood form, to try to ensure that patients have grasped the information provided, and to help the patient clarify his or her own parameters for the decisions.

Decisional Capacity

Decisional capacity can be described as a "socio-cultural construct" (Dunn et al. 2007), consisting of intrapersonal elements, aspects related to the quality of the consent process (deriving from the information-sharing component as well as from the professionalism of the physician), and the complexity of the information and the decision at hand. For example, figuring out whether or not to undergo electroconvulsive therapy for severe, psychotic depression is a difficult decision. On the one hand, the disease process itself as well as other individual factors (such as age and cognitive functioning) may substantially impair patients' abilities to make a fully informed, meaningful choice about this treatment; on the other hand, empirical evidence suggests that many people with severe depression may commonly have adequate abilities to make such a decision. Thus, a judgment of capacity cannot reside in the diagnosis alone nor in the severity of the illness; a targeted assessment, which can be aided by capacity assessment tools designed to help guide such evaluations, is the most valid way to determine a patient's capacity to make a specific decision at a specific time. At times, particularly when a clinical situation is rapidly fluctuating or progressing, the best course of action (while also ensuring that the patient is safe) is to try to delay a decision to permit greater clarity, because the clinical circumstances may change (e.g., a manic patient becomes more stable or a delirious patient's delirium resolves). There is thus often a need to reassess capacity, which is best viewed not as a static trait but, rather, as a state that may fluctuate over time depending on various individual, clinical, and contextual factors.

The phrase *decision-making capacity* differs from the term competency in that competency to perform a specific function or for a particular life domain is a legal determination made through a judicial or other legal process. It should be noted, however, that some legal jurisdictions have different standards for establishing competency (Appelbaum and Grisso 1995; Grisso and Appelbaum 1995; Grisso et al. 1995). *Decisional capacity* refers to a determination made by a clinical professional with knowledge of and experience in assessing the key abilities necessary for making a specific medical decision.

Decisional capacity has been defined by experts as consisting of four standards (Appelbaum and Grisso 1995; Grisso and Appelbaum 1995; Grisso et al. 1995). The first ability, communication of a preference, is the least stringent standard, requiring that a person be able to express or state a decision. This standard was originally conceived as a basic physical ability to communicate—a capability that is sometimes lost when a patient is experiencing catatonia or in patients who are comatose, poststroke, or post–spinal injury. Some have come to view this standard differently and as relating to the ability to communicate a stable choice, and there are certainly circumstances in which even this standard is not met—for example, a patient with delirium whose attention waxes and wanes, affecting her ability to focus on a discussion of her treatment options or a patient who is ambivalent or erratic by virtue of his illness process.

The second standard, understanding or comprehension of the information necessary for the specific decision at hand, is primarily a cognitive ability and has been shown to be correlated with cognitive functioning in people with a variety of psychiatric illnesses (Carpenter et al. 2000; Kovnick et al. 2003; Moser et al. 2002; Palmer et al. 2005). Cognitive disorders such as dementia clearly affect the ability to understand relevant information (Kim et al. 2001). It is important to note additionally that sociocultural factors, such as literacy, numeracy, and educational background, clearly influence the ability to understand health decision information. It is thus critical that psychiatrists strive to communicate health information in ways that can be more readily understood by patients (Roberts 2016).

The third ability or standard is appreciation. This generally is considered to refer to the patient's awareness of the implications and significance of the information provided or the choice being made for the patient's own life circumstance. Appreciation is a concept tightly linked with the psychiatric notion of insight, a patient's knowledge that his or her symptoms are abnormal or the product of illness. Insight is often eroded in diverse mental illnesses, personality disorders, and disabling conditions. Lack of insight may create a situation in which an individual has an understanding of factual information but cannot apply it to his or her own situation, in which case appreciation would be lacking. An example is the patient who can demonstrate an understanding that an untreated infection could lead to death but who believes that this information does not apply to him—for example, because he has supernatural powers that will protect him.

The capacity for appreciation is seen as the most personal, the most influenced by individual values and experiences, and thus is often the most difficult to assess in clinical contexts. The basis for an apparent lack of appreciation might be religious beliefs or idiosyncratic personal beliefs or values; thus, it has been more difficult to derive consensus about what constitutes lack of appreciation. It has also been more difficult to operationalize in the form of standardized questions, because it is a less factually based standard. Nonetheless, it is important to try to assess the degree to which a patient integrates the information about the decision with his or her own values and personal beliefs.

Some recent models of decisional capacity argue for the identification of the ability to value (see Figure 2–6), which Roberts (2016) situates as one dimension of the capacity for appreciation. Valuing ability is defined as the ability to weigh information in accordance with one's life choices, preferences, and values. This criterion incorporates prior evidence that some patients who demonstrate capacity in the intellectual domains of decision-making may not act in full accordance with their demonstrated theory of self, due to the countervailing presence of a severe affective disorder, new treatment, or other impairment. Therefore, the evaluation of appreciation capacity involves the careful weighing of multiple factors and requires a physician to remain attuned to his or her own sources of bias in the form of value and belief judgments.

The fourth standard is the ability to reason, that is, to weigh information, comparing options and considering their consequences. An assessment of reasoning abilities should include evaluating whether the patient understands the consequences of alternative treatment choices and also of no treatment. A patient does not need to be able to calculate prob-

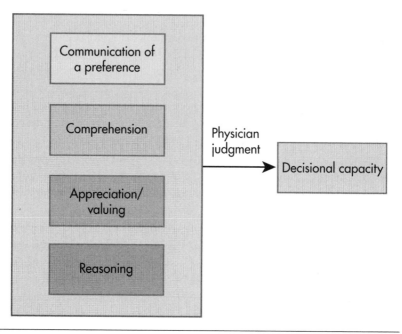

FIGURE 2–6. Framework for evaluating medical decision-making capacity.

abilities but should be able to weigh options. Patients also need not come to the "rational" choice as a result of their reasoning process, and their capacity to reason should not be judged according to the content of their values and beliefs. A patient who refuses treatment but whose understanding, appreciation, reasoning, and indication of a choice are adequate has the right to refuse treatment. Involuntary treatment is predicated, in part, on the absence of intact decision-making capacity, and thus careful assessment of these component abilities is vital in evaluating the appropriateness of implementing involuntary treatment for a given patient.

Voluntarism

The third key part of informed consent is voluntarism. Being able to make an authentic, free decision—a decision that is most concordant with an individual's values, history, and circumstances—is a fundamental aspect of autonomy. Four spheres, or domains of influence, have been proposed as a framework for thinking about those issues that may affect an individual's ability, in a given set of circumstances, to make a voluntary decision (Roberts 2002b). These domains include developmental factors; illness-related factors; psychological, cultural, and religious factors; and external features and pressures (Figure 2–7). For example, an adolescent who is asked to volunteer as a healthy control for a research study on a disease afflicting his sibling may be influenced by numerous factors that could impair his voluntarism, including his youth and relative immaturity; feelings of guilt, anger, concern, competitiveness, and/or love toward his sibling; religious and cultural beliefs regarding the meaning of disease and the importance of helping family members and society; and overt or covert pressure from family members, treating physicians, or research personnel.

The existence of such influences does not mean that voluntary decisions are not possible; rather, awareness of possible influences on decision-making can help clinicians tune in to and explore issues they may not have previously considered as affecting their patients' choices. The clinician's attention to upholding voluntarism also represents acts of beneficence and justice. As with other ethical principles, voluntarism is rooted in a sociocultural consensus of the rights of individuals to self-determination, and it "involves philosophical ideals of freedom, independence, personhood, and separateness" (Roberts 2002b, p. 705). Yet, there are also unresolved issues related to how voluntarism applies in various contexts (including both treatment and research), and voluntarism remains an understudied ethical principle and topic compared with decision-making capacity.

Treatment Refusal

Autonomous individuals have the right to refuse mental health or medical treatment, even when doing so is counter to the advice of clinicians. Many ethical dilemmas arise in the health care setting because of treatment refusal, such as rejecting psychotropic medications and requesting to leave the hospital against medical advice. In these circumstances, the clinician's duty to act beneficently is in conflict with the duty to respect the patient's autonomy. Managing dilemmas caused by treatment refusal requires clinicians to be knowledgeable about the requirements for informed consent and particularly the concepts of decision-making capacity and voluntarism. The sliding scale for consent (Figure 2–5) applies to these situations, in that more rigorous standards for consent are required to refuse a low-risk, life-saving treatment compared with a high-risk, low-benefit treatment (Drane 1984).

Alternative Decision-Making and Advance Directives

In cases in which an individual is deemed through a clinical assessment or legal decision to lack the ability to make a particular decision or set of

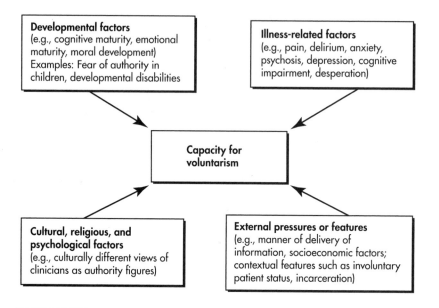

FIGURE 2–7. Conceptual model of voluntarism: four domains of potential influences.

Source. Adapted from Roberts 2002b.

decisions related to his or her care, a surrogate, proxy, or alternative decision-maker is asked to step in and make choices for that person. Alternative decision-making has received some empirical attention in the ethics literature, with the perhaps surprising finding that alternative decision-makers' choices do not closely align with what the patient would have decided for himself or herself (Sachs et al. 1994). Alternative decision-makers are, in fact, asked to do what is a very challenging task: make a treatment or research decision on behalf of another person, often in the absence of any information about the patient's wishes in such a situation.

Advance directives are documents that describe an individual's wishes regarding future care in the event that the person loses decisional capacity. Advance directives are typically used to help in end-of-life decision-making. The existence of an advance directive does not necessarily increase the accuracy of an alternative decision-maker's choices.

Psychiatric advance directives may be useful for persons with mental illnesses that cause fluctuating or progressive impairment. For example, a patient with a history of severe bipolar disorder or recurrent psychotic depression may create an advance directive requesting hospitalization and involuntary medication treatment if he or she becomes incapable of decision-making during a future relapse. Psychiatric advance directives represent a means for patients with chronic and severe illnesses to maintain control over their treatment despite periods of incapacity. Advance directives are used only when patients lack decisional capacity, and patients can change their advance directives at any time.

In the context of psychiatric treatment and research, the use of psychiatric advance directives remains quite limited in the United States (Murray and Wortzel 2019), although there appears to be increasing interest in developing guidelines and policies for these mechanisms in both contexts (Srebnik et al. 2004, 2005). In the final analysis, policies regarding alternative decision-making and advance directives must adhere to and advance the same fundamental ethical principles that are requirements for individually based decision-making.

Ethical Use of Power

The relationship between clinician and patient is inherently one of inequity. Relative to the population at large, the mental health professional holds a position of power because of his or her education, socioeconomic standing, role as healer and keeper of confidences, and, in the case of psychiatrists, the special powers granted by the state to involuntarily hospitalize patients and to stand as a gatekeeper to health care services such as prescribed medications. Conversely, individuals who seek mental health care are relatively disempowered compared with the general population. Neuropsychiatric disorders may impair one's abilities to reason, feel, and behave in an effective manner. Most individuals enter treatment at a time of great personal vulnerability, and some psychotherapeutic treatments may encourage further regression as a step toward eventual healing. Individuals are likely to already face sources of compounded inequity and distress based on race, gender, sexual or cultural identity, socioeconomic status, or other attributes. In these cases, there is an immediate risk of inequity being reinforced through bias in clinical decision-making, in forms such as misdiagnosis and misperceptions of severity of illness (Dudley et al. 2016). Such a highly unequal power relationship can leave the weaker party less able to advocate for his or her interests and needs and thus more potentially vulnerable to exploitation.

The most egregious ethical violations in the history of psychiatry have been blatant abuses of power. Some have involved sociopathic practitioners who exploit their patients for financial gain, sexual gratification, or sadistic pleasure (Gabbard and Lester 1995). Others have involved entire communities of psychiatrists who have allowed their skills and legal powers to be misused to harm patients. In Nazi Germany, psychiatrists killed thousands of patients in mental hospitals in the name of eugenic goals (Gottesman and Bertelsen 1996). Psychiatrists in the former Soviet Union diagnosed political dissidents as suffering from dubious "mental disorders" and subjected them to unnecessary treatments, including long-term, involuntary hospitalization (Bloch and Reddaway 2019).

Involuntary Treatment

Far more subtle but nonetheless important ethical issues surround the use of power in high-risk situations by well-meaning and thoughtful clinicians. An example of such a high-risk situation is psychiatrists' legally authorized use of involuntary treatment (e.g., inpatient hospitalization, outpatient commitment, or involuntary medication treatment), which is sometimes necessary in the care of patients whose mental illness makes them a danger to themselves or others. Involuntary treatment is a clear example of conflicting ethical principles: the obligation to respect patient autonomy and the obligation of nonmaleficence. Choosing not to override a patient's treatment refusal is an expression of respect for patient autonomy, but blind adherence to a patient's wishes about treatment may not be ethically justifiable, and may, in fact, cause harm. The suicidal patient who refuses hospitalization, the patient who expresses homicidal ideas, and the patient whose mental illness seriously jeopardizes his or her health (e.g., the psychotically depressed patient who refuses to eat due to a somatic delusion) are all examples of patients for whom involuntary treatment can be necessary and justifiable.

In American jurisprudence there have been two main theories of the justification for involuntary commitment. The first is *parens patriae*, literally the "father of the people," which is the concept that mental, medical, and legal professionals act out of beneficence to commit patients against their will to protect their well-being (Appelbaum and Gutheil 2020). Underlying this theory is an assumption that severely psychotic, addicted, or suicidal patients are often not truly decisionally capable and that involuntarily hospitalizing such patients enables their autonomy to be restored. This is a therapeutic and clinical criterion that seeks to prevent further decompensation and to treat mental illness. Police power is legal warrant that justifies curtailing the liberty of patients in the case of immediate, foreseeable, and preventable danger to self or others. Police power is limited by state and U.S. law and is based on the dangerousness criteria that threat of harm to oneself or others in society requires involuntary commitment. The history of psychiatry has seen an oscillation between these two theories, depending on complex political and cultural developments. Involuntary commitment of individuals with mental illness involves both parens patriae and police power (Appelbaum and Gutheil 2020).

Legal statutes and mechanisms for providing treatment on an involuntary basis vary from state to state. The ethical use of involuntary treatment in such situations has been a matter of much discussion among psychiatrists, legal scholars, the public, and policy makers (Appelbaum and Gutheil 2020; Bartlett 2003; Levenson 1986–1987; Rosenman 1998). Indeed, a major transformation in the United States mental health care system occurred in the latter half of the twentieth century, when many involuntary, long-term patients in state psychiatric hospitals were released and transferred to community settings (Burnham 2006). Although some civil rights advocates and psychiatrists have argued that any involuntary treatment is an unethical violation of individual rights (Szasz 1976), a middle ground has emerged, supported by most psychiatrists as well as by major patient advocacy organizations (e.g., NAMI [National Alliance on Mental Illness]), using the guideposts of clear and specific indications for involuntary treatment (as opposed to merely the presence of a serious mental disorder). These include careful assessment, documentation, and review of the justification for involuntary treatment and ongoing monitoring and reevaluation of treatment progress and the involuntary status (Appelbaum and Gutheil 2020; Roberts 2016).

Involuntary Outpatient Treatment

In the outpatient setting, involuntary treatment poses special challenges. Deinstitutionalization and a fragmented mental health care system have led to a crisis of lack of access to quality, continuous care. As a result, individuals with mental illnesses living in the community frequently fall through cracks in the system. The safety of some of these individuals may be in jeopardy for reasons of lack of access or nonadherence to treatment.

In recognition of the needs of many seriously mentally ill individuals for outpatient treatment and spurred by the tragic death of a young woman in New York City, a mandatory outpatient treatment program was signed into law in New York State in 1999 (New York State Office of Mental Health 2005). Known as Kendra's Law, this legislation provided mechanisms for identifying and providing care to individuals with a treatment history of nonadherence who were unlikely to engage in treatment voluntarily and whose current behavior indicated that without assisted outpatient treatment, they were at risk of clinical deterioration likely to result in harm to themselves or others. Although most states in the United States have assisted outpatient treatment statutes in some form, the programs vary widely in terms of the adequacy of their extent of programming, resources, and funding. And although concerns about the ongoing sustainability of these programs are likely to continue (Cripps and Swartz 2018), it is crucial to note that assisted outpatient treatment programs have been associated with improvements in a number of life domains for participants (New York State Office of Mental Health 2005; Swanson and Swartz 2014).

Overall, the ethical use of involuntary therapies, regardless of setting, must be approached with care and with careful regard for the balancing of duties that should characterize assessments of the need for involuntary treatment. Clinicians hold great power in their relationships with patients, and lines can be crossed in sometimes subtle ways. The ethical use of power in therapeutic relationships is a topic of central importance for mental health professionals at all levels. Table 2–9 summarizes key strategies for providing ethical care in high-risk situations, such as involuntary treatment.

Physician-Assisted Dying and Euthanasia

In recent years, the topic of physician-assisted dying (also known as medical aid in dying or physician-assisted suicide) and the related (but distinct) practice of euthanasia have become contentiously debated issues in the United States and internationally.

Physician-assisted dying refers to a physician providing either the means or information necessary for a patient to end his or her life. Euthanasia refers to the termination of life by a physician (Table 2–10). From ethical and legal points of view, assisted dying and euthanasia are distinct from withholding or withdrawing care necessary for continued life. Additionally, assisted dying and euthanasia are viewed as different from administering medications to relieve pain or to bring greater comfort, as the primary intention in this case is not to end the patient's life. Arguments in favor of assisted dying and euthanasia include respect for autonomy and compassion for patients who are suffering, and arguments against these practices relate to sanctity of life, the role of physicians as healers, and fears of abuse. Fears of abuse have been especially salient in the context of individuals living with mental illness, including intellectual disabilities and neurodevelopmental conditions, severe affective disorders, psychotic disorders, and neurocognitive disorders.

In the United States, physician-assisted dying is now legal in some form in eight U.S. states and the District of Columbia (Meisel 2020). Euthanasia remains illegal across the country. Laws that decriminalize or

TABLE 2–9. Working therapeutically in the setting of involuntary treatment

Understand treatment refusal as a possible expression of distress.

Ascertain the reasons for refusal.

Allow the patient to discuss his or her preferences and fears.

Explain the reason for the intervention in simple language.

Offer options for the disposition of treatment.

Appropriately enlist the assistance of family and friends.

Request support from nursing and support staff.

Assess decisional capacity and, if necessary, have recourse to the courts.

Attend to side effects—both long- and short-term, serious and bothersome.

Employ emergency treatment options when available.

Work to preserve the therapeutic alliance.

Enlist treatment guardians when appropriate.

Source. Adapted from Roberts and Dyer 2004.

legalize physician-assisted dying typically focus on issues such as the presence of a curable, progressive, or terminal illness; the intractable pain or other symptoms of the patient; the consistent and repeated request by the patient; and the decisional ability and voluntariness of the patient. It should be noted that one of the major concerns of those opposed to these laws is that psychiatric or psychological evaluation is rarely required and instead is left to the judgment of the attending physician.

Although a number of European countries permit assisted dying and even euthanasia for psychiatric and neurocognitive disorders, concerning data have been reported about the use of "safeguards" to protect these individuals (e.g., Kim et al. 2016; Mangino et al. 2020; Thienpont et al. 2015). In Canada, eligibility for euthanasia, originally available only for individuals with "reasonably foreseeable natural death," may expand to include individuals with psychiatric illnesses (Herx et al. 2020). If this expansion occurs, commentators worry, ethical concerns include the following: conflict between the patient's desire for an end to suffering on the one hand and limitations on access to specialized psychiatric care on the other; the implicit message that individuals with chronic and/or severe psychiatric illnesses have lives not worth living; the limits of supposed "safeguards" surrounding euthanasia; the erosion of the ethical principle of nonmaleficence; and contributions to provider moral distress and burnout (Herx et al. 2020).

TABLE 2–10.   Definition of physician-assisted dying and
euthanasia

Term	Definition	Legality (United States)
Physician-assisted dying	A physician provides the means and/or information necessary for a patient to end their life.	Legal in some states
Euthanasia	A physician directly acts to end a patient's life.	Illegal in all states

It should be noted that the American Psychiatric Association, in response to concerns about the spread of these laws, released a position
statement in 2016 stipulating that "a psychiatrist should not prescribe or
administer any intervention to a non-terminally-ill person for the purpose of causing death" (American Psychiatric Association 2016).

Moreover, providing physician-assisted dying or euthanasia conflicts
with the physician's duty to do no harm (nonmaleficence). The AMA
Code of Medical Ethics states that a physician "(a) Should not abandon a
patient once it is determined that a cure is impossible; (b) Must respect
patient autonomy; (c) Must provide good communication and emotional
support; and (d) Must provide appropriate comfort care and adequate
pain control" (American Medical Association, Council on Ethical and
Judicial Affairs 2006). Withholding or withdrawing life-sustaining treatment with patient consent is not considered physician-assisted dying.

The extremely challenging and even polarizing topics of assisted dying and euthanasia are certain to continue to be relevant for mental
health providers. An awareness not only of the laws governing one's jurisdiction, but also of the ethical issues involved, will be vital for all mental health clinicians in the foreseeable future. When a patient requests
assisted dying or euthanasia, the clinician should clarify the reason or
reasons for the request and take actions to help address the concerns in
another manner. For example, is the patient experiencing suicidal ideation due to an untreated or partially treated psychiatric or physical condition that is bringing unbearable pain? The request for aid in dying does
not free the clinician of the legal and ethical responsibility of providing
an appropriate evaluation and standard of care. The clinician should further attempt, with the patient's consent, to mobilize resources that may
improve the patient's existence and circumstances and should confer
with colleagues, for example, on the local ethics committee or with the
hospital attorney.

Torture and Interrogation

Torture was defined by the World Medical Association in 1975 as "the deliberate, systematic or wanton infliction of physical or mental suffering by one or more persons acting alone or on the orders of any authority, to force another person to yield information, to make a confession, or for any other reason." Physician participation in or facilitation of torture is not ethically acceptable and is explicitly prohibited by medical ethics codes, by the American Psychiatric Association, and by guidance of the United Nations. Physician participation in torture in military situations has been characterized as a dual-loyalty conflict, that is, a physician's sense of loyalty to a nation conflicts with a physician's duty to provide care and protect those entrusted to his or her care. This ethical argument has been rejected on the basis that the physician's positive duty based on beneficence and nonmaleficence holds greater significance.

The American Psychiatric Association, in its 2006 Position Statement on Psychiatric Participation in Interrogation of Detainees, defined interrogation as "the deliberate attempt to elicit information from a detainee for the purposes of incriminating the detainee, identifying other persons who have committed or may be planning to commit acts of violence or other crimes, or otherwise obtaining information that is believed to be of value for criminal justice or national security purposes" (American Psychiatric Association 2006). The American Psychiatric Association prohibits direct participation in interrogation, as such participation conflicts with physicians' primary obligation to promote the well-being of patients. However, the American Psychiatric Association's position currently permits psychiatrists to "provide training to military or civilian investigative or law enforcement personnel on recognizing and responding to persons with mental illnesses, on the possible medical and psychological effects of particular techniques and conditions of interrogation, and on other areas within their professional expertise"; for example, psychiatrists may use their professional expertise to educate law enforcement and to prevent individuals with mental illness from being treated unjustly.

Female Genital Mutilation

The American Medical Association (2017) condemns the practice of female genital mutilation (FGM) as a form of child abuse. In the United States, 39 states have legislation prohibiting FGM (Batha 2021). State laws require child abuse to be reported to local authorities, and this mandate includes FGM. Psychiatrists should be aware of the practice of FGM throughout the world and should know the risks associated with the procedure, which may include hemorrhage, infection, chronic pain, painful urination, urinary tract infections, reproductive tract infections, cysts, and keloids, as well as the legal and social consequences of the procedure (World Health Organization 2018). Health care professionals have an obligation to educate themselves about FGM and discuss FGM with female patients. The World Health Organization has released a handbook on the care of individuals living with FGM, which provides guidance on how to discuss FGM with patients (World Health Organization 2018). Individuals who have undergone FGM are at increased risk for PTSD and other mental disorders (Behrendt and Moritz 2005).

Human Trafficking

Human trafficking (also known as "labor trafficking" or "sex trafficking") is a human rights abuse that inflicts devastating physical and psychological harm on victims and their loved ones. In its 2004 Convention Against Transnational Organized Crime, the United Nations defined human trafficking as "the recruitment, transportation, transfer, harboring or receipt of persons, by means of the threat or use of force or other forms of coercion, of abduction, of fraud, of deception, of the abuse of power... for the purpose of exploitation" (United Nations 2004). Human trafficking subsists in the systematic silencing of its victims through direct threats to life, material, and psychological security; the deprivation of basic means by which to understand their abuse as such; and the means to make their abuse known. Many victims of human trafficking are thus deprived of medical care or are unable to report their circumstances verbally in clinical settings. As experts with a trained sensitivity to and duty to care for individuals suffering from abuse, health care professionals have a special responsibility to identify individuals impacted by human trafficking and to refer them to the necessary medical, psychiatric, social, and legal services. Health care professionals who treat victims of human trafficking should have a sophisticated and broad understanding of its physical and mental health consequences (see Coverdale et al. 2020). The failure to detect signs of human trafficking leads to the perpetuation of these exploitative systems and the revictimization of abused individuals.

Confidentiality

Respect for the privacy of patients' personal information has been an established ethical duty of physicians for millennia and is an essential ethical obligation of all the modern mental health disciplines. In *The Oath*, Hippocrates stated the ethical duty of confidentiality as follows: "What I may see or hear in the course of treatment... in regard to the life of men

...I will keep to myself, holding such things to be shameful to be spoken about" (Edelstein 1943, p. 6). Patients entrust their clinicians, especially their therapists, with the most intimate details of their lives, often telling their mental health providers things they have never told—or would never tell—anyone else. Effective treatment, and in particular, effective psychotherapy, would not be possible if patients did not feel free to disclose intensely personal information under the assumption of confidentiality.

From the standpoint of U.S. law, clinician-patient confidentiality is a legal right granted to patients. Confidentiality is also an obligation for physicians and other clinicians that requires them to keep patient information private, unless they are legally compelled to make a disclosure or the patient waives the privilege. Although this may sound straightforward, in practice there are many gray areas in which a professional's legal and ethical duties may conflict. In remote rural settings, where clinicians and their patients are also neighbors, lifelong friends, and even relatives by blood or by marriage, confidentiality poses extraordinary challenges (Roberts et al. 1999). This is true in other small communities in which individuals have multiple and overlapping roles (Roberts 2016).

Psychiatrists may protest a specific legal mandate to provide otherwise protected patient information if they believe that the disclosure would be unethical. Such disagreements have led to numerous court cases, and the legal protection of confidentiality between patients and psychotherapists has thus evolved over the last 50 years, culminating in a 1996 U.S. Supreme Court decision recognizing the legal privilege between patient and psychotherapist (*Jaffee v. Redmond* 1996). With the Health Insurance Portability and Accountability Act (HIPAA) of 1996, specific protections for personal health information, including a higher level of protection for psychotherapy notes, were also enacted. Currently, patient records should be kept confidential even after the patient's death. The records of patients in substance abuse treatment programs are accorded an even higher level of protection in light of the greater stigma attached to substance abuse and the elevated interest in addiction by some segments of society. Once a patient is involved at any stage in therapy at an addictions program, that participation cannot be disclosed without explicit consent or very limited and specific conditions, such as crime committed on the premises (Lopez 1994). It behooves clinicians working in addictions to familiarize themselves with these more stringent requirements for confidentiality.

What remains unclear, however, is whether, to what degree, and how special privacy protections for mental health treatment will continue to be guarded in an emerging era of electronic health records, digitized medical information, and a push toward national health identifiers. Based on recommendations from the American Psychiatric Association, a good rule of thumb is not to place the following types of information in psychotherapy notes that can be accessed in the electronic medical record: "intimate personal content or facts; details of fantasies and dreams; process interactions; sensitive information about other individuals in the patient's life; the therapist's formulations, hypotheses, or speculations; topics/themes discussed in therapy sessions" (American Psychiatric Association 2002, p. 1).

Additionally, the movement toward "open notes" (increasing patients' access to their entire medical record) raises new issues about the extent to which mental health records may receive additional or special safeguards. Although a common approach now is the implementation of "break the glass" protocols for providing access to mental health records, such safeguards still allow many different providers access (Shenoy and Appel 2017). Awareness (in a general sense) of who has access to the documentation in a patient's electronic medical record will continue to be vital for all mental health providers.

There is a broad recognition of several limits on confidentiality. When patients consent to specific, limited disclosures of their information (e.g., for third-party payment or for a court proceeding), disclosure may occur. In these instances, the amount of information to be revealed should be the minimum amount necessary for the specific situation; that is, a rigorously upheld "need to know" approach. Patients should be informed of limits to confidentiality when entering treatment (although there is disagreement about how best to enact this duty). Patients should not be asked to sign a blanket waiver of general consent to disclosure, because many patients would not want all of their personal mental health information being disclosed to a third-party payer, for example.

There are other instances when a nonconsenting patient may have the privilege of confidentiality suspended based on the provider's overriding duties to others. These situations typically involve breaching patient confidentiality to protect third parties in cases of child or elder abuse or threatened violence. The notion that psychiatrists have a "duty to protect" members of the public from the violent intentions of their patients was demonstrated by the legal case *Tarasoff v. Regents of the University of California* (1976). From an ethical standpoint, the *Tarasoff* ruling gives more weight to the importance of beneficence (preventing harm to a third party) than to fidelity and confidentiality (protecting the confidences of one's own patient).

In general, however, mental health patients should reasonably be able to expect that the information they tell their clinician will be kept confidential and that disclosure will not occur without their consent. Unfortunately, several studies have shown that many patients are not informed about specific safeguards for their confidentiality and that many do not seek treatment out of fears about lack of confidentiality. A useful list of do's and don'ts for safeguarding patient confidentiality related to specific issues has been compiled by Roberts et al. (2002a) and is shown in Table 2–11.

Overlapping Roles, Dual Agency, and Conflicts of Interest

By virtue of their skills and training, mental health professionals are naturally invited to participate in a variety of roles in the medical community and in society. Psychiatrists and psychologists, nurses, and social workers are educators of students, residents, and interns; administrators of academic programs and health care systems; clinical researchers and basic scientists; and consultants to industry. Because the ethical duties required by one role may not align precisely with the duties of another role, clinicians in multiple roles may face ethical binds. The conflicts of interest that arise are not necessarily unethical, but they must be managed in a way that allows the psychiatrist to fulfill professionalism expectations and maintain a fiduciary relationship with patients. There are many strategies for helping to ensure that role conflicts do not distort the judgments of professionals, such as disclosure and documentation, focused supervision and oversight committees, and retrospective review.

Some mental health professionals have primary or secondary professional duties that may not be fully congruent with the beneficence and altruism obligations of the physician. Such conflicts are sometimes referred to as *dual agency situations*. A clear example is the forensic psychiatrist or psychologist who may be asked to evaluate a death row inmate to determine whether he or she is "sane enough" to be executed (Roberts and Dunn 2019).

Ethical binds occur with many other types of dual roles. For example, mental health researchers who also provide clinical care for participants may struggle to maintain the integrity of the doctor-patient relationship in the face of the demands of the research protocol. Similarly, medical trainees, supervisors, and administrative psychiatrists may find that their roles as students, teachers, and managers challenge their ability to put the needs of patients first (Roberts 2016). In public health settings, psychiatrists may find it challenging to balance fidelity to individual patients with the legitimate need to be good stewards of social resources and distribute them fairly (Snyder Sulmasy et al. 2019). U.S. military and Veterans Affairs mental health clinicians also face conflicts in determining fitness for duty

TABLE 2–11. Nine do's and don'ts for protecting confidentiality

Confidentiality issue	Don't	Do
Patient information	Assure your patients that whatever they tell you is confidential.	Provide accurate information to your patients about the realities of confidentiality in your clinical care situation.
Medical records	Assure your patients that the medical record—whether printed or electronic—is confidential.	Explain that the purpose of the medical record is to be read so that optimal care may be given.
Accessing records	Access records that are not necessary for patient care or access records for individuals who are not your patients.	Retrieve background medical information appropriate for clinical responsibilities arising in the care of your established patients.
Stigmatizing conditions	Avoid discussing the difficult issues that surround stigmatizing disorders.	Strategize explicitly with your patients about potential confidentiality problems.
Tailoring the charts and gaming the system	Use these protective practices without considering the consequences.	Consider how to reconcile accuracy and privacy in all forms of documentation.
Significant others	Talk to significant others without permission from the patient.	Remember to inquire about patient's important relationships.
Law and professional standards	Break the law or violate professional standards in the process of respecting confidentiality.	Actively work to change laws and policies regarding confidentiality that you think are unethical.
Lifelong learning	Neglect your commitment to lifelong learning, including ethics.	Continue to learn about professional aspects of medicine and share your knowledge with colleagues.
Consultation	Feel that you are on your own when confronting difficult confidentiality questions.	Seek consultation and direction from other sources: books, articles, continuing medical education, websites, ethics consultants, and ethics committees.

Source. Adapted from Roberts et al.: "Ethics in Psychiatric Practice: Essential Ethics Skills, Informed Consent, the Therapeutic Relationship, and Confidentiality." *Journal of Psychiatric Practice* 8(5):290–305, 2002. Used with permission.

and eligibility for compensation (Schneider and Bradley 2018). Managing these multiple roles requires clinicians to recognize the potential for ethical binds, institute safeguards when possible, and fully inform patients of the dual role and its implication for patient care (Roberts 2016).

Financial conflicts of interest pertaining to patient care represent another key ethical issue in mental health. Conflicts of interest matter because they may compromise a clinician's primary commitment to the health and well-being of patients. The conflict may compromise the judgment of the clinician, and there is greater potential for negative outcomes for patients when compromised or bad decisions are made by clinicians with conflicts (Lo 2020a). Among the most obviously unacceptable conflicts of interest are those in which physicians or other mental health professionals have a clear-cut financial arrangement that could adversely influence how they treat patients. For example, fee-splitting arrangements in which a psychiatrist is paid to refer patients to a consultant are unethical because the payment may compromise the psychiatrist's judgment about the clinical merits of the referral. In a similar fashion, accepting lavish bonuses from hospitals for referring patients suggests that the physician's professional judgment may be co-opted. Professionals who work in integrated health care systems, managed care, or accountable care organizations may also experience tensions between the obligation to provide competent care and incentives to meet various metrics and demonstrate value-based care. Enduring guidelines for ethical practice in organized settings established in 1997 by the American Psychiatric Association require that managed care psychiatrists disclose such incentives to patients (American Psychiatric Association 2001a).

The possibility of conflicts of interest arising from accepting gifts or other forms of support from industry has fueled significant controversy across the House of Medicine. An early meta-analysis of 29 studies on physician-pharmaceutical company interactions demonstrated that physicians' attitudes toward a medication and/or their prescribing practices were influenced by having personal contact with pharmaceutical sales representatives, attending sales presentations, attending continuing medical education conferences sponsored by pharmaceutical companies, and using industry funding for travel and housing expenses to attend professional meetings (Wazana 2000). Over the past 20 years, appreciation of the impact of gifts from industry has grown as the field of implicit bias has been studied. Critics of gifts from industry emphasize how gifts impair objectivity and introduce greater bias in decisions and in the evaluation of medical information. Gifts from industry also diminish the public trust and belief in the field of medicine as dedicated to patient well-being. Ethicists and psychologists alike raise the issue of how gifts set up the expectation of a quid pro quo arrangement, whether implicitly or explicitly, and create a distorting sense of personal obligation that may interfere with good judgment.

Currently, various organizations within medicine differ in their approaches and guidelines for dealing with relationships with industry, but nearly all state explicitly that conflicts of interest must be avoided or managed. At minimum, clinicians should disclose gifts and reassure patients that the goal of their relationship is to promote the health and well-being of the patient. Clinicians furthermore should be aware of issues that may concern patients (e.g., patients may note that the name of the medication being prescribed by their clinician matches the name on the pen being used to prescribe it). Attending to such concerns and learning about and working within the guidelines specified by one's professional organizations and work setting are important aspects of delivering care in the current clinical environment. Academic departments of psychiatry, psychology, social work, and nursing are increasingly playing important roles in educating future mental health professionals about ethical issues involved in relationships with the pharmaceutical industry. A spectrum of opinion exists in contemporary guidelines regarding the ethical acceptability of accepting gifts and hospitality from private industry, allowing private industry to fund conferences and scholarships for trainees, and clinicians' use of samples, particularly in a public mental health setting. There is growing consensus that ethical handling of relationships with industry should be covered in psychiatric ethics education and policy development, providing current and future clinicians with the ability to constructively address the role of the pharmaceutical industry, for example, or digitally based commercial activities, in clinical care and research.

The arrest of Charles Lieber of Harvard University—linked with nondisclosure of personal and research funds he received from Wuhan University of Technology—is an important example of how truth telling, disclosure, and conflict of interest intersect. In this situation, Lieber's relationship with a foreign entity while Lieber's laboratory received NIH funding raised many concerns (U.S. Department of Justice 2020b).

Social Stigmatization of Mental Illness and Advocacy

Stigma sits at the intersection of several ethical issues in mental health. Stigma is a barrier to equitable care, both at the individual (care-seeking) and systemic (care-providing, financing) levels.

Stigma may affect students' decisions to enter mental health professions, and it may influence an individual practitioner's ability to "do good" throughout his or her career because of barriers and challenges experienced by patients who are stigmatized. Providers of all specialties need to be particularly attuned to their own feelings toward mental illnesses and patients. Most mental health professionals have at some point or another felt the sting of stigma simply by working in the field.

Mental illness diagnoses place patients at risk of receiving inadequate medical treatment. For instance, a large study found a significantly lower likelihood of receiving a coronary revascularization procedure after acute myocardial infarction among patients with a psychiatric diagnosis compared with those without such a diagnosis (Druss et al. 2000). Insurance parity for covering mental health remains elusive, despite the massive strides made by the field in demonstrating treatment effectiveness and cost effectiveness of providing care.

Stigma may impede patient autonomy by interfering with individuals' abilities to enact personal wishes for care and recovery. Studies have documented the role of stigma as a barrier to accessing care, specifically among some cultural and ethnic minority groups (Ojeda and McGuire 2006; Schraufnagel et al. 2006; U.S. Department of Health and Human Services 2001). Research has also demonstrated the impact of stigma on the self-esteem of people with mental illnesses (Link et al. 2001) and the perceptions and effects of stigma on family members (Ostman and Kjellin 2002; Phelan et al. 1998). Moreover, stigma has ongoing complicating effects on individuals' mental health treatment, such as in individuals dually diagnosed with substance abuse and mental illness (Committee on the Science of Changing Behavioral Health Social Norms 2016; Link et al. 1997).

Many view stigma as a call to action for mental health providers. Certain professional ethics codes, such as those of the American Psychiatric Association and the American Medical Association, state that a physician "shall recognize a responsibility to participate in activities contributing to an improved community" (American Medical Association, Council on Ethical and Judicial Affairs 2006, p. liv). Many psychiatrists feel ethically compelled to speak out as advocates and champions for people with mental illness and against social injustice that harms psychiatric patients, such as mental health insurance nonparity, discrimination, and public policies that neglect the needs of individuals with mental illness.

Responding to Colleague Impairment or Misconduct

As professionals, mental health care clinicians are expected to behave ethically toward their colleagues individually and collectively. The AMA's

Principles of Medical Ethics explicitly states that physicians should deal honestly with colleagues, "respect the rights" of colleagues, and "strive to report physicians deficient in character or competence, or engaging in fraud or deception" (American Medical Association, Council on Ethical and Judicial Affairs 2006, p. xxi) (see Table 2–5). Whereas the first two statements in the ethics code encourage collegial behavior, the third suggests the importance of self-governance in the medical professions and the need to report colleague misconduct and impairment.

Misconduct can be defined as professional violations or acts that violate ethical standards. Impairment is the inability to practice medicine because of physical or mental illness or deterioration, or the excessive use of drugs or alcohol (Belitz 2020). An impaired psychologist is defined by the American Psychological Association as someone whose condition may result in ineffective interventions and harm toward the patient or others (American Psychological Association 2006). Extreme stress is the primary cause of distress and impairment in the health professions (Belitz 2020).

In addition to the legal obligation to report an impaired colleague, there are also legal duties, governed by applicable law. These duties overlap but are not always the same (Figure 2–8).

In recent years, there has been a growing evidence base around how to predict whether an individual is at risk for subsequent professionalism issues, misconduct, or ethics complaints. In a recent study by Krupat et al. (2020), researchers looked at the future career problems of 108 medical students at Harvard Medical School and Case Western Reserve University School of Medicine who had appeared before their school's professionalism review committees for problem behaviors between 1993 and 2007. This study was especially valuable because the researchers included a control comparison group of 216 medical students who were matched by sex, minority status, and year of graduation. The study found that students who appeared before their schools' review committees were over five times more likely to undergo disciplinary review during residency and nearly four times more likely to be required to undergo counseling or added oversight, compared with controls. In clinical practice, nearly 10% of those who had problems as students had been sued or sanctioned, which was twice the proportion of the controls. This study follows on earlier work by Colliver et al. (2007), Papadakis et al. (2004, 2005), Stern et al. (2005), and Murden et al. (2004) and is evidenced more fully in a major review by Fargen et al. (2016). Such studies matter in that they provide a way to identify individuals who may employ maladaptive coping mechanisms when under the stresses of training and clinical practice; such studies may also help to rally appropriate supports to prevent

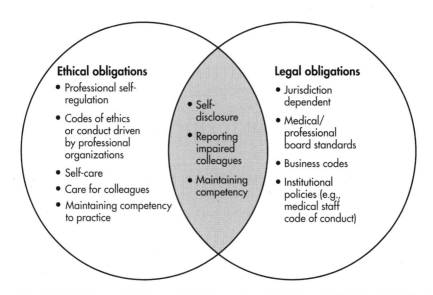

FIGURE 2–8. Overlapping ethical and legal obligations related to provider impairment.

Source. Reprinted from Gengoux G, Zach SE, Derenne JL, et al.: *Professional Well-Being: Enhancing Wellness Among Psychiatrists, Psychologists, and Mental Health Clinicians.* Washington, DC, American Psychiatric Association Publishing, 2020, p. 154. Copyright © 2020, American Psychiatric Association. Used with permission.

professionalism or ethics errors, or to arrange for quick intervention to prevent harm to patients and to support compassionate approaches for the health professionals.

Glen Gabbard, in his book *Sexual Exploitation in Professional Relationships* (Gabbard 1989), and Peter Yellowlees, in his book *Physician Suicide: Cases and Commentaries* (Yellowlees 2019), describe cases of psychiatrists and other physicians and health professionals who find themselves in psychological pain and unable to perform their clinical work up to the standards of the profession. Their narrative accounts illustrate how boundary crossings can progress to transgressions or how inattention to patient care needs can result in mistakes, which in turn can lead to further clinical care problems and poor patient outcomes; in addition, the clinician may feel distressed, hold on to self-critical or even self-loathing cognitions, and experience fear of professional repercussions. All of these events and experiences can contribute to impairment. Cognitive impairment may also arise for psychiatrists and psychologists who have among the longest careers in the health professions. Psychiatrists not uncommonly work into their 70s and even into their 80s, and according to the

AMA Physician Masterfile database are among the "oldest" specialty physicians, based on average age. Cognitive impairment may be especially difficult to appreciate, both by the affected clinician or by others, and is accompanied by considerable embarrassment and shame (Belitz 2020). Such psychosocial concerns may cause others to be hesitant to report concerns about impairment.

Even when physicians or other clinicians feel "prepared" to report colleagues they perceive as impaired or incompetent, however, a number of barriers appear to affect willingness to report (Belitz 2020; DesRoches et al. 2010). These range from concerns about stigmatizing one's colleague, believing the problem or situation will resolve on its own, and overidentification with one's colleague, to worries about retribution, believing that nothing would result from reporting, and assuming that someone else will deal with the issue. Some argue that findings of reluctance to report impaired colleagues suggest that clinicians need greater education in professionalism and that those who do report require greater assurance of protection (Wynia 2010).

The early roots of this harmful code of silence were suggested by Roberts et al.'s (2000a) study of over 1,000 medical students at nine medical schools. When participating students were asked to consider hypothetical scenarios involving medical students with severe illnesses such as uncontrolled diabetes, suicidal depression, and substance dependence, approximately one-third of participants said they would protect the student's privacy rather than actively intervene or report the problem.

To help mental health professionals overcome their reluctance to report a colleague's improper or worrisome behavior, Overstreet (2001) has suggested a useful four-step procedure for working through the issue. First, the clinician should become informed about the reporting requirements of his or her state. In some locales and for some professions, there is a legal mandate to report colleague misconduct, with penalties for failure to do so. Second, the clinician should seek to more fully understand the situation, including how his or her own feelings may complicate both the ability to observe the colleague's behavior objectively and to report it. Third, the clinician should identify all the options that fulfill the duty to "strive to expose" the misconduct. Just as there is a range of clinician misbehaviors, there can be a range of appropriate responses. These may include speaking privately with the colleague about one's concerns, informing the colleague's supervisor or administrative chief, filing an ethics complaint with the professional organization's district branch, and/or notifying the state licensing board. Finally, the clinician should choose the most appropriate option or options as a critical step, knowing that others are available should the situation persist (Overstreet 2001).

A reporting provider is not expected to make a definitive judgment about whether or not a colleague is practicing competently. Problematic professional behavior is investigated by appropriate professional bodies such as the American Psychiatric Association, the American Psychological Association, and state licensing boards. Many states have enacted laws regarding physician impairment designed to encourage appropriate treatment and recovery rather than approaches that may be seen as merely punitive. To understand reporting obligations and consider whether to intervene with or report an impaired colleague, providers may be guided by the practices shown in Table 2–12 (see also Gengoux et al. 2020).

TABLE 2–12. Considerations for reporting impaired colleagues

1. Learn the relevant jurisdiction's (state or province) and licensing board's reporting requirements.

2. Understand your obligations under your institution's code of conduct as well as your professional code of conduct.

3. Understand the different roles and responsibilities of licensing boards and physician/provider health programs.

4. Consider both patient safety and the well-being of yourself and your colleagues as an integral part of your professionalism and ethical obligation.

5. Realize that there are supports available for yourself and your colleagues, and that these supports do not necessarily result in disciplinary or punitive actions by licensing boards.

6. Identify your institution's or organization's resources for reporting or inquiring about an impaired colleague. Physician wellness committees, ombudspersons, and other resources are in place at most organizations.

7. If you do become concerned about a colleague, trainee, or supervisor, the following options are all potentially useful, bearing in mind that different states have varying policies:

   • Consult with a trusted colleague about next steps.

   • Talk to your colleague about seeking help, as being proactive is most likely to lead to positive (and not punitive) outcomes.

   • Consult with your health system's physician/provider wellness committee.

   • Consult with your local, regional, or state physician health program about how to encourage your colleague to get help or how to refer your colleague.

Issues in Multidisciplinary Practice

Mental health practice is increasingly multi- and interdisciplinary, with most psychiatrists and psychologists practicing in a team environment in which relationships with colleagues can create ethical challenges as well as greatly enrich patient care. The common practice of split treatment—in which the medical practitioner manages psychotropic medications and the psychologist or social worker provides therapy—requires ongoing coordination, careful monitoring of confidentiality concerns, avoidance of splitting, and mutual respect for the complementary skills of each clinician (Lazarus 2001). Similarly, supervision of nurses and other midlevel practitioners by doctoral clinicians also warrants a participatory leadership style with genuine appreciation for the contribution of each member of the team in delivering high-quality patient care if conflicts are to be avoided. Nurses and social workers may feel they have less social prestige and clinical power and therefore may struggle when confronted with what they perceive as unethical conduct on the part of a supervisor. Just as with trainees, these practitioners must have independent lines of communication to appropriate authorities in which they can voice their concerns in a safe and supportive environment. For instance, a primary care provider may inappropriately ask a psychologist without prescribing privileges to suggest an antidepressant medication for a patient with social phobia (Austin et al. 2005). Or a psychiatrist may request that a social worker perform a diagnostic assessment for bipolar disorder, which the social worker feels is beyond his or her competence.

Finally, each of the unique mental health disciplines has its own orientation—for instance, nurses have historically valued patient-centered care and advocacy; physicians have traditionally been educated under a more science focused biomedical model; and social worker training often has emphasized more systems-based and culturally oriented perspectives. If a clinician is not attentive to these nuances, colleagues may feel diminished, patients may feel confused, and conflicts may be generated among individuals who come from professional disciplines that differently prioritize certain values of importance in patient care. For the optimal treatment of individual patients, it is ethically incumbent on all clinicians to understand and appreciate these different viewpoints, integrate them, and employ all team members' skills to provide the most competent, compassionate, and comprehensive approach to mental health care.

Despite their differences in theoretical orientation and practice style, all mental health clinicians are united in their experience of moral distress in the face of economic, administrative, and institutional demands that they feel compromise the fundamental ethic of patient care.

Issues in Novel Modes of Prediction, Evaluation, and Treatment

As advances in the basic, translational, and clinical research continue to reveal new avenues and applications for the prediction, evaluation, and treatment of mental illnesses, professionals in mental health fields are likely to encounter a number of novel ethical issues. These range from the application of machine learning to health data or social media to predict symptoms, syndromes, or behaviors (e.g., onset of depression, risk for future suicide attempts); genetics and genomics; novel somatic therapies or novel uses of known agents (e.g., psychedelics); "digital" mental health; and even brain-machine interfaces. Psychiatry has a long history of novel approaches that have stoked initial excitement at the potential benefits for patients. However, this excitement has often come to be tempered by recognition of unintended, unforeseen, or frankly harmful consequences of the modality. Thus, "novelty" in mental health research and treatment poses its own set of ethical issues (Figure 2–9).

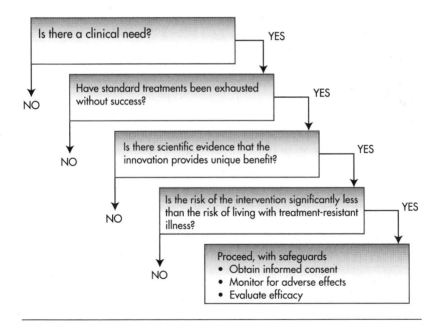

FIGURE 2–9.   Decision tree for ethical use of clinical innovation.

Reprinted from Hoop JG, Layde J, Roberts LW: "Ethical Considerations in Psychopharmacological Treatment and Research," in *The American Psychiatric Publishing Textbook of Psychopharmacology*, 4th Edition. Edited by Schatzberg AF, Nemeroff CB. Washington, DC, American Psychiatric Publishing, 2009, p. 1490. Copyright © 2009, American Psychiatric Publishing. Used with permission.

Social Media, Electronic Footprints, and Digital Health

The maintenance of ethics and professionalism in the digital age is increasingly seen as an important task for professionals, as online platforms and media bring new opportunities and challenges for providers to navigate (Mostaghimi and Crotty 2011; Torous and Roberts 2017).

All psychiatrists need to make conscientious and informed choices about whether, how, what, and how much to interact and disclose online. Given that the majority of psychiatry trainees, and an increasing number of physicians, have social media accounts, outright avoidance or rejection of social media has become impractical. Moreover, these sites now play integral and positive roles for many physicians as facilitators of social interaction. Furthermore, if psychiatrists act carefully and proactively, they can maintain appropriate boundaries, ethics, and professionalism online. Suggested guidelines center around basic issues of trust, privacy, professional standards of conduct, and awareness of potential implications of all digital content and interactions (Gabbard et al. 2011). Simply put, online expression should be viewed as "the new millennium's elevator," where psychiatrists have little control over who hears what they say (Mostaghimi and Crotty 2011, p. 561).

Prediction

Emerging methods of prediction are bringing to the forefront a range of ethical questions that have only recently begun to be examined. Such methods include, for example, machine learning and artificial intelligence for use in prognostication about illness course or for prediction of specific behaviors (including suicide attempts). In the instance of prognostication, machine learning may affect the patient-clinician relationship in unexpected ways, for example, by influencing treatment decision-making or allocation of resources (Char et al. 2018). Algorithmic bias poses great risk in machine-aided decision-making, as it can operationalize biases already at work in human decision-making under the guise of sophistication. Transparency about when algorithms are being used (i.e., veracity), how such algorithms affect patient confidentiality, appropriate communication (i.e., informed consent), and bias safeguards (e.g., ecological validity of training data, choice of learning model) are therefore crucial to the ethical implementation of such tools. However, consensus about how to achieve these ideals remains sparse, including for mental health applications (Martinez-Martin et al. 2018).

The use of machine learning to predict self-harm or suicide attempts provides another example of an emerging tool—one that carries both ethical weight and yet is of urgent public health importance. Recent work examining the accuracy of suicide risk prediction algorithms demonstrated that such strategies, when applied to available electronic health records, significantly increased the accuracy of prediction over traditional methods (Barak-Corren et al. 2017; Walsh et al. 2017). Although such methods of prediction are as yet in their early stages, the proliferation of research on this issue raises a host of ethical issues—from privacy of medical records, to potential harms and stigma, to the question of whether, how, and what kinds of additional monitoring or intervention are appropriate or necessary for individuals deemed at high risk.

Another form of suicide risk prediction—the essentially unregulated domain of "social suicide prediction" (Marks 2018; Notredame et al. 2019)—harnesses data from online and other digital activities (e.g., texting) to predict the risk of self-harm. Large companies such as Facebook have already implemented algorithms for this purpose, including protocols for escalating surveillance of users deemed high risk and initiating "wellness checks" by local police or other public safety or health officials.

Ethical issues in this brave new world of algorithmic risk prediction abound. There is no ethical review of these practices, which are essentially "trade secrets" held by these companies. Furthermore, as noted by Marks (2018), it is unclear whether sharing such risk prediction (e.g., labeling a consumer "suicidal" because of their online data) could adversely affect these individuals:

> Because most companies predicting suicide are not covered entities under HIPAA, their predictions can be shared with third parties without consumer knowledge or consent. Transferring or selling suicide prediction data to advertisers, data brokers, and insurance companies can promote discrimination against consumers who are labeled suicidal.

Furthermore, as Marks argues, wellness checks initiated by these companies' algorithms may ultimately result in involuntary hospitalization. It is unknown how frequently this occurs, as these data are not made public. This potential threat to autonomy has been minimally addressed by the companies themselves.

In contrast, some have argued that these kinds of algorithms—even with their flaws and limitations—represent a vast improvement over the present ability of individuals, their loved ones, the health care system, and the public to identify risk for, and ultimately prevent, suicide (Toomey 2019). A robust public debate is needed on the question of whether, when, and by what means our online lives and data should be allowed to be used to justify intrusions or even suspensions of our individual liberty. Numerous additional ethical questions raised by these kinds of tools will also need to be addressed.

Evaluation

Ethical issues accompany the advent of any new diagnostic and evaluative tools. In mental health, advances in genetics, genomics, and other biomarkers (e.g., neuroimaging) hold the potential, some believe, to transform the practice of psychiatry by bringing psychiatry into the realm of "precision medicine." For example, work on neural circuits has evolved to the point of proposing a taxonomy of circuits that contribute to mental disorders (Williams 2016).

Precision psychiatry will raise issues of autonomy (does the patient fully comprehend and voluntarily agree to the use of the diagnostic tool or method?); beneficence (i.e., will such novel diagnostic schema have clear benefits for the patient?); nonmaleficence (are there any foreseeable harms of the new methods?); and justice (is access to novel diagnostic or evaluative methods fair and nonexploitative of vulnerable populations?).

Another example of novel evaluative methods involves psychiatric genetic testing. Psychiatric genetic testing may have a number of possible goals, including predictive testing, diagnostic testing, testing that may aid treatment decision-making (e.g., pharmacogenomics testing), or testing to aid in reproductive decision-making (Hoge and Appelbaum 2012). A review of studies that examined the perspectives of patients, family members, and psychiatrists regarding psychiatric genetic testing found strong interest in diagnostic and predictive testing among patients and family members, as well as substantial interest in predictive testing for offspring. However, a number of concerns were endorsed about the possibility of discrimination based on genetic testing (Lawrence and Appelbaum 2011).

Additional ethical issues are emerging as digital medicine and digital health tools rapidly proliferate. For example, there are now apps to help patients self-monitor their symptoms, digital technologies for medication adherence tracking, and predictive analytics relevant to mental health. From an ethical perspective, novel digital health tools ideally will be used as an adjuvant strategy in support of the goals of the therapeutic relationship (Torous and Roberts 2017). Modern psychiatric practitioners should become knowledgeable about the digital apps and digital engagements of their patients and discuss these tools with them, including potential value and potential liabilities. For instance, a patient may use a daily diary app, tracking symptoms and behaviors. This diary may be positively incorporated into the therapeutic process with the clinician. A patient may be uncertain or unaware, however, of how passive data collection through devices, apps, and programs may be encroaching on his or her privacy; this topic may be important to consider for its implications on the patient's life and well-being.

Treatment

At present, psychiatric researchers are exploring a range of novel therapeutic approaches to address unmet needs in patients with mental illness. For example, investigations are ongoing into the potential use of psychedelic compounds (e.g., psilocybin) for treatment-resistant depression. Novel neurosurgical approaches are also being evaluated for their efficacy in treating psychiatric conditions (including addictions, eating disorders, and neurocognitive disorders). These endeavors raise ethical issues that invoke all of the ethical principles and tensions described previously—from the need to ensure that a patient with treatment-resistant depression enrolling in a novel therapeutics trial provides informed, authentic consent; to ensuring that protocols (whether in the research or treatment context) are designed with adequate safeguards for both known potential risks, as well as unforeseen adverse events; to disseminating accurate, judicious information about the known benefits and risks of these emerging therapies.

Caring for Complex Patients

Mental health clinicians are often called on for their strengths and relevant skill set in caring for complex or "difficult" patients, such as persons with addiction, personality disorders, relentless and complex physical and mental health issues, and social problems. Although it is true that mental health training does provide more education in the management of these patients, such patients continue to be among the most challenging groups in all of health care and require the exercise of heightened self-awareness and self-care on the part of the mental health clinician to avoid countertransference reactions or emotional exhaustion.

Complex patients raise ethical concerns because they aggressively test the therapeutic relationship and because their behaviors can be trying for even the most compassionate and tolerant clinician, who may become reactive rather than therapeutically responsive (Table 2–13). The complex patient is thus a setup for ethical violations and compromises. Consider the patient who refuses to be seen by a Black or African American physician, a Muslim psychiatrist, a gender-nonconforming psychologist, or an American Indian social worker. Consider the violent pa-

TABLE 2–13. Steps in managing complex patients

Step 1	Understand yourself.
	• Be aware of your biases and responses.
	• Understand why certain types of patients upset you.
	• Realize you are not a "bad" doctor if you have negative feelings about some patients.
	• Recognize that everyone has trouble managing some patients.
Step 2	Understand your patient.
	• Every difficult behavior is a form of communication.
	• Every complex patient is trying to express real fears and needs.
Step 3	Think, don't react.
	• Remember your duty to help and not harm.
	• Focus on medical and psychiatric issues you can treat.
	• Strive to be empathic, consistent, and stable.
Step 4	Form an alliance.
	• Find something you can agree on.
	• Educate the patient about your limits and responsibilities.
	• Reinforce positive behavior, and don't reward negative behavior.
Step 5	Treat whatever is treatable.
	• Screen for medical conditions.
	• Screen for mental disorders.
	• Use therapy and medication to treat problems.
Step 6	Avoid traps of wanting to...
	save the patient and be idealized.
	reject the patient and not be hurt.
	punish the patient.
	do anything to help the patient so the patient won't hurt himself or herself.
Step 7	Get help.
	• Seek consultation.
	• Foster team consensus.
	• Encourage the patient to participate in support groups.

TABLE 2–13. Steps in managing complex patients *(continued)*	
Step 8	Handle your emotions.
	• Find constructive ways of venting frustration.
	• Prepare yourself for seeing complex patients.
	• See managing complex patients as a clinical skill to master.

Source. Adapted from Roberts 2016.

tient who threatens a clinician in the emergency department; it is easy to be dismissive of this patient's health needs, of the pain he reports having, or of his need for increased medications.

A therapeutic approach to such diverse complex patients involves three steps. First, it is important to recognize what makes certain patients problematic. This is obvious in certain patients, such as those who are experienced as unreasonable, threatening, "medication seeking," "manipulative," or unlikable. Other patients, such as patients who are fellow professionals or family members or who have other attributes that make them too similar or too close to the clinician are also difficult, although this may be harder to recognize initially. Categories of patients that both theory and research have identified as problematic are those too different or similar from the clinician, which can lead to over- or underidentification. Chronically suicidal patients who invite retaliation or abandonment are difficult to treat, as are patients with unexplained somatic symptoms that can trigger overtreatment with medications or underdiagnosis of physical and mental health problems. Patients who reject help or are noncompliant and those who are angry, threatening, dying, or known to be sexually exploitative of a partner or partners can all elicit frustration, disgust, and even stronger negative countertransference reactions in even the most seasoned and dedicated clinician. These issues may be hardest for early career health professionals—significant numbers of students have reported in several studies and in past Association of American Medical Colleges Medical School Graduate Questionnaires the problem of patients behaving in an intimidating, aggressive, or racist manner, suggesting that these problems are neither rare nor isolated. Sometimes the behavior is overt, and sometimes it is a product of implicit bias. In this first step, it is important to identify the nature of the "difficult" behavior and, to the extent possible, whether it is an intentional and controlled behavior or if it is not.

Second, it is essential to view the difficult behavior as a clinical sign, that is, as a marker of an underlying, clinically important factor or process.

In other words, being difficult has a differential diagnosis. For example, being irritable or amotivational or untrusting may relate to an undiagnosed anxiety, addiction, or affective disorder. A personality style that is informal and appears to invite boundary crossings (such as the performance of favors or "special treatment" rather than care that follows standard practices) may be an indication of other health care issues, such as poor self-care at best and self-harmful behaviors (e.g., prescription drug misuse) at worst.

The third step is to think before acting; the clinician should pause before reacting to the complex patient, as shown in Figure 2–10. If a clinician feels unsafe in caring for a threatening or physically imposing patient who is demanding discharge against medical advice, for instance, then he or she should try to arrange for greater safety to permit a complete evaluation before simply allowing the patient to leave the clinical facility.

Mental health professionals caring for complex patients are advised to seek consultation frequently and widely, to provide careful documentation of their decisions, to arrange for productive outlets for their own distress, and to stay attuned to their own biases. Reminding oneself that complex patients are suffering and that even the worst and most disruptive behavior is a form of communication may be helpful in holding steady in the therapeutic setting. Through consistent, calm, and compassionate efforts, most patients—even very difficult patients—can be helped to attain a better quality of life and lessened distress.

Caring for Special Populations

Culturally Diverse Patients

The ethical principle of respect for persons is demonstrated by working competently and sensitively with individuals from different backgrounds. Cultural humility and culturally inclusive skills and knowledge are therefore increasingly seen as an important component of mental health professionalism. Both the Accreditation Council for Graduate Medical Education (2018) and the American Psychological Association (2003) specifically mention sensitivity to cultural issues as features of professional behavior and practice. DSM-5 highlights the cultural formulation as critical to excellence in psychiatric care. Early on, Tseng and Streltzer (2004) defined *cultural competence* as consisting of the therapeutic use of three personal qualities: cultural sensitivity (an appreciation of human diversity), cultural knowledge (an awareness of factual information about human cultures), and cultural empathy (the ability to make an emotional connection with another's cultural perspective). Culturally compe-

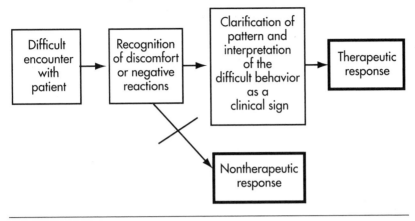

FIGURE 2–10.   Responding therapeutically to the complex patient.

Source.   Adapted from McCarty and Roberts 1996.

tent mental health practitioners use these three abilities therapeutically by noticing when and how cultural issues affect the therapeutic relationship, by determining whether an individual's problems are related to his or her heritage, and by suggesting culturally relevant therapeutic interventions (Table 2–14).

Even among individuals from the same cultural background, there may be profound differences in beliefs about mental illness and the utility of psychotropic medications and the "talking cure" (Hoop et al. 2008). More challenges may arise when there is a cultural mismatch between patient and practitioner. Language difficulties are the most concrete barrier to be surmounted. Professional translators should be used to avoid the loss of confidentiality that would occur if a family member or other nonprofessional were asked to translate.

The obligation to deal with a patient's cultural beliefs and practices in a respectful manner may become ethically challenging if a patient's culturally sanctioned treatment preferences are not congruent with standard practice in Western medicine. Because Western medical culture places high value on the worth of the individual, and therefore on autonomy, tensions may arise when treating adults from a culture that views the family as the essential unit of society. For example, the family of a competent adult patient may feel entitled to view the confidential treatment record or to make decisions for the patient regarding the disclosure of diagnosis. Clinicians must clarify how the patient would like such issues to be handled. For example, when beginning a diagnostic workup for brain pathology, a psychiatrist might ask the patient what his or her

TABLE 2–14. Speaking with patients from different cultural backgrounds than your own

Explore and remain mindful of the presence of cultural differences and similarities.

Be aware of assumptions and biases related to cultural aspects of the situation.

Seek to understand the values of the patient and family and their potential origins.

Listen carefully, use open-ended questions, and reflect back to the patient what you have heard.

At different moments in the discussion, try to summarize what you have heard and request feedback or clarifications.

Offer reassurance and encouragement, especially when discussing difficult or more sensitive topics.

Enlist interpreters when needed; avoid engaging family members as interpreters to preserve the focus on the patient.

Seek consultation with an advisor or local expert with greater knowledge or relevant lived experience.

Acknowledge when you do not feel you understand or know enough in the situation, seek greater shared understanding.

If a topic comes up that you are uncomfortable with, bring another team member into the conversation.

preference would be for being informed if the workup showed serious clinical findings. Similarly, when beginning individual psychotherapy with an adult with family-centered values, a counselor might explore with the patient his or her wishes regarding sharing private material with others.

LGBTQ+ Patients

Lesbian, gay, bisexual, transgender, and queer (LGBTQ+) individuals are at greater risk for poor mental health outcomes (Drescher et al. 2019). Mental health clinicians should remain aware of their own perceived ideas regarding "normal" and "abnormal" sexual behavior and gender expression and the potential moral underpinnings of these beliefs (Yarbrough 2018). Attempting to determine the "cause" of a patient's sexual orientation or gender identity is countertherapeutic. The APA has also long opposed conversion therapy (American Psychiatric Association 2018), given that attempts to change an individual's LGBTQ+ identity are discriminatory and harmful, absent of scientific evidence, and not in line with the duties of the mental health professional. The field of psychology has developed 28 recommendations for measuring and evaluating LGBTQ+ cultural competence (Boroughs et al. 2015). Mental health clinicians should seek consultation when personal bias or limited knowledge threatens to interfere with the evaluation of an LGBTQ+ patient.

LGBTQ+ patients may require greater assurances of confidentiality (Drescher et al. 2019). Family may be unaware of the patient's identity; engaging with a patient's family or friends does not require disclosing the patient's gender or sexual identity without the patient's permission. The broadly homophobic and transphobic nature of society may lead some LGBTQ+ individuals to hide their sexual or gender identities or lead some to blame their identity, rather than life circumstances, as the cause of their distress.

Asking patients directly for their preferred pronouns and preferred name and then referring to patients in this way demonstrates respect for persons (Lane-McKinley 2018; Yarbrough 2018). In gender-affirming therapy, clinicians provide a safe space for patients to identify who they are, outside of external relationships and social pressures (Yarbrough 2019). Gender-diverse patients are at heightened risk for suicide because of minority stress and also face lack of access to competent care (Yarbrough 2019). LGBTQ+ and gender-diverse patients who are also members of an ethnic or racial minority are especially likely to experience unequal treatment in health care settings. Mental health professionals can help to ensure that all individuals receive an appropriate standard of care (Drescher et al. 2019).

Children and Adolescents

Providing mental health care for children and adolescents is a clinically complex endeavor, in which diagnostic and treatment issues are shaped by the child's cognitive, social, and emotional development and by the relationships between the child and his or her parents and other caregivers. These complexities give rise to specific ethical challenges, particularly in the realm of confidentiality and consent for treatment.

In general, individuals do not have the legal standing to consent to medical treatment or research participation unless they have reached the age of majority, below which the consent of a parent or guardian is required. However, a growing number of states now allow minors to legally consent to mental health, substance abuse, or reproductive health treatment. In 2000, 20 states and the District of Columbia permitted minors to consent to outpatient mental health treatment, and 44 states and the District of Columbia allowed children to consent to drug and alcohol treatment (Boonstra and Nash 2000). Practitioners should seek legal advice about their jurisdiction's requirements for consent.

Children who are below the age of consent for treatment may nonetheless be capable of providing assent, defined as an affirmative agreement to the decision made by the guardian and not merely a failure to disagree (Arnold et al. 1995; Office for Human Research Protections 2005; Rosato 2000). The capacity to assent or dissent in a truly autonomous manner depends on the developmental stage of the child. Children under age 7 years generally are viewed as incapable of making treatment decisions. As a child's age and cognitive abilities increase, however, clinicians should pay increasing attention to obtaining the child's assent and, for adolescents, consent. A child in mid- to late adolescence can probably make reasoned decisions about treatment (Hurley and Underwood 2002; Nurcombe 2002). This does not absolve the clinician from obtaining consent from the child's guardian, if that is legally required; instead, consent should be obtained from both parent and child.

Clinicians should also consult state law to understand regulations pertaining to confidentiality protections for children and adolescents. Legal guardians typically have significant rights in this area, including the right to view the medical record of an adolescent capable of consenting to treatment, although in some states it is possible to withhold information if it is judged to be detrimental to the patient. At times, it may be in the best interests of the young person for the clinician to disclose private information to the guardian over the objections of the patients. To avoid irreparable damage to the therapeutic relationship, it is important for treatment providers to be explicit about how personal information will be handled in the treatment relationship and about what kind of information (i.e., indications of risky or self-injurious behavior) will be shared with the guardian. Parents and guardians should also be informed about clinicians' legal mandate to report suspected child abuse (duty to report). Failure to report suspected abuse is a breach of mental health professionals' professional and legal responsibilities.

Groups With Overlapping Vulnerabilities

People with mental illness often have overlapping vulnerabilities, such as poverty, homelessness, medical illness, and minority status (Roberts 2016). The mental health professional has a duty to act respectfully, in a manner that fosters health and recovery and protects against poor outcomes. The mental health professional should respect individuals' fundamental rights and, wherever possible, advocate for patients with disabilities and additional sources of vulnerability.

ETHICAL ISSUES IN PROFESSIONAL TRAINING

Trainees in the health professions encounter many significant ethical dilemmas. The first is the core idea of "using" patients to learn skills while becoming a clinician. Some skills in psychiatric training are not highly invasive, such as speaking with a patient or family members, but even this example can be difficult when usual boundaries of social discourse are crossed. Conversations of a personal nature—learning about a patient's sexual health or intimate relationships, a patient's childhood, or a patient's fears, self-critique, or hopes—cover sensitive and meaningful issues. Performing a physical examination, performing procedures, and engaging in clinically significant and legally significant procedures (e.g., an involuntary commitment hearing) have great impact on the patient's life. Receiving care in training institutions can be frustrating and stressful for the patient, and it is difficult for trainees to feel correct or comfortable in such circumstances. Being honest with patients, seeking informed consent for treatment, obtaining appropriate supervision, acknowledging the limits of one's ability and training, and avoiding taking on too much responsibility are steps that can help ensure that the experience is ethically acceptable and is understood and consented to by patients. Other ethical issues arise when trainees are abused by their teachers or by patients, when their abilities are misrepresented to patients by others, or when trainees make errors of judgment or make technical mistakes. For these reasons, careful supervision by teachers and efforts to remain self-aware are essential.

The ethical obligations of mental health care faculty toward trainees involve many of the same requirements as relations with colleagues, plus the added obligations of a "fiduciary-like" relationship with trainees. The connection between faculty member or supervisor and trainee, although not identical, has some similarities to the doctor-patient relationship. In both, there is a power differential, the possibility of transference feelings, and in some cases the potential for the "weaker" party to be exploited. This exploitation could take many forms, from being asked to run errands to sexual relations. Sexual relationships between supervising clinicians and trainees are recognized as potentially unethical, because of the potential negative impact on the trainee, the patients whose care is being supervised, and the training program as a whole (American Psychiatric Association 2010).

The 2019 Medical School Graduate Questionnaire (N=19,933) conducted by the Association of American Medical Colleges found that more than 60 respondents reported having been asked to exchange sexual favors for grades or other rewards during medical school (Association of American Medical Colleges 2019). More than 700 respondents reported being subject to unwanted sexual advances, and more than 750 respondents reported being required to perform personal services.

Psychiatry, psychology, and social work training involve specific ethics related to the need for trainees to provide care that may be beyond their current level of expertise. For instance, the new psychiatry intern responsible for evaluating the suicide risk of a patient in an emergency room and the inexperienced psychology or social work intern with a severely regressed therapy patient must provide care outside their current zone of competence to learn skills that will benefit future patients. The process in some ways requires treating patients as a means to an end— a violation of the principle of respect for persons—and yet the thorough training of these mental health professionals is clearly beneficent from a public health standpoint. Handling this ethical dilemma requires the informed consent of patients as willing participants in the educational setting, as well as safeguards to ensure that trainees practice only marginally beyond their current capabilities and with adequate supervision.

As noted by McCullough and colleagues (2020), trainees in the health professions must occasionally take up reasonable personal risk to fulfill beneficence-based ethical obligations to patients. Professional training should therefore prepare trainees to discern risk and provide disciplined, ethical care given the understanding of risk. These skills require the capacity to acknowledge fear, to distinguish between reasonable and unreasonable risk, and ultimately to accept reasonable risk. Professional training should also communicate the complementary significance of risk determinations that are derived collectively by experts. For example, during a pandemic, training should draw from ethical standards established in response to past disease outbreaks, as well as from the "living memory" of faculty who encountered them in their own professional formation. In cases in which standardized ethical guidelines must be communicated to trainees, "reasonable risk" should be defined in consultation with multiple stakeholder groups, including medical educators and academic and organizational leadership.

ETHICAL ISSUES IN MENTAL HEALTH RESEARCH

The suffering of persons with mental illnesses, the distress of their families and friends, and the social and economic impact of psychiatric diseases on society justify heroic research efforts. Many currently available treatments, although providing some benefits, do not cure the disorder in question; moreover, although providing some relief, treatments may be accompanied by difficult-to-tolerate or long-term side effects. Additionally, there is a great need in mental health and in medicine more generally for data about the effectiveness of various treatments in broader, more representative samples and in more real-world contexts and settings. Moreover, as neuroscientific advances move mental health research into increasingly novel territory, additional ethical challenges are certain to emerge.

Concerns regarding the ethics of psychiatric research have centered on issues of scientific design (e.g., the use of medication washout periods, the use of placebo controls), research safeguards (institutional review practices, study monitoring, and debriefing), and informed consent (Dunn and Roberts 2005). The nature of psychiatric illnesses—which may cause some individuals to have impaired decision-making abilities, to have decreased insight into the need for and potential benefits of treatment, and to be subject to involuntarily imposed treatments—has raised ethical concerns about the recruitment and enrollment of those with serious psychiatric disorders into clinical research protocols.

Because mental illnesses are highly stigmatized, research involving individuals with psychiatric illnesses historically has received intense public scrutiny (Kong and Whitaker 1998a, 1998b, 1998c, 1998d; National Bioethics Advisory Commission 1998). In some cases, heightened concerns and attention are justified. On the other hand, blanket restrictions or protections targeting psychiatric research or people with psychiatric diagnoses considering research enrollment have repeatedly been shown to be unjustified. Diagnostic-driven restrictions are problematic for several reasons. First, a substantial amount of research has now been amassed demonstrating that problems with informed consent are frequently due to a combination of factors (e.g., overly complex and lengthy consent forms, inadequate efforts to ensure that information provided during the consent process is actually understood) and not just impaired decision-making capacity (Dunn and Jeste 2001; Flory and Emanuel 2004). Indeed, in certain circumstances, such as acute medical illness (Raymont et al. 2004), or in desperate or catastrophic circumstances (Dermatis and Lesko 1990; Roberts 2002b), individuals who were previously decisionally capable may be vulnerable and unable to give informed consent.

When individuals with mental illnesses lack an adequate understanding of informed consent, educational interventions have been shown to enhance comprehension, generally up to the level of non-ill comparison subjects (Carpenter et al. 2000; Moser et al. 2006). A corollary of this finding is a concern held by numerous psychiatric research ethics investigators—namely, that the danger in seeking perfect or near-perfect comprehension of consent from people with mental illnesses considering research participation holds these populations to an unreasonable standard, one that is not asked of people with medical illnesses or of healthy people who enroll in research trials.

Concerns about both the potential vulnerability of research subjects with psychiatric illness and the risks of further stigmatizing those with mental illness by developing policies and practices in the absence of empirical research on these issues have thus fueled numerous research groups' endeavors to examine specific, ethically relevant issues in psychiatric research (Dunn and Roberts 2005; Dunn et al. 2006a). These studies, taken as a whole, have affirmed that patients with serious neuropsychiatric disorders are generally able to provide adequate informed consent for research, that enhancements to consent procedures result in improved understanding of research consent, and that participants' motivations for enrolling in psychiatric research are very similar to those of people with medical illnesses.

The shared societal and scientific need for the ethical participation of research volunteers has led to the extension of empirical research into the factors that influence individuals' decisions to enroll or not enroll in research. Such research aims to minimize the possibility of exploitation in research, proceeding from the understanding that a risk of exploitation exists in any situation characterized by an asymmetry of power or information, regardless of intent or internal rigor of study design. Decision-making factors are defined as having ethical "valence," in that they represent incommensurable aspects of personal valuation, yet are amenable to ethical analysis and optimization when conceived as a multivariable system.

A substantial body of prior work has identified numerous factors that affect a potential participant's decision-making (Kaminsky et al. 2003; Roberts et al. 2006). Some of these, called "positive valence" factors (e.g., altruism; salience of the condition under study; accurate understanding of study procedures, risks, and benefits), are appropriately influential as the individual weighs their decision. Conversely, "negative valence" factors may tilt an individual's decision toward participation for more ethically problematic reasons (e.g., desperation, lack of access to care or other resources, threats to voluntarism) (Grady 2001; Roberts 2002b, 2016). Other examples of negative valence factors include familial pressure, false hope, the lure of financial incentives, informational asymmetry, and presence of the therapeutic misconception. The Roberts Ethical Valence Model, as shown in Figure 2–11, synthesizes some recent findings on the attitudes, preferences, and values embedded in research decision-making.

Research on the decision-making of prospective volunteers takes the implicit logical positivist position that ethical valence factors are of indeterminate ethical status until they are empirically studied, and that their analysis should therefore be decoupled from their normative connotations. This position is supported by evidence that some factors commonly viewed as "good" or "protective" (e.g., optimism) may present paradoxical sources of vulnerability (Jansen et al. 2016).

This novel model of ethical research holds that ethically sound participation decisions are grounded in rigorous and authentic informed consent, in which informed consent is predicated on the condition that positive valence factors are optimized, while at the same time appropriate and robust safeguards are put in place to address negative valence factors. However, minimal research has examined the full range of potential positive and negative valence factors in combination nor has any prior work evaluated the overall impact of these factors on participation decisions of people with mental illness and addiction. Because all risks cannot be eliminated or protected against, the safeguards for such research must themselves be particularly well founded, especially when involving potentially vulnerable populations. Yet, important research on these devastating conditions should not be hindered because of biases about people with mental illness and addiction (Michels 1999, 2004).

Attention to the detailed application of ethical principles to psychiatric research is vital not just for the protection of patient volunteers—it is also critical to upholding and enhancing public trust in research, which has come under increased strain in recent decades. As psychiatric research expands and takes on more potentially ethically fraught areas of inquiry, there will be a growing need for the field to develop ethically sensitive and nuanced approaches to research (Appelbaum 2004; Biesecker and Peay 2003; Dinwiddie et al. 2004; Wilson and Stanley 2006). Unfortunately, specific guidance on how to deal with these issues and other issues in psychiatric research is lacking in federal laws and regulatory guidelines. Two novel frameworks for evaluating the ethics of clinical research protocols have been recently articulated. Emanuel and colleagues (2000) describe seven required aspects of ethical clinical research (Table 2–15), including value, scientific validity, fair subject selection, favorable risk-benefit ratio, independent review, informed consent, and respect for enrolled subjects. The basis of each of these requirements can be discerned in research ethics codes. For example, the first requirement, value, reflects the second point of the Nuremberg Code (Emanuel et al. 2000).

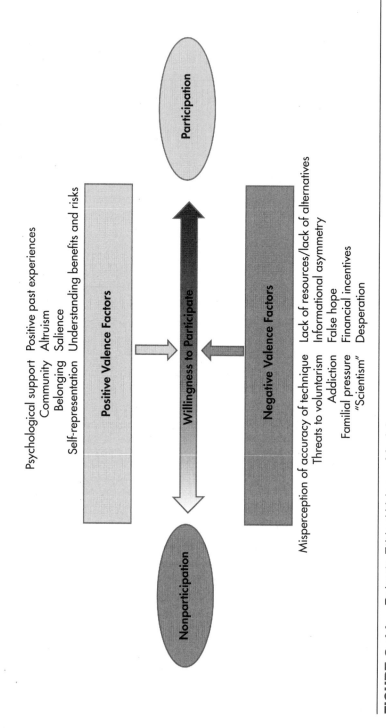

FIGURE 2-11. Roberts Ethical Valence Model.

TABLE 2–15.   Requirements for ethical clinical research

Value	Research must have the potential to lead to improved knowledge or health and must answer a nontrivial question.
Scientific validity	Methods must be scientifically rigorous.
Fair subject selection	Communities and people should not be exploited for research purposes; inclusion criteria and study sites should be determined with these principles in mind. Burdens and benefits of research participation should be equitably distributed.
Favorable risk-benefit ratio	Risks of research should be minimized. Potential benefits (to individuals and knowledge gained for society) should be enhanced and should exceed risks.
Independent review	People not associated with the research must evaluate it and have the authority to monitor it and, if necessary, terminate it.
Informed consent	Consent to research must be voluntary and must follow a complete discussion of the research.
Respect for enrolled subjects	Respect for the privacy of enrolled participants and ongoing monitoring of participants must occur throughout the research period.

Source. Adapted from Emanuel et al. 2000.

Roberts (1999) has also enumerated a framework for investigators to identify ethical dimensions and potential pitfalls in research protocols, emphasizing the need for investigators to view consideration of these ethical aspects as a critical, proactive endeavor. The Roberts Research Protocol Ethics Assessment Tool method suggests research protocols be analyzed on 24 topics in the following categories: scientific merit and design issues; expertise, commitment, and integrity issues; risks and benefits; confidentiality; participant selection and recruitment; informed consent and decisional capacity; and incentives and other issues. Table 2–16 provides an outline of questions that may be reviewed in seeking to identify, clarify, and resolve ethics issues relevant to mental health research.

TABLE 2–16.   Questions to consider regarding the
ethical acceptability of psychiatric research
protocols

1. Scientific issues

   • Is the study scientifically valuable?

   • Will the hypotheses be tested adequately?

   • Can the design yield meaningful data?

   • Does the protocol employ accepted scientific methods?

2. Research team and institutional issues

   • Does the investigative team have enough expertise and institutional and other support to successfully complete the experiment?

   • Are the researchers aware of research ethics issues and potential problems related to the protocol?

   • Are they in good standing within the scientific and professional communities?

   • What conflicting roles and conflicts of interest exist in relation to this protocol? How will they be dealt with?

   • Are the documentation features of the protocol adequate to monitor procedures and the professional accountability of the research team?

3. Design issues related to risk and benefit

   • Does the design minimize experimental risks to participants? Do alternative designs pose less risk?

   • Does the protocol pose excessive risk to individual participants, the community, and/or larger society?

   • If participants are likely to have emerging symptoms as a result of protocol involvement, have appropriate mechanisms for following symptom progression been developed? Are there clear criteria for disenrollment, and have alternative mechanisms for treatment been provided?

   • What benefits exist for participants? Is the likelihood of benefit accurately described?

   • Is it expected that any benefits derived from the protocol will be applicable to the specific population being studied?

4. Confidentiality

   • Is participant information carefully safeguarded during the collection, storage, and analysis stages of the study?

   • Is the participant aware of potential disclosure obligations of the researchers?

TABLE 2–16. Questions to consider regarding the ethical acceptability of psychiatric research protocols *(continued)*

4. Confidentiality *(continued)*

   • Are research records kept separate from clinical records? If not, is there a sound justification for this practice?

   • Are there important overlapping relationships between investigative staff and participants?

   • How will such relationships be dealt with in terms of confidentiality protections?

5. Selection, exclusion, and recruitment issues

   • Does the process of selection, exclusion, and recruitment ensure that members of vulnerable populations are included in a manner consistent with federal guidelines and only if essential to the study's scientific hypotheses?

   • Are understudied populations inappropriately excluded from participation (i.e., are selection and recruitment practices potentially biased)?

   • Is the recruitment process itself noncoercive?

6. Informed consent and decisional capacity issues

   • Is the consent form concise, readable, accurate, and understandable?

   • Does the informed consent disclosure process include all relevant information, such as the following:

     — The study's purpose and the nature of the illness or the phenomenon being studied

     — Who is responsible for the scientific and ethical conduct of the study

     — Why the individual may be eligible for participation

     — The proposed intervention and its associated risks and benefits and their relative likelihood

     — Alternatives to participation

     — Key study design features (e.g., placebo use, randomization, medication-free intervals, frequency of visits, confidentiality, plans for use of data)

   • Is there reasonable assurance of adequate decisional capacity of participants with respect to the ability to understand, analyze, and appreciate the meaning of the research decision?

TABLE 2–16. Questions to consider regarding the ethical acceptability of psychiatric research protocols *(continued)*

6. Informed consent and decisional capacity issues *(continued)*

- If participants have (or are at risk for) diminished decisional capacity at any time during protocol participation, are efforts to identify and follow the participant's capacity in place? Have specific interventions intended to enhance or restore the diminished capacity been built into the protocol?

- Does the protocol include an appropriate mechanism for advance decision-making by the participant or for identifying an alternative decision-maker for the participant? Is it clear when the advance directive or alternative decision-maker should be put into effect?

- Is there reasonable assurance that individuals will not experience coercive pressure to participate in the project or continue in the project?

7. Incentive issues

- Are incentives for participation sufficient and timed so that they compensate research participants without being coercive?

- If health care is an incentive, how will the patient's health care needs be met if disenrollment becomes necessary?

8. Institutional and peer/professional review issues

- Is the institutional context sufficient to allow the research to be conducted successfully?

- Has the protocol undergone appropriate scientific and ethical review?

- Should the protocol undergo any additional review steps (e.g., by community leaders)?

- Does the protocol have features (e.g., very high risk, very vulnerable participants) that merit ongoing external monitoring?

9. Data presentation issues

- Will the presentation of the data describe the ethical safeguards employed in the protocol?

- Will the presentation of the data meet current ethical standards (e.g., authorship, accurate disclosure of conflicting roles and conflicts of interest)?

- Will participants' identities be adequately protected in data presentation?

Source. Reprinted from Roberts LW, Geppert CM, Brody JL: "A Framework for Considering the Ethical Aspects of Psychiatric Research Protocols." *Comprehensive Psychiatry* 42:351–363, 2001. Copyright 2001, with permission from Elsevier.

FUTURE DIRECTIONS AND CONCLUSION

For the past several decades, major topics of ethical reflection in the mental health professions have included boundary issues in psychotherapy, informed consent, and involuntary treatment. More recently, several new avenues for ethical inquiry have opened. First, technological advances continue to create new and unforeseen ethical challenges. For example, scientific research in computer science, genetics, and molecular and cellular neuroscience holds the potential to produce new technologies for diagnosing predispositions to mental illness and providing more individualized treatments. Both the risks and the benefits of such diagnostic testing could be substantial, and empirical and conceptual ethics research is needed to guide its proper use. Another example is presented by emerging invasive treatments (including surgical interventions) for disorders such as severe depression. Issues pertaining to patient selection, informed consent for both research and treatment options, and maintenance of an ongoing therapeutic relationship with such patients are just beginning to be described. In addition, attitudes toward psychiatric futility and assisted suicide are changing, as are laws in other nations and in states across the United States.

Unprecedented developments in pharmacology, neuroimaging, informatics, and genetics, among other fields, will require adaptation and expansion of the age-old virtues and principles of medical ethics. Mental health clinicians in the twenty-first century and beyond must grapple with issues that were once the domain of science fiction. Should we use genetic manipulation to prevent schizophrenia? What is my professional duty when patients with serious mental disorders choose to use alternative medications rather than evidence-based treatments? How do I ethically respond to the increasing influence of direct-to-consumer advertising, the use of digital strategies and artificial intelligence, including robotic applications, in therapy, and internet pharmacies? These challenging questions and those we cannot even yet imagine, which will surely emerge in the coming decades, emphasize the need not so much to teach mental health clinicians a body of ethical knowledge but to train them in critical reasoning, literature searching, ethical problem solving, and patient-centered care.

Finally, mental health professionals as well as their practice settings and patterns have changed considerably over the last three decades. Mental health professionals in the United States are now more diverse. Many practice in managed care settings, in group practices, or within governmental agencies. It seems reasonable to expect that such sweeping changes would be reflected in the mental health profession's ethical and professional standards in the future. Although based on enduring principles of human morality, the application of bioethics principles is a dynamic enterprise, evolving with changes in the scientific, social, and cultural landscapes.

In summary, ethics is intrinsic to the practice of mental health care and related professional activities. This is perhaps more obvious in the high stakes situations that arise in the care of suicidal patients or in research involving the most seriously mentally ill in our society. Ethics is also fundamental to the everyday, more routine work of mental health professionals and trainees. With every decision, there is intent and there is action or inaction—all with ethical meaning and ethical impact. In these ways and through our ongoing attempts to become more discerning, more self-aware, and more respectful and inclusive of others, we embody ethics for our patients, our profession, and ourselves.

CONSIDER AND REFLECT

Case 1. A 19-year-old has been isolated at home for several weeks after graduating from high school. Her plans for college shifted because of her family's financial situation and because of an infectious disease pandemic. She made one phone call in an effort to get mental health care, but could not find sufficient privacy in her home, which is a small apartment. She reached out to a high school friend whose father is a psychiatrist and asked if it would be possible to text the psychiatrist from time to time and to get a prescription for antidepressant medications.

- What ethical issues and conflicts are present in this clinical scenario?
- What contextual factors are influencing the situation and the decision and options available to the psychiatrist?
- What kinds of potential risks exist for this psychiatrist in providing care in this particular situation?
- How might you handle this situation? What are the most important next steps for the psychiatrist?
- What other expertise or resources may be introduced to help or address ethical issues or professionalism challenges in this situation?

Case 2. A 68-year-old psychiatrist is the sole mental health professional in a multispecialty group practice. The group practice has become increasingly busy: the volume of referrals to the psychiatrist has grown dramatically and the kinds of patient care situations have become much more severe since a local inpatient unit was closed. The psychiatrist is concerned about stress and has noticed that his notes are not as complete and that he awakens at night, worrying over questions he forgot to ask or problems he failed to address in caring for patients the previous day.

- What ethical issues and conflicts are present in this clinical scenario?
- What contextual factors are influencing the situation and the decisions and options available to the psychiatrist?
- What kinds of potential risks exist for patients and for this psychiatrist in this particular situation?
- How might you handle this situation? What are the most important next steps for the psychiatrist?
- What other expertise or resources may be introduced to help or address ethical issues or professionalism challenges in this situation?

Case 3. An addiction psychiatry trainee is on a 3-month rotation in which she provides care for patients in a general mood disorders clinic. She notices that one of the teaching attending psychiatrists seldom asks about addiction-related issues and never asks about safety in the home when evaluating patients. She wishes to raise concerns, especially regarding female patients with multiple health issues, but feels very intimidated by the attending psychiatrist who always seems stressed, irritable, and quick to offer a harsh or negative comment.

- What ethical issues and conflicts are present in this clinical scenario?
- What kinds of potential risks exist for patients and for the psychiatry trainee in this particular situation?
- How might you handle this situation? What are the most important next steps for the psychiatry trainee?
- What other expertise or resources may be introduced to help or address ethical issues or professionalism challenges in this situation?

Case 4. A psychiatrist accepts a telehealth contract to provide consultations on psychiatric patients who come to emergency rooms in a five-county region. The psychiatrist has a full-time "day job" but felt he could handle the extra work and hoped to be able to pay off his school debt more quickly by accepting the added role. The emergency rooms are located in urban and rural community hospitals, which are typically understaffed, and the number of patient evaluations per contracted shift may range from 4 to 18. The psychiatrist loves the work and feels he is helping to identify patients who are in the greatest immediate need for psychiatric expertise. He also enjoys working with his emergency medicine colleagues, even in this limited way, but worries that a brief telehealth visit does not really help patients in the long run and is just a "band aid" on an inadequate system.

- What ethical issues are present in this clinical scenario?
- What inherent risks exist in this situation?
- What other expertise or resources may be introduced to help or address ethical issues or professionalism challenges in this situation?
- How are the psychiatrist's roles as clinician, colleague, and advocate relevant in this scenario?

Case 5. A medical student rotating through a psychiatry emergency/crisis clinic for a third-year clerkship becomes extremely distraught after seeing a patient (with the attending psychiatrist) who described her experience surviving childhood sexual abuse. Recognizing the student's distress, the chief resident meets with the student who describes being upset by the patient's personal story and the attending psychiatrist's manner, which the student feels was "insensitive" because of the psychiatrist's efforts to direct the patient to the "here and now."

- What ethical issues are present in this clinical scenario?
- What inherent risks exist in this situation?
- What other expertise or resources may be introduced to help or address ethical issues or professionalism challenges in this situation?
- How are the student's, attending psychiatrist's, and chief resident's roles and professional duties influencing the ethical dimensions of the situation?
- How might you handle this situation, if you were the chief resident? What are the most important next steps?

Case 6. A psychologist and a psychiatrist co-lead a group for patients shortly after they have been discharged from the inpatient unit affiliated with their academic department. The psychologist notices that the psychiatrist occasionally arrives late to the group meeting, which occurs after lunch, and seems distracted or "checked out." Twice the psychologist smelled alcohol on the breath of the psychiatrist.

- What ethical issues are present in this clinical scenario?
- What inherent risks exist in this situation?
- What other expertise or resources may be introduced to help or address ethical issues or professionalism challenges in this situation?
- How are the psychologist's and psychiatrist's roles relevant in this scenario?
- How might you handle this situation, if you were the psychologist? What are the most important next steps?

Case 7. A psychiatrist wishes to conduct a quality assurance project that will involve reviewing the electronic medical record of recent psychiatric inpatients to verify the presence of appropriate documentation of sexual history, suicidality, and substance use. The psychiatrist is hoping that eventually there will be an interesting research project to come out of the quality assurance work.

- What ethical issues are present in this clinical scenario?
- What inherent risks exist in this situation?
- What other expertise or resources may be introduced to help or address ethical issues or professionalism challenges in this situation?
- What issues should the psychiatrist consider in setting up appropriate safeguards for the quality assurance project? And if it becomes a research project? What are the most important next steps?

PART II

QUESTIONS AND ANNOTATED ANSWERS

CHAPTER 3

CORE CONCEPTS IN ETHICS AND PROFESSIONALISM

3.1

For each of the following descriptions, choose the most appropriate ethical concept. Each answer option may be used once, more than once, or not at all.

    A.   Autonomy.
    B.   Compassion.
    C.   Fidelity.
    D.   Nonmaleficence.
    E.   Veracity.

    ____   Honesty; conveying information and meaning truthfully and without deceit
    ____   Empathy; possessing the capacity for "suffering with" another individual
    ____   Faithfulness; remaining dedicated to the goals of patient care
    ____   "Do no harm"; seeking to avoid harm toward others
    ____   "Self-rule"; having the capacity to make and enact decisions for oneself

Autonomy is the capacity to make and enact decisions for oneself. *Compassion* relates to the idea of "suffering with" another person—being genuinely empathic. *Fidelity* is the notion of remaining dedicated, or "faithful," to the goals of patient care and to the therapeutic task in working with a patient or client. *Nonmaleficence* is the duty to avoid doing harm. *Veracity* refers to truth telling or honesty. (Beauchamp and Childress 2001; Boyd et al. 1997) *Answers 3.1: E, B, C, D, A*

3.2

A psychiatrist and a psychologist together advocate for insurance coverage "parity" for mental illnesses, providing the rationale that mental illnesses are prevalent, severe, and stigmatized and that they do not receive the insurance benefits that medical illnesses receive in our society.

Which of the following ethical concepts is the primary ethical rationale behind the argument advanced by this psychiatrist and psychologist?

- A. Beneficence.
- B. Compassion.
- C. Justice.
- D. Nonmaleficence.
- E. Veracity.

The bioethics principle underlying the argument offered by the two mental health professionals in this scenario is justice. *Justice* refers to the equitable distribution of resources across society to address an issue of importance to society, that is, the public health. The observations that mental illnesses are prevalent, stigmatized, and not insured at the same level as other illness types are especially pertinent to the justice-based argument. The psychiatrist and psychologist also mention that mental illnesses are severe. This suggests that the two also may be motivated by beneficence, compassion, and nonmaleficence, but these are not the primary rationales behind the argument made in the scenario. (Beauchamp and Childress 2001; Roberts 2016) *Answer 3.2: C*

3.3

A psychiatrist attends a neighborhood picnic and is approached by an acquaintance who was a psychology major in college and wants to "run something by her" regarding a friend. The psychiatrist learns that the friend (with whom the psychiatrist does not have a therapeutic relationship) is depressed and has occasionally spoken of a wish to die. The friend is in treatment with another provider.

Which of the following is the psychiatrist's most appropriate first step?

- A. Clarify her role with the acquaintance.
- B. Contact the person's treatment provider and offer professional assistance.

C. Do and say nothing, because she has no professional relationship with the person who may harm himself.
D. Do and say nothing, because the information is incomplete and thirdhand.
E. Report the information to the authorities, just in case.

On one hand, psychiatrists always have the duty to act with respect and professionalism in relation to a person with mental illness. In this situation, however, no doctor-patient relationship has been established in which the psychiatrist would be enabled to act or intervene on behalf of the individual. To act on an informal basis, in fact, could create unexpected and adverse consequences for the individual.

On the other hand, doing and saying nothing is not the optimal first response in this situation because the neighborhood acquaintance may not understand the boundaries surrounding the psychiatrist's professional role in society and the doctor-patient relationship. The psychiatrist should clarify her role with the acquaintance. She may also wish to help the acquaintance identify other relevant mental health resources in the area.

It is important to note that although a psychiatrist may perceive herself to be off the clock and not actively serving in her role as a psychiatrist, others may not perceive her as such. It is permissible and even recommended to keep one's personal and professional roles separate when possible. Nevertheless, one must bear in mind that laypersons may not make such distinctions and that one's role may need to be clarified from time to time. (American Psychiatric Association 2006; Anfang and Appelbaum 1996)
Answer 3.3: A

3.4

For each of the following descriptions, choose the most appropriate term. Each answer option may be used once, more than once, or not at all.

A. Assisted suicide.
B. Active euthanasia.
C. Both assisted suicide and active euthanasia.
D. Neither assisted suicide nor active euthanasia.

_____ A voluntary request by a decisionally capable individual to be provided with the means (e.g., medication) to commit suicide

____   Legal across the United States in 2020
____   Endorsed by the American Medical Association in 2020
____   A physician administers a lethal dose of medication
____   Legal in certain situations in some countries (e.g., the Nether-
          lands) for more than a decade
____   Ethically the same as withholding treatment that allows a ter-
          minally ill patient to die
____   Ethically the same as providing medication to alleviate pain
          and resulting in patient death

Assisted suicide refers to a decisionally capable individual self-administer-
ing a means to commit suicide that is provided by a physician (Materstvedt et al. 2003). *Euthanasia* is a form of physician-assisted death in
which the physician acts with compassionate intent to end the life of a person with an incurable and progressive disease that will cause imminent
death. *Active euthanasia* refers to euthanasia in which a deliberate "act"
is taken to end a person's life; usually this act is the administration of a
lethal dose of medication (Meisel 2020). *Withholding treatment* involves
not starting a treatment that might prolong a patient's life, whereas *withdrawing treatment* involves stopping a treatment that might prolong a patient's life. Both withholding and withdrawing treatment may be referred
to as *passive euthanasia*. Physicians have a duty to do no harm (nonmaleficence), to respect patient autonomy, and to provide adequate pain control (American Medical Association 2020). Physician-assisted suicide is
legal in eight U.S. states and the District of Columbia at the time of this
writing, but euthanasia is illegal across the country (Meisel 2020). Both
assisted suicide and active euthanasia have been legal in certain situations in some countries for more than a decade (Quill 2018). For example, in the Netherlands, both were legalized by the Termination of Life on
Request and Assisted Suicide (Review Procedures) Act, which took effect
in 2002. Neither assisted suicide nor active euthanasia is endorsed by
the American Medical Association in 2020. (American Medical Association, Council on Ethical and Judicial Affairs 2016a) *Answers 3.4: A, D,
D, B, C, D, D*

3.5

A psychiatrist sits on the pharmacy and therapeutics committee of a
public hospital. A new antidepressant has just received approval from
the U.S. Food and Drug Administration, but research indicates that it offers little benefit over existing agents and that it is much more expensive

than older medications no longer under patent protection. The pharmaceutical representative offers the psychiatrist a 3-year supply of free samples of the drug for his own practice if he agrees to lobby the committee to make the medication a first-line treatment for depression on the formulary.

Which of the following is the most appropriate response to the offer and its ethical justification?

A. Agree, because adding the drug to the formulary will not hurt the hospital, and the free samples will help many of the psychiatrist's patients.
B. Agree, because research indicates the medication is as effective as older drugs and, although expensive, it offers the hospital's patients another treatment alternative.
C. Refuse, because this offer compromises the psychiatrist's role as a member of a committee dedicated to balancing patient care and stewardship of public resources.
D. Refuse, because it is unethical to accept free medication samples.
E. Refuse, because the arrangement has the appearance of a conflict of interest, even though it is not improper.

Health care professionals are increasingly confronting potential conflicts of interest stemming from relationships with industry. A crucial professional skill for all clinicians is the ability to recognize and respond to these conflicts in an ethically sound manner. In this case, the psychiatrist is contemplating acting as both an agent of the pharmaceutical company in promoting a preferential place on the formulary for its product and a trustee of the public's good, which are potentially contradictory roles. If the psychiatrist's primary moral duty as a member of the pharmacy and therapeutics committee is to develop a formulary that provides for optimal patient care while wisely using scarce health care resources, then there is a clear conflict with the action of lobbying for a drug that has no clinical superiority but is more expensive than existing alternatives. Furthermore, the arrangement to receive free samples is a special deal outside the normal contractual bidding mechanism that must be disclosed to fellow committee members. Even if the psychiatrist agreed only to give his honest assessment of the drug's benefits to the formulary committee and to fully disclose his arrangement with the drug company, the special deal might compromise his judgment and his ability to provide accurate, objective information. (Field and Lo 2009; Roberts 2016; Snyder Sulmasy et al. 2019) *Answer 3.5: C*

3.6

Decisional capacity has been conceptualized as having four component capacities. Which of the following constitutes the set of these capacities?

A. To appreciate, to communicate, to reason, to understand.
B. To appreciate, to reason, to translate, to understand.
C. To communicate, to infer, to reason, to translate.
D. To infer, to reason, to speak, to understand.
E. To reason, to speak, to translate, to understand.

Informed consent is one of the most critical ethical and legal safeguards in clinical care and human research. Informed consent is the process through which a physician (or a designated colleague) helps shepherd informed, deliberate, and authentic decision-making by an individual. It often, but not always, is signified by a written document that is signed by the individual (or by a legally acceptable or authorized decision-maker).

The informed consent process exists within a particular context (e.g., an acute, high risk decision; a routine, low risk decision; a voluntary, minimal risk research decision) and consists of three necessary aspects: information sharing, decisional capacity, and voluntarism capacity.

The information to be shared should encompass the nature of the illness or health condition; the reason for the decision at the time; the risks, benefits, alternatives, and anticipated consequences of the decision (or an alternative decision); and related issues. Decisional capacity involves the following: 1) the ability to communicate a preference, 2) the ability to understand, 3) the ability to reason, and 4) the ability to appreciate the decision. The last element, appreciation, is linked to insight and to the personal values of the patient/participant. Voluntarism capacity is the ability to make an authentic decision, free from coercive influences and involves the following: 1) developmental capacity, 2) illness-related factors, 3) psychological issues and cultural and religious values, and 4) external pressures. (Roberts 2002b; Roberts 2016) *Answer 3.6: A*

3.7

A psychiatrist has been in private practice for 15 years and treats patients with psychotherapy as well as psychopharmacology. A patient he has been treating for bipolar disorder has deteriorated after not having responded to lithium, valproic acid, or carbamazepine. The psychiatrist has not prescribed one of the newer anticonvulsants or antipsychotics for the patient's condition because he has not kept up to date on the efficacy of newer medications, but he believes that one of those agents may be helpful to the patient.

Which of the following is the best course of action for the psychiatrist to take, given the patient's clinical deterioration?

A. Attend a dinner talk on the latest treatments for bipolar disorder.
B. Develop a self-directed learning program on newer medications.
C. Discuss with the patient the need for the psychiatrist to obtain consultation on medications.
D. Suggest the patient find a psychiatrist specializing in psychopharmacology.
E. Transfer the patient to a younger psychiatrist for medication management, and focus on treating this patient with psychotherapy.

Part of a physician's professionalism, which, in turn, is part of the profession's social contract, is to keep up to date with new developments in the clinical care of patients. There is also an expectation for physicians to assess their own abilities and learn throughout their careers. If gaps are recognized, physicians should take steps to remedy them. These expectations also fall under the practice-based learning and professionalism competencies adopted by accreditation and certification authorities. Because the patient's condition is deteriorating, the psychiatrist should quickly obtain consultation. Referral or transfer would be options under less urgent conditions, but the physician should take pains to ensure that the new provider is capable of meeting the patient's clinical needs without abandoning the patient. Industry-sponsored dinner talks are generally not unbiased sources of information and should not be a clinician's sole source of new information. (American Board of Psychiatry and Neurology 2020; Sah and Fugh-Berman 2013) *Answer 3.7: C*

3.8

For each of the following descriptions, choose the most appropriate term. Each answer option may be used once, more than once, or not at all.

A. Discrimination.
B. Implicit bias.
C. Neither discrimination nor implicit bias.

_____ Intentional unjust treatment of people on the basis of race, age, or gender

_____ Unintentional unjust treatment of people on the basis of race, age, or gender

_____ An employer not hiring a job candidate with an uncontrolled seizure disorder for a role driving a bus

_____ An employer not hiring a job candidate to drive a bus because of the candidate's having a family history of depression

Discrimination is defined as the intentional unjust treatment of individuals on the basis of some actual or perceived characteristic, whereas implicit bias is defined as the unintentional unjust treatment of individuals on the basis of some actual or perceived characteristic (see Chapman et al. 2013; Sue et al. 2007). The Americans with Disabilities Act prohibits employers from discriminating against qualified individuals with disabilities (U.S. Department of Justice 2020a). Choosing to not hire a candidate because the candidate cannot adequately perform the functions of the position is neither discrimination nor implicit bias. *Answers 3.8: A, B, C, A*

3.9

A first-year medical student is looking for a patient to interview as part of the course "Introduction to the Patient." While looking through charts for a suitable person on a medical inpatient unit, she discovers that one of her classmates has been hospitalized overnight. She is deeply concerned about her fellow classmate and wants to provide emotional support. Which of the following is the best course of action for this first-year student?

A. Approach the classmate-patient directly to give emotional support.

B. Ask a unit staff person what the medical issue is before approaching the classmate-patient to give emotional support.

C. Thumb through the chart to see what the medical issue is before approaching the classmate-patient to give emotional support.

D. Send a card to the classmate-patient, but do not look at the chart or speak with staff.

E. Do not look at the chart, speak with staff, or approach the classmate-patient in any way.

This scenario represents an inadvertent breach of confidentiality. The first-year student should not seek to learn anything further about the classmate-patient, nor should she mention it to others. If in another, more personal, setting, the student learns about the classmate's illness, then it may be appropriate to send a note or card or to approach the classmate personally. (Lane et al. 1990; Roberts et al. 2001b) *Answer 3.9: E*

3.10

A military psychologist attached to the U.S. detention center at Guantanamo Bay is involved in the interrogation of Al-Qaeda terrorism suspects. The psychologist attempts to determine if the detainees have any phobias that could be exploited to encourage the suspects to divulge information about planned terrorist attacks.

Which of the following is the ethical concept that is most clearly violated by such a practice?

A. Do no harm.
B. *E pluribus unum.*
C. Protect innocent lives.
D. Respect for autonomy.
E. Respect for persons.

Practices at the Guantanamo Bay detention facility have been criticized for their failure to recognize that medical personnel are not to misuse their specialized knowledge and training under any circumstances. Members of professions with duties to benefit and to refrain from harming patients cannot ethically use their specialized knowledge to find and exploit vulnerabilities in prisoners simply by defining the work that occurs in a detention setting as a nonclinical role.

The United Nations' *Principles of Medical Ethics Relevant to the Role of Health Personnel, Particularly Physicians, in the Protection of Prisoners and Detainees against Torture and Other Cruel, Inhuman or Degrading Treatment or Punishment* states that health care personnel may not engage, actively or passively, in any acts that contribute to torture or other cruel treatment. The United Nations principles further hold that it is unethical for health care personnel—including psychiatrists and psychologists—to engage in professional relationships with detainees other than relationships that evaluate, protect, or improve detainees' physical and mental health. Medical personnel who act in a way that is harmful to prisoners, such as by increasing the possibility that a vulnerable person will be subjected to something feared, rather than acting to alleviate the harm of a phobia are acting unethically. (Abeles 2010; Bloche and Marks 2005a, 2005b; United Nations 1982) *Answer 3.10: A*

3.11

Patients are sought for enrollment in a clinical trial of a new medication. During an initial conversation with the research physician, a patient with severe symptoms agrees to participate in the proposed study, stating, "Yes, of course I'll sign up. I'll do anything to help myself. I've just got to feel better." The patient's statement is most consistent with what misconception of some research participants?

A. All volunteers are allowed to participate in research.
B. Medical research is a purely altruistic activity.
C. Recruiting physicians exert pressure on potential participants to enroll.
D. Research participants are certain to receive better treatments than are clinically available.
E. Research protocols fully safeguard participants.

A common misconception concerning medical research is that clinical protocols are certain to provide research participants with direct therapeutic benefits. In reality, investigational therapies often fail to show significant advantages over standard treatments. Moreover, to be ethical, under most circumstances studies are structured to answer the unresolved question of whether or not a particular intervention is helpful—that is, the condition of equipoise is necessary for an ethically sound scientific design.

The overestimation of the benefits of research participation has been termed the *therapeutic misconception*. Among both psychiatric and non-psychiatric research participants, the therapeutic misconception leads to inappropriate expectations regarding the degree of individualization of the treatment and the nature or likelihood of therapeutic benefit. Research participants demonstrating this misconception may be unrealistically optimistic about the benefits of the experimental intervention. Often these individuals also minimize the risks associated with the experimental agent. Investigators themselves may be influenced by the fallacy as they recruit participants or enroll them in specific arms of a trial.

To minimize the impact of the therapeutic misconception, researchers must use the informed consent process to educate potential participants about the goals of the trial (i.e., to seek to answer a scientific question) and how they differ from the goals of clinical care (i.e., to seek to benefit the individual patient). Potential participants must be thoroughly informed about the elements of the research protocol that involve risks and about nonroutine procedures and should be carefully educated about the concepts of randomization and blinding, if applicable. (Appelbaum and Grisso 1988; Jansen et al. 2016; Lidz et al. 2004; Roberts et al. 2004a, 2004c) *Answer 3.11: D*

3.12

For each of the following descriptions, choose the most appropriate ethical principle. Each answer option may be used once, more than once, or not at all.

    A. Advocacy.
    B. Compassion.
    C. Justice.
    D. Scope of practice.
    E. Veracity.

    ____ Accurately documenting the medical and psychiatric history of the patient
    ____ Providing sufficient treatment for the pain experienced by a terminally ill patient
    ____ Referring a complex patient to a subspecialist with greater expertise

Veracity refers to truth telling or honesty, which is most directly relevant to the idea of accurately documenting the medical and psychiatric history of the patient. *Compassion*—the notion of acting with kindness and "suffering with" one's patient—will help ensure that the terminally ill individual has sufficient pain control. *Scope of practice*, or *area of expertise*, is the phrase used in the health professions to demarcate the set of clinical activities for which one is adequately prepared and is able to provide an appropriate standard of care. (Beauchamp and Childress 2001; Roberts 2016; Roberts et al. 2011) *Answers 3.12: E, B, D*

3.13

An unmarried male psychiatry resident has been treating an unmarried female patient for 18 months in psychodynamic psychotherapy. The resident finds himself increasingly sexually attracted to the patient. In the final session of the therapy, he mentions his desire to the patient. She states that she is also attracted to him. The resident suggests that they wait

6 months after the termination of psychotherapy and then meet to consider starting a relationship.

Which of the following is true about this situation?

A. Because of the decision to delay a personal relationship for 6 months after the termination of therapy, the ethical issue of a boundary violation does not exist.

B. Because the resident waited until the final session to discuss his attraction with the patient, the resident's revelation is not a serious ethical lapse.

C. Because the attraction is mutual, it is not unethical for the resident to pursue a relationship with his former patient.

D. If the resident does not bill the patient for the planned meeting 6 months after the termination of the psychotherapy, this meeting will be ethically acceptable.

E. This scenario describes an unacceptable boundary violation.

Sexual relations between therapists (e.g., psychiatrists, psychologists, other mental health professionals) and their patients are prohibited by professional organizations and violate criminal statutes in some jurisdictions. The power differential between healer and patient coupled with the strong transference feelings that arise during psychotherapy make patients extremely vulnerable to exploitation by their therapists. Current understanding of the strength and longevity of transference feelings suggests that future romantic relationships between a therapist and ex-patient are also tainted by the prior therapeutic relationship. Almost all authorities now agree that such a relationship could lead to unethical sexual exploitation of the ex-patient by the therapist and hence must be forbidden. In this case, the resident's unethical behavior is not mitigated by any of the circumstances of the case—including the apparent mutuality of the attraction and the decision to wait 6 months before starting a relationship.

Two virtues are especially important in ethical arguments that justify an absolute prohibition of doctor-patient sexual relationships: self-effacement and self-sacrifice. *Self-sacrifice* is the habit of taking reasonable risks to one's self-interest. Physicians are expected to accept reasonable levels of risks to their personal well-being, health, and even life in the care of patients. Forgoing the pursuit of sexual attraction or the satisfaction of sexual desire is, in the larger order of things, a relatively small sacrifice of self-interest for the physician to make. Thus, self-sacrifice places stringent demands on the physician when it comes to sexual relationships with patients. *Self-effacement* means making oneself inconspicuous and is a virtue related to humility and modesty. Self-effacement obligates a physician to put aside his or her own feelings about a patient's sexual attractiveness without denying the reality of such feelings. Self-effacement and self-sacrifice combine to obligate the physician to have and to routinely display moral and physical discipline in response to feelings of sexual attractiveness in the context of the doctor-patient relationship, that is, to put such feelings aside and never to act on them. It follows that pursuing feelings of sexual attraction in the context of the doctor-patient relationship counts in all cases as a vice of mere self-interest, which is wholly antithetical to the professional virtues of self-effacement and self-sacrifice. (American Psychiatric Association 2010; Fisher 2004; Gabbard 2002; Norris et al. 2003) *Answer 3.13: E*

3.14

A psychiatrist practices at a community mental health center that serves several small rural communities. He lives near the mental health center and is the only psychiatrist in the region. A local community leader asks the psychiatrist to treat her for depression. The leader and the psychiatrist regularly see each other at community events and serve together on a public committee.

What should the psychiatrist do to manage his overlapping relationships ethically with the community leader?

A. Establish confidentiality parameters and guidelines for out-of-session encounters.

B. Request that the community leader cease all public interactions with the practitioner.

C. Request that the community leader sign a "no confidentiality" agreement.

D. Schedule appointments away from the mental health center to conceal the therapeutic relationship.

E. Under no circumstances treat the community leader, because overlapping relationships are never ethical.

Overlapping or multiple relationships occur when a clinician has a professional therapeutic relationship with a patient while also having another relationship or role with that individual. Although overlapping relationships are common in small communities, the practitioner is obligated to maintain professional and therapeutic boundaries with the patient and to abstain from a therapeutic relationship if there is likelihood that the relationship will impair the practitioner's clinical capabilities or cause the individual any harm. Although these relationships are complex, they are not inherently unethical. The psychiatrist is required to discuss the boundaries of the professional relationship, the limits and scope of confidentiality, and the role of each in the professional relationship. The patient's expectations of the psychiatrist in other settings or roles (i.e., out-of-session encounters) need to be explored. Any differences between the psychiatrist's and patient's perceptions need to be clarified and reconciled. (American Psychiatric Association 2010; Roberts 2016; Simon and Williams 1999; Stockman 1990) *Answer 3.14: A*

3.15

Which of the following statements is closest to the definition of human subjects research, according to the U.S. Department of Health and Human Services regulatory standards?

A. Systematic collection of data with the intent to contribute to generalizable knowledge.
B. Systematic collection of data on living persons with the intent to contribute to generalizable knowledge.
C. Systematic collection of data on persons, living or dead, for any purpose.
D. Systematic collection of identifiable data on persons, living or dead, for any purpose.
E. Systematic or nonsystematic collection of data on persons, living or dead, for any purpose.

The terms *human subjects* and *research* are defined in the U.S. Department of Health and Human Services Code of Federal Regulations, Section 46.102. These definitions are used to determine whether or not an activity is governed by federal protections for human subjects and whether it requires approval by an appropriate institutional review board (IRB) (Roberts 2016).

The code defines *research* as follows:

Research means a systematic investigation, including research development, testing and evaluation, designed to develop or contribute to generalizable knowledge. Activities which meet this definition constitute research for purposes of this policy, whether or not they are conducted or supported under a program which is considered research for other purposes. For example, some demonstration and service programs may include research activities. (U.S. Department of Health and Human Services 2018)

The code defines who is a human subject for purposes of research protection as follows:

> *Human subject* means a living individual about whom an investigator (whether professional or student) conducting research i) obtains information or biospecimens through intervention or interaction with the individual, and uses, studies, or analyzes the information or biospecimens; or ii) obtains, uses, studies, analyzes, or generates identifiable private information or identifiable biospecimens. *Intervention* includes both physical procedures by which information or biospecimens are gathered (e.g., venipuncture) and manipulations of the subject or the subject's environment that are performed for research purposes. *Interaction* includes communication or interpersonal contact between investigator and subject. *Private information* includes information about behavior that occurs in a context in which an individual can reasonably expect that no observation or recording is taking place, and information which has been provided for specific purposes by an individual and that the individual can reasonably expect will not be made public (e.g., a medical record). (U.S. Department of Health and Human Services 2018)

Answer 3.15: B

3.16

Which of the following statements is correct regarding the American Medical Association's position on ritual genital cutting or mutilation of female minors by physicians in the year 2020 in the United States?

A. Prohibited in all states.
B. Prohibited in some states.
C. Allowed in all states with parental consent.
D. Allowed in some states with parental consent.
E. Allowed in some states with minor's consent.

Genital mutilation of female minors is not a culturally accepted practice in the United States. Female genital mutilation (FGM) is considered abusive and must be reported to authorities. The American Medical Association's position on FGM is as follows:

> [The American Medical Association] (1) condemns the practice of FGM; (2) considers FGM a form of child abuse; (3) supports legislation to eliminate the performance of female genital mutilation in the United States

and to protect young girls and women at risk of undergoing the procedure; (4) supports that physicians who are requested to perform genital mutilation on a patient provide culturally sensitive counseling to educate the patient and her family members about the negative health consequences of the procedure, and discourage them from having the procedure performed. When possible, physicians should refer the patient to social support groups that can help them cope with societal mores; (5) will work to ensure that medical students, residents, and practicing physicians are made aware of the continued practice and existence of FGM in the United States, its physical effects on patients, and any requirements for reporting FGM; and (6) is in opposition to the practice of female genital mutilation by any physician or licensed practitioner in the United States. (American Medical Association 2017)

The United States District Court for the Eastern District of Michigan ruled the federal law prohibiting FGM unconstitutional in 2018. As of this writing, 39 states have anti-FGM legislation (Batha 2021). *Answer 3.16: A*

3.17

In a public hospital support group for patients with schizophrenia, religion comes up as a topic. One patient says, "God takes care of us all." Another patient says, "There is no God." The members of the group are not aware that the group facilitator is devoutly religious, with a deep faith in God. Which of the following is the facilitator's best course of action?

A. Explain to the group that this topic is inappropriate for discussion in a public hospital.

B. Without explanation, quickly change topics, because this is a no-win situation.

C. Openly share with the group his own belief in God and make an honest attempt to persuade those who disagree.

D. Without divulging his own views, facilitate discussion about whether God exists and explore issues (e.g., hope, spirituality) that may be relevant for mental health.

E. Without divulging his own views, subtly introduce evidence that supports the existence of God.

Professionalism requires group therapists and facilitators to show appropriate respect for the beliefs and values of each group member. In this setting, attempting to impose one's own religious beliefs on the group members is an inappropriate use of the facilitator's role. The most appropriate action is to encourage a respectful and open discussion in which each group member has an opportunity to express his or her own beliefs. As long as the facilitator can manage his own strong feelings about the topic so that they do not impair his clinical abilities, there is no need to move the group to a less controversial subject, because developing the ability to tolerate disagreement can be healthy and beneficial for the group participants. (American Psychiatric Association 2001a, 2010; Roberts 2016) *Answer 3.17: D*

3.18

A psychologist at a Veterans Affairs (VA) medical center has been treating a 26-year-old former airman who was medically discharged because he developed major depression. In the psychologist's therapy notes, he assigns the patient a Global Assessment of Functioning (GAF) score of 55. The airman obtains a copy of his medical records and learns of the score. He returns angrily to the psychologist and demands that the score be lowered because he is applying for "service-connected" compensation for his depression, and it will not likely be granted with such a high score. The psychologist believes that the score is accurate. Which of the following is the most ethically appropriate course of action?

A. Do not change the score, but provide an explanatory narrative for reviewers that describes the man's continued problems.
B. Explain to the patient that the GAF score should not be used in compensation determinations.
C. Inform the patient that if his GAF is 55, then he is functioning too highly to be eligible for compensation.
D. Lower the documented GAF score so that the patient can receive compensation.
E. Lower the documented GAF score so that the patient does not leave treatment.

The therapeutic relationship is often challenged by requests to provide an "objective" assessment of a patient's disability or capacity to return to work. Ideally, such an assessment involves familiarity with the patient's work history, interviews of collateral informants, and a skeptic's awareness of the possibility that the patient may desire secondary gain. These demands may be, and often are, incompatible with the physician's primary responsibility in a treatment relationship. In fact, forensic or independent evaluations entail obligations to the compensation system or other third parties that may be harmful to the patient or his treatment. Separation of the forensic assessment and clinical roles is an accepted strategy for maintaining primary allegiance to the patient. When the separation of roles is not possible, clinicians must attempt to manage them ethically.

In this case, although the GAF was designed as a clinical rather than a regulatory or institutional measure, the VA (and other organizations, such as the Social Security Administration) uses the score to make disability determinations. However, it would be unethical for the psychologist to alter an accurate clinical judgment to enable a patient to obtain a financial benefit. The ideal option would have been to discuss with the patient the possibility of such a conflict at the beginning of treatment. Failing that, the clinician should not change the score if he believes it is clinically correct. He can be helpful to the patient without compromising his clinical integrity by explaining to the patient the dual uses of the assessment, encouraging continued treatment, and writing a narrative for compensation reviewers that describes the patient's deficits as accurately and fairly as possible. (American Academy of Psychiatry and the Law 2005; Herlihy and Corey 2014; Mischoulon 1999) *Answer 3.18: A*

3.19

A deeply religious patient with severe bipolar disorder is referred to a resident psychiatrist for treatment. Before the initial evaluation, the resident reviews the patient's prior treatment notes, noticing a pattern of "extreme hyperreligiosity" during manic episodes and a history of involuntary hospitalizations. During the evaluation, the patient begins by asking the resident, "Do you worship God?" Which ethics skill or skills are required in this clinical situation?

A. The ability to anticipate potentially ethically problematic or risky situations.

B. The ability to identify ethical principles involved in a particular patient's care.

C. The ability to identify one's scope of practice and work within those boundaries.

D. The ability to understand that one's own background and beliefs may influence one's care of patients.

E. All of the above.

Anticipating ethically problematic or risky situations is a core ethics skill for mental health professionals. In this circumstance, after reviewing the case history, the resident may expect that ethically high risk situations such as involuntary hospitalization may occur in the future. The ability to identify and apply the ethical principles involved in a particular patient's care is another essential ethics skill. In this scenario, the resident may reasonably predict that cultural issues as well as the possibility of involuntary hospitalization may complicate the therapeutic relationship. A third core ethics skill is realizing one's limitations in clinical competence. The resident should ensure that adequate attending supervision is available to assist in the treatment of this patient with a chronic and severe illness. Another key ethics skill pertinent to this case is the ability to understand how the clinician's own background and beliefs may affect patient care. In this case, self-awareness and self-examination may prevent this resident's own religious beliefs from subtly influencing the treatment of this patient. (American Psychiatric Association 2001a; Roberts 2016) *Answer 3.19: E*

3.20

According to Jonsen et al.'s (2002) four-topics method of clinical ethical decision-making, which of the following is not one of the four issues that should be carefully considered when working through clinical ethical dilemmas?

    A.   Clinical indications.
    B.   Commitment to improving access to care.
    C.   Patient preferences.
    D.   Quality of life.
    E.   Socioeconomic/external factors.

Clinical indications, patient preferences, socioeconomic/external factors, and quality of life are the four major components described in Jonsen et al.'s (2002) model for ethical decision-making. By carefully assessing the clinical indications of a case, the clinician fulfills his or her responsibility to the medical well-being of the patient. Evaluating and responding to patient preferences expresses respect for persons, helps the clinician better understand the patient, and strengthens the therapeutic alliance. Quality-of-life issues pertain to the physical, mental, and social elements of life satisfaction for each patient. Socioeconomic/external factors involve treatment costs, access to care, family situations, and other circumstantial agents that affect a patient's quality of care. The commitment to improving access to care is a meritorious idea but is not part of the decision-making model outlined by Jonsen and colleagues (2002). (Roberts 2016) *Answer 3.20: B*

3.21

Identify the experiment conducted in the twentieth century that selectively exploited the disadvantaged and/or minority population specified below. Each answer option may be used once, more than once, or not at all.

A. Human radiation experiments.
B. Jewish Chronic Disease Hospital Study.
C. Nazi hypothermia experiments.
D. Tuskegee Syphilis Study.
E. Willowbrook Hepatitis Studies.

___ Educationally and economically disadvantaged African American men
___ Hospitalized elders with advanced Alzheimer's disease
___ Institutionalized young people with developmental disabilities
___ Jewish concentration camp prisoners
___ Navajo people of the southwestern region of North America

It is important for all clinical researchers to be familiar with historical examples of research abuses. These scandals and the public reactions to them have shaped society's ideas about what is ethical and permissible in research with human beings and what is not. Notorious cases of research abuse also drove the creation of important regulations and ethical guidelines for research, including the *Belmont Report*, the *Declaration of Helsinki*, the *Nuremberg Code*, and the U.S. Department of Health and Human Services *Code of Federal Regulations* that govern research. Furthermore, research protocols involving members of some of these groups are now understood to require special safeguards for participants because history has demonstrated that they may be "vulnerable populations" at risk for abuse in the research setting. (Amdur and Bankert 2002; Council for International Organizations of Medical Sciences 2016; Levine et al. 2004) *Answers 3.21: D, B, E, C, A*

3.22

A well-known actor is filming a movie in a small resort community. During the shooting, she falls and breaks her leg. The movie crew rushes her to a nearby hospital emergency department. X-rays indicate fractures of her tibia and fibula that require immediate surgical intervention. While the local orthopedic surgeon is preparing to operate on the actor, a television reporter and video crew arrive at the hospital. With cameras rolling, the reporter asks the nurse in the triage area about the actor. How should the nurse respond?

A. Because the public has the right to know about the health and well-being of public figures, the nurse should inform the reporter that the actor is being prepared for surgery but avoid giving details about the injury that might violate her privacy.

B. To protect the actor's privacy, the nurse should tell the reporter that the actor is not at the facility.

C. The nurse should ask the reporter to turn off the cameras and then provide information about the actor's condition only with the assurance that it is off the record.

D. The nurse should decline to answer any questions and refer media inquiries to the hospital public affairs department.

E. Because of the special nature of this case, the nurse should refer the reporter to the orthopedic surgeon to make the decision about whether and how to inform the press.

This is an example of a VIP (very important person) patient whose public persona may create special challenges in the treatment situation. It can be very tempting for caregivers to show just how much they are "in the know" when dealing with celebrities, politicians, and other public figures. However, VIP patients have the same right to privacy and privilege of confidentiality as other patients. In this scenario, the nurse's obligation is to say nothing about the patient ("neither confirming nor denying"). The nurse should not overtly lie or deceive. The nurse may, to minimize disruptions, refer the media to the hospital public affairs department. (Dewald and Clark 2001; Lo 2020b) *Answer 3.22: D*

3.23

Overlapping roles naturally occur in many settings and may produce conflicts of interest that may adversely affect the decisions of professionals as they seek to fulfill their primary obligations in these roles simultaneously.

Which of the following overlapping roles may cause conflicts of interest?

A. Administrator and clinician.
B. Colleague and clinician.
C. Investigator and clinician.
D. Neighbor and clinician.
E. All of the above.

Overlapping roles can set up ethical problems, including role conflicts and conflicts of interest. These problems and conflicts arise because of the nonalignment of duties and interests that exist within the coexisting roles. Sometimes the nonalignment results in no or very minor effects, but sometimes the consequences can be serious and threaten or distort the judgment of the professional. In such situations, the interests of the patient or participant or student may be overridden by other interests.

Overlapping personal and professional roles are common in small communities, ranging from rural towns to medical schools to religious or cultural groups. Examples of overlapping roles include a rural physician who provides health care to a neighbor and close friend and a psychiatrist in a medical school who is involved in occasional teaching and works in the student mental health clinic.

Other kinds of overlapping roles in professional settings can also be potentially problematic, as in the case of the clinician who provides prescriptions to a colleague without formally evaluating the colleague and establishing a clear therapeutic relationship. Physician investigators who provide care, perform trials, and may derive financial or academic benefit from those activities also represent an overlapping role situation. In this circumstance, there may be pressures that interfere with scientific obligations as well as obligations to patients and participants.

It is very important to note that not all overlapping roles are unethical but, rather, that they introduce ethical risks that should be anticipated and managed appropriately. (American Psychological Association 2003; Roberts 2016) *Answer 3.23: E*

3.24

Match the ethical theory with the most appropriate phrase.

A. Casuistry.
B. Deontological.
C. Utilitarian.
D. Virtue-based.

_____ Emphasizes consequences: "the ends justify the means"
_____ Emphasizes the character of the moral agent
_____ Emphasizes the role of adherence to duty
_____ Emphasizes the particulars of a situation

Utilitarianism refers to an ethical theory supported by the writings of Jeremy Bentham (1748–1832) and John Stuart Mill (1806–1873). Utilitarian philosophy posits that the most ethical actions and rules are those that bring about the greatest good for the most people, that is, those actions that have the greatest utility (Saxena 2019). *Virtue ethics* defines as ethical the actions of virtuous people (Crowden and Gildersleeve 2019). *Deontology* posits that decisions ought to be made based on adherence to moral norms ("doing what is right") (Alexander and Moore 2016). *Casuistry* describes a bottom-up approach to ethical decision-making, in which ethicists focus first on the details of a particular case rather than overarching rules and principles. Casuistry also highlights the importance of ethical reasoning by analogy with similar cases from the past. (Arras 2010) *Answers 3.24: C, D, B, A*

3.25

A 10-year-old Mexican American boy is referred to treatment by a school counselor because of his behavior at school. The parents speak Spanish but do not speak English. The boy is fluent in both languages. The therapist does not speak Spanish and is unfamiliar with Mexican culture.

Under what conditions should the therapist agree to work with the family?

A. The therapist should never work with the family; the linguistic and cultural differences are too great.
B. The therapist can work with the family if she has the boy act as an interpreter for the parents and asks the family to explain cultural differences as the therapy progresses.
C. The therapist can work with the family if she has the boy act as an interpreter for the parents and consults with a colleague who is knowledgeable about Mexican culture.
D. The therapist can work with the family if she employs a competent interpreter to translate for the parents and asks the family to explain cultural differences as the therapy progresses.
E. The therapist can work with the family if she employs a competent interpreter and consults with a colleague who is knowledgeable about Mexican culture.

To whatever extent it is possible, clients should be able to receive services in their preferred language, an approach that helps fulfill the ethical principle of respect for persons. Therapists who lack the linguistic skill necessary for the provision of services have an obligation to refer the client to a mental health professional who is linguistically, culturally, and clinically competent to work with the client. The second alternative is to employ a professional interpreter who is culturally sensitive to the client's values and beliefs. Hospitals that receive U.S. federal funding are required to have translators available for patients with limited proficiency in English. When translators are not available in person, telephone-based translation services can be used. Family members and friends cannot be used in this role because this practice encroaches on (or may violate) the boundaries and safeguards necessary for a trusting therapeutic relationship.

In the context of therapy, at no time should a child be expected to interpret for the parents. This disrupts the roles and hierarchies of the family system because the child is given disproportionate power and the adults' parenting functions are compromised. This places the child in a conflictive position; the child is expected to honestly interpret for the parents and therapist and to protect his or her personal interests and role in the family. If a child is being emotionally or physically abused by the parent or someone the parent trusts, the child is placed in an untenable and nontherapeutic position if he is asked to interpret for the parents. (American Psychological Association 1990, 2003; Chu et al. 2016) *Answer 3.25: E*

3.26

A psychiatrist is treating an adolescent patient for bipolar disorder. During a meeting with the patient's father, the father states that he too has been diagnosed with bipolar disorder but has just stopped his medications because he is uninsured and cannot afford them. The psychiatrist feels strongly that the father's stability would greatly contribute to the son's well-being, so she writes a prescription in the son's name for the father's medication. The father's medications will therefore be paid for by the son's insurance. Several years later, the patient makes an ethics complaint to the American Psychiatric Association charging the psychiatrist with "unprofessional behavior." The American Psychiatric Association district branch ethics committee concludes that there are numerous ethical problems with the psychiatrist's actions. Which of the following is *not* identified as an important ethical breach?

A.   The psychiatrist prescribed for the father although she had no established treatment relationship with him.

B. The psychiatrist's action may have raised questions in the patient's mind about the psychiatrist's trustworthiness, harming the therapeutic alliance.

C. The son's records stated that he is on medications he is not receiving, creating the possibility for maleficence.

D. Because the psychiatrist's action was essentially stealing from the insurance company—a fraudulent activity—the patient's continued insurance coverage was put at risk.

E. The psychiatrist did not obtain the son's consent to write the prescription.

Although the psychiatrist's intentions may have been good (supporting the son by supporting the father), her action was unethical largely because it violated the fidelity of the psychiatrist's treatment relationship with the son. The ethical principle of fidelity requires that physicians remain faithful to the therapeutic relationship with their patients and to the goals of patient care. Writing a prescription for another person in the patient's name was a dishonest act, and asking for the son's consent would compound the problem by making the son complicit in the act. The remaining choices (A–D) all describe significant ethical concerns raised by the psychiatrist's action, which could have resulted in harm. For example, should the son present in an emergency room with an overdose, records would state that the patient is on medications he is not taking, potentially leading to misinformed, harmful treatment. The psychiatrist could have handled the situation appropriately by referring the father to a charity or low-fee clinic. This would establish a treatment relationship in which options for low-cost medication could be pursued, such as through pharmaceutical company indigent programs. Although this case is somewhat unusual, inappropriate prescribing is not uncommon. In one study, 11% of physicians disciplined by a state medical board were disciplined for inappropriate prescribing practices (Morrison and Wickersham 1998). (American Psychiatric Association 2001a) *Answer 3.26: E*

3.27

A Scottish physician ethicist wrote the first modern medical ethics text in the English language. His approach to medical ethics was based in part on defining professional virtues and on the concept of sympathy developed by David Hume (1711–1776).

Which of the following individuals is this Scottish physician ethicist?

A. Benjamin Rush.
B. John Gregory.
C. Thomas Percival.
D. Tom Beauchamp.
E. H. Tristram Engelhardt Jr.

John Gregory's (1724–1773) writings on medical ethics were brought to North America by his students, including Benjamin Rush (1746–1813), and were translated into French, German, Spanish, and Italian. He introduced into modern medical ethics the virtues-based concept of the physician as moral fiduciary of the patient. Thomas Percival (1740–1804), also influenced by Gregory, wrote *Medical Ethics* in 1803, from which the American Medical Association code of ethics of 1847 was largely adopted. Tom Beauchamp and H. Tristram Engelhardt Jr. are contemporary medical ethicists. (Coverdale et al. 2011) *Answer 3.27: B*

3.28

For each of the following scenarios, choose the most appropriate medicolegal term. Each answer option may be used once, more than once, or not at all.

A. Durable power of attorney for health care.
B. Living will.
C. Power of attorney.
D. Psychiatric advance directive.
E. Testamentary will.

_____ A patient with bipolar disorder, who is currently stable but has had many manic episodes, documents her preferences for medications and hospitalization in the event she becomes psychotic.

_____ A young mother diagnosed with metastatic breast cancer wishes to name her husband as her health care proxy in case she is too ill to make medical decisions.

A number of legal documents enable individuals to state their wishes and help ensure that these preferences will be honored. A patient with mental illness completes the psychiatric advance directive when he or she is stable and possesses decisional capacity. The psychiatric advance directive may cover preferred hospitalizations, treatments, or persons to make decisions should the patient become ill and unable to make his or her own decisions. Although the legal status of such psychiatric advance directives varies according to jurisdiction, psychiatric advance directives have been shown to improve doctor-patient relationships and to enhance autonomy. The Patient Self-Determination Act of 1990 requires hospitals to inquire on admission if patients have or wish to complete advance directives. All 50 states have provisions honoring advance directives.

A living will enables patients while decisionally capable to specify their treatment preferences should they lose capacity. Besides setting out treatment preferences, a durable power of attorney for health care also appoints a surrogate decision-maker to make decisions for the patient when he or she is not able to do so. A power of attorney appoints an agent to make financial and other types of decisions other than medical ones for an incapacitated person. A testamentary will indicates the disposition of assets and possessions after the death of the person making the will. (Gutheil and Appelbaum 2019; Edelstein et al. 2019; Simon 1992) *Answers 3.28: D, A*

3.29

A severely depressed patient who fails to improve on a serotonergic antidepressant medication is hospitalized. The psychiatrist stops the medication and promptly commences treatment with a monoamine oxidase inhibitor antidepressant medication, without remembering that doing so is contraindicated. The patient develops serotonin syndrome. On recovery, the patient asks his physician why he became so ill.

What is the psychiatrist's most appropriate response?

A.   Do not admit to the error, because such a disclosure would unnecessarily worry the patient about other aspects of care.

B.   Do not admit to the error, because doing so is a form of self-disclosure that may lead to other boundary violations.

C.   Do not admit to the error, because doing so may create legal liability for the hospital and the nurses as well as for the physician.

D.   Explicitly acknowledge and explain the error and its consequences.

E.   Tell the patient that he had an adverse reaction to the medication and express general regret about what happened.

Although it can be extremely difficult for physicians to admit to making mistakes, disclosing errors to patients conveys respect for the patients and maintains public trust. When surveyed, almost all patients report that they would want even minor errors disclosed to them. Patients also report that they would more likely sue if the physician had not informed them of an error than if the physician voluntarily admitted the error immediately after committing it. Disclosure also allows the patient to be fully informed about the need for clinical monitoring, tests, or treatment to mitigate the harms the error caused. Finally, the practice of nondisclosure of errors damages the credibility of the profession as a whole because the public may come to believe that physicians are more concerned with protecting themselves than fulfilling their ethical responsibility of veracity, or truth telling. In this case, the physician clearly made an error and the patient suffered a serious harm. Under these circumstances, the physician's responsibility to the patient should prevail over any self-interest in concealing the error—even if that self-interest is masked by rationalization that disclosure will harm the patient or third parties. (Hérbert et al. 2001; Institute of Medicine 2006; Lo 2020b) *Answer 3.29: D*

3.30

A young man who has been living out of state for the past several years returns to the small town where he grew up. He presents to a local clinic asking for a refill on a prescription medication to treat what he describes as "irritable bowels." When the clinic doctor mentions that the particular medication is typically used to treat diarrhea associated with HIV infection, the patient denies being HIV positive.

Which of the following options would be the clinic physician's best next step?

A. Agree to provide the prescription if the patient allows the doctor to contact the patient's previous physician to obtain medical records.
B. Agree to provide the prescription and surreptitiously contact the patient's previous physician to obtain medical records.
C. Show the patient written information about the drug and insist that he tell the truth about his medical history if he wants to receive a prescription.
D. Prescribe the medication without pursuing the matter further.
E. Refuse to treat this patient because of the potential malpractice liability.

In this situation, the physician needs accurate information about the patient's history to make appropriate recommendations and interventions. It is possible that the medication has been prescribed for an off-label indication, but it is also possible that the patient is HIV positive and is reluctant to disclose that fact to a clinician in the town where he grew up. The ethical principles of beneficence and respect for patient autonomy require that the physician obtain prior records so that he can provide appropriate care for this patient and that the physician obtain the patient's consent for the requested information. Of the options provided, option A presents the most expeditious way to obtain needed clinical information while respecting patient autonomy. (American Psychiatric Association 2001a; Beauchamp and Childress 2001) *Answer 3.30: A*

3.31

A recent immigrant elder with depression presents for treatment at a community mental health center. He is monolingual and does not speak English. The psychiatrist on duty speaks English but does not speak the native language of the patient.

Which of the following individuals is the best interpreter in this situation?

- A. A bilingual radiation technician.
- B. A bilingual patient who is in the waiting room and is known to the psychiatrist.
- C. A bilingual daughter of the patient.
- D. A sister of the patient who is fluent in the patient's native language and has some ability in English, but is not fluent.
- E. An administrative staff member who is fluent in English and has some ability in the patient's native language, but is not fluent.

In this difficult situation the bilingual radiation technician is the best interpreter. The technician has been trained in patient privacy and understands that there are clinical reasons behind the questions the psychiatrist might ask the patient. It is best if the translator is physically present; the psychiatrist will be able to get a sense of the patient's nonverbal behavior while being confident that the verbal translation is accurate. The next best interpreter in this situation is the administrative staff member. Despite the staff member's limited facility in the native language and his or her nonclinical background, the patient may be better able to disclose concerns or symptoms that he would be embarrassed to disclose in front of family members who might serve as interpreters. It is possible that the family members who could serve as interpreters in this scenario (i.e., a daughter or sister) may be contributing to the distress of the patient in some manner. This boundary concern precludes their being invited into the interpreter role, although they may provide collateral information about the patient and his life circumstances and health situation. Asking another patient to interpret is not appropriate under all but the most exceptional circumstances because it undermines the focused therapeutic relationship with the translator-patient. (Tseng and Streltzer 2004) *Answer 3.31: A*

3.32

"What I may see or hear in the course of the treatment or even outside of the treatment in regard to the life of men, which on no account one must spread abroad, I will keep to myself, holding such things shameful to be spoken about." This statement about physicians' duty of confidentiality is attributed to which of the following individuals?

     A.   Aristotle.
     B.   Galen.
     C.   Hippocrates.
     D.   Plato.
     E.   Pythagoras.

The quote is from the Oath of Hippocrates. Although it was not likely written by Hippocrates himself, most historians believe it emerged from the Hippocratic School around the fifth century B.C. The injunction to physicians to respect confidentiality is thus one of the oldest and most consistent of all ethical principles in medicine. Galen was a famous Roman physician, Pythagoras was a Greek philosopher who probably influenced the Hippocratic ethics, and Aristotle and Plato were also Greek philosophers. (Edelstein 1967) *Answer 3.32: C*

3.33

A Vietnam veteran with active symptoms of posttraumatic stress disorder threatens to shoot his supervisor at work with his hunting rifle because the supervisor has changed his job duties. The veteran is involuntarily committed to a psychiatric facility by his psychiatrist. Which of the following court cases is most relevant to the psychiatrist's action?

A. *Addington v. Texas* (1979).
B. *Cruzan v. Director, Missouri Department of Public Health* (1990).
C. *Lake v. Cameron* (1966).
D. *O'Connor v. Donaldson* (1975).
E. *Tarasoff v. Regents of the University of California* (1976).

This scenario describes a situation to which the *Tarasoff* guidelines would apply. The *Tarasoff* rulings indicate that psychiatrists must act to protect identifiable potential victims of reasonably predictable violence (*Tarasoff v. Regents of the University of California* 1976). In this case, a patient with a weapon has threatened an identified victim and has a disorder that increases the risk of carrying out the threat. To treat or hospitalize this patient would likely comply with *Tarasoff* guidelines. If the threat persisted, notifying the potential victim and law enforcement would be appropriate. Certain states interpret the *Tarasoff* requirements as both a duty to warn and to protect, so clinicians must be aware of the requirements of their jurisdiction.

The other court cases are relevant to other aspects of clinical care. *O'Connor v. Donaldson* (1975) established that the state could not confine a nondangerous individual who is able to survive outside the hospital with the help of loved ones or the community. *Addington v. Texas* (1979) established that the burden of proof for civil commitment is "clear and convincing evidence," a more stringent standard of proof than preponderance of the evidence required to prevail in civil cases but a less stringent standard of proof than beyond a reasonable doubt required for criminal conviction. *Cruzan v. Director, Missouri Department of Public Health* (1990) refers to end-of-life decision-making, including the withdrawal of a feeding tube from a patient in a persistent vegetative state. *Lake v. Cameron* (1966) pertains to the least restrictive alternative for treatment. (Stern et al. 2018) *Answer 3.33: E*

3.34

In the former Soviet Union, individuals who held beliefs contrary to those advanced by the official government were routinely institutionalized for mental illness. Curtailing the freedom of these individuals is widely recognized as a violation of fundamental human rights.

Which of the following ethical principles is most relevant to this issue?

A. Beneficence.
B. Confidentiality.
C. Fidelity.
D. Respect for persons.
E. Veracity.

In many oppressive political regimes throughout history and presently throughout the world, individuals have been institutionalized for mental illness because they have held views or have engaged in behaviors that are different from local, regional, or broader societal expectations. This stance is seen as a violation of the ethical principle of respect for persons, the core ideal that serves as the foundation of the profession of psychiatry. A diagnosis of mental illness involves multiple elements, including a significant behavioral or psychological pattern in a person associated with distress, disability, and heightened risk of suffering, death, or loss of freedom. A mental illness is not merely an expectable, culturally sanctioned response to a particular event nor is it a behavioral difference or conflict, unless this element is symptomatic of dysfunction (i.e., impairment in social, occupational, or other important areas of functioning). (Bloch and Reddaway 2019; Post 2004) *Answer 3.34: D*

3.35

For each of the following scenarios, identify the principal ethics method used to minimize potential role conflicts and conflicts of interest. Each answer option may be used once, more than once, or not at all.

A. Defined limits of interests that may be involved in a role conflict.
B. Open disclosure of potential role conflicts and conflicts of interest.
C. Separation of roles, including withdrawal from certain decisions or activities.
D. Strict oversight of potential role conflicts and conflicts of interest.

_____ A psychiatric researcher who serves as an institutional review board (IRB) member is asked to leave the room when a departmental colleague's work is discussed by the IRB committee.

_____ An academic psychiatrist is required to document his sources of income and research funding when submitting an empirical manuscript.

_____ A $5,000 cap is placed on the amount of money that an individual faculty member may invest personally in a work project.

_____ A psychiatrist is required to acknowledge his participation in a speakers' bureau supported by a pharmaceutical company prior to giving a psychopharmacology presentation.

_____ A neutral committee is appointed by the dean of a medical school to review the involvement of specific faculty members in a new academic-private entrepreneurial partnership on an ongoing basis.

_____ A medical school adopts the policy that academic faculty who are involved in key teaching roles cannot provide direct health care to medical students.

Professionals often serve in a variety of roles, and the interests and responsibilities associated with these roles may come into conflict. There are a number of methods for minimizing these conflicts. Public disclosure of potential role conflicts and conflicts of interest is a method that relies most clearly on the principles of truth telling and honesty. This is common practice in the publication of manuscripts or the presentation of clinical or scientific material. A more rigorous approach involves very clear role separation, including withdrawal from certain decisions or activities. This approach emphasizes the clear demarcation of professional boundaries and ensures that there is no ambiguity in the responsibilities carried by a professional in a particular role. In recent years, active management and strict oversight of potential overlapping roles and conflicts of interest are methods that have been adopted in many institutions. In some settings, there may be policies and procedures that circumscribe the extent to which an individual may have interests at stake in a particular role, for example, limiting the investments of a faculty member. (Field and Lo 2009; Roberts 2016; Warner and Roberts 2004) *Answers 3.35: C, B, A, B, D, C*

3.36

Which of the following is the best description of self-regulation in the profession of medicine?

A. Abiding by an approved code of ethics.
B. Ensuring competence and character of self and other practitioners.
C. Mastering a specialized body of knowledge and skill.
D. Passing a certifying examination.
E. Pursuing lifelong learning.

Society grants physicians the ability to self-regulate, that is, to determine who meets the qualifications to be admitted to the profession and to sanction those members who do not live up to the standards of the profession either through incompetence or unethical behavior. Option B is the most inclusive description of self-regulation, but all of the options listed reflect an aspect of medicine as a profession. The members of professions such as law, clergy, or medicine have mastered a specialized body of knowledge and skills that must be sustained through ongoing learning. Intrinsic to this special expertise is substantial power, which must be used in the best interests of patients and society. The exercise of this power is governed by a code of ethics. (American Medical Association, Council on Ethical and Judicial Affairs 2005; Roberts 2016; Snyder Sulmasy et al. 2019) *Answer 3.36: B*

3.37

For each of the following scenarios, identify the most appropriate organizational entity responsible for consultation and oversight. Each answer option may be used once, more than once, or not at all.

    A.   Data and safety monitoring board.
    B.   Department chair.
    C.   Hospital ethics committee.
    D.   Institutional review board.
    E.   State medical board.

    _____   A psychology intern serves as a research assistant for a federally funded grant. The intern is concerned that the principal investigator is not obtaining informed consent for study participation in the manner outlined in the protocol.

    _____   A social worker serves on the oncology service providing care for a patient who has been diagnosed with terminal lung cancer. The patient does not wish to have "anything scary or painful" done that will prolong his life. After multiple discussions with the social worker and the patient, the attending physician refuses to write a "do not resuscitate" order, saying that it is "premature" and against the physician's personal religious beliefs.

The abilities to identify ethical dilemmas and to seek appropriate consultation represent key skills for all mental health trainees. A number of institutional, professional, and government organizations are in place to review, mediate, resolve, and oversee ethical problems in health care and research. An IRB would be the appropriate organization to investigate the situation described in the first vignette in which the principal investigator is not adhering to protocol procedures to safeguard participants. IRBs exist in any facility or system where research using government funds is conducted and in many private sector organizations.

The hospital ethics committee would be the proper venue to take the dilemma presented in the second vignette. The Joint Commission (formerly Joint Commission on Accreditation of Healthcare Organizations) requires that each health care facility have an ethics committee or ethics consultation service available to clarify and address ethically important conflicts arising in patient care. (American Hospital Association 1990; Hester 2001; Lo 2003; Snyder Sulmasy et al. 2019) *Answers 3.37: D, C*

3.38

A 9-year-old boy is brought to treatment by his parents because of his oppositional behavior. The father reports using corporal punishment as a means of disciplining his son. The therapist tells the father that corporal punishment has not proven to be an effective form of discipline. The father informs the therapist that corporal punishment is part of the tradition of disciplining children among the family's ethnic group.

What best describes the therapist's ethical obligation(s)?

A. Accept the father's cultural explanation and ask him to further educate the therapist about the ethnic minority group's traditions and cultural practices.

B. Accept the father's cultural explanation and set it aside as no longer a clinical issue.

C. Consult with a colleague who is knowledgeable about the specific ethnic minority group's traditions to increase the therapist's sensitivity and competence, and inform the parents about their state's definition of child abuse and the therapist's role as a mandatory reporter.

D. Consult with a colleague who is knowledgeable about the specific ethnic minority group's traditions to increase the therapist's sensitivity and competence and use this as a guide for treatment.

E. File a report to the local children's protective services agency because spanking and other forms of corporal punishment always constitute child abuse.

Clinicians have a responsibility to be sensitive to and knowledgeable about the cultural and ethnic differences that exist among their client populations. More specifically, clinicians are expected to recognize and appreciate the perspectives of culturally different clients and how these perspectives inform their values, psychological processes, and behaviors. Providers must recognize the limitations of their cultural competence and use consultations and educational experiences to expand their competence.

Concurrently, clinicians in the United States are legally mandated to report child abuse to the appropriate state agency. This obligation transcends the cultural differences that may exist between the client and therapist. However, the provider is expected to educate the client and family about their state's definition of child abuse and the provider's duty to report child abuse. Providers are encouraged to not allow their personal prejudices to dictate their perceptions and clinical judgment. There is a dual responsibility to be sensitive to cultural differences and to protect children from harm. (American Psychological Association 1990, 2003)
Answer 3.38: C

3.39

A 43-year-old father of three is taken to a psychiatric hospital by local authorities. The man had left his home in the middle of the night and was found wandering in the snow dressed only in pajamas. In the emergency department, the man appeared delusional, often remarking that "they" were going to incarcerate him forever, preventing him from seeing his family again. He told the attending psychiatrist that during his brief wandering he contemplated ending his life but that God told him to return to his family because they needed him. About 10 minutes into his evaluation, the man demanded to be discharged so that he "could be the father his family wanted him to be."

Which of the following issues is at stake in the clinical assessment of this patient?

A. Advanced directives.
B. Decisional capacity.
C. Justice.
D. Scope of practice.
E. Veracity.

Although several of these issues may arise throughout the course of treatment, B is the best answer choice in this situation. Decisional capacity is an assessment based on a specific individual's symptoms, prior experiences, personal values, and other features. It encompasses four main abilities: expression and communication, comprehending relevant information, reasoning and rationalization, and understanding consequences. It is important to note that competency is a legal determination of decision-making capacity that is made by a court—it is not a clinical assessment. Veracity is the ethical virtue of truth telling. Advanced directives are documents specifying medical decisions and preferences for an individual's future health care. Justice is a bioethical principle focusing on nondiscrimination and the equitable distribution of benefits and burdens in society. Scope of practice is a medical term used to identify the set of clinical activities for which the health care professional can provide an appropriate standard of care. (Roberts 2016) *Answer 3.39: B*

3.40

Professionalism in medicine requires that the interests of patients are placed before the personal self-interest of the health care provider. Professionalism thus involves addressing and resolving to whatever extent possible any potential, perceived, and actual conflicts of interest. Techniques for managing conflicts of interest include which of the following?

A. Disclosure to relevant "stakeholders," for example, patients, colleagues, employers.
B. Oversight by a committee charged with evaluating and resolving conflicts.
C. Recusal or withdrawal from certain roles or decision processes related to roles.
D. Separation of roles that produce potential conflicts of interest.
E. All of the above.

All of the techniques listed may be employed in managing conflicts of interest, which may produce pressures that distort decision-making and the ability to fulfill all of one's professional obligations inherent to each of the roles. Depending on the seriousness of the issues at stake, all of these techniques may be employed and, indeed, necessary for sufficient management of conflicts. Historically, disclosure—often with firm financial benchmarks—has been the principal method for managing conflicts. Disclosure alone has increasingly been recognized as insufficient to prevent consequential conflicts of interest. For this reason, role separation, oversight, guidelines, and recusal/role withdrawal are gaining in their importance in managing conflicts of interest in many circumstances. (Field and Lo 2009; Roberts 2016) *Answer 3.40: E*

3.41

A 4-year-old child is found to have a glioblastoma in the posterior aspect of his brain. The child's family practices the Christian Scientist faith. On the basis of their religious beliefs, the parents decline the medical team's recommendation for chemotherapy for the child.

What are the most significant opposing ethics principles that the medical team must balance in this case?

   A.   Respect for autonomy versus altruism.
   B.   Respect for autonomy versus beneficence.
   C.   Respect for autonomy versus confidentiality.
   D.   Respect for autonomy versus self-effacement.
   E.   Respect for autonomy versus veracity.

The primary conflict for the clinicians in this case is respect for autonomy (i.e., respect for the parents' right to make their own decisions about the welfare of their family) versus beneficence (i.e., the physicians' duty to do good by treating the child's tumor). Altruism and self-effacement both involve placing personal interests aside to serve the best interests of others; these are not the central conflicts of this scenario. Similarly, confidentiality (protection of the personal information of patients, to the limits of the law), and truth telling (veracity) are not the central challenges in this case. (Beauchamp and Childress 2001; Roberts 2016) *Answer 3.41: B*

3.42

A hospital ethics committee was asked to comment on a clinical case that presented an ethical dilemma. Committee members discussed similar clinical cases they had encountered, called other hospitals in the region to see how they had handled such situations, searched the medical and legal literature for other examples, and interviewed the patient and family members before making their recommendations.

Which model of ethical decision-making is best described in the example above?

A.   Care-based model.
B.   Patient-centered model.
C.   Principle-based model.
D.   Rule-based model.
E.   Value-based model.

There is more than one valid method for ethics committees to evaluate the cases that come before them and arrive at a consensus about the best course of action. It is often useful for committee members to be explicit and intentional about their methods. In this case, the committee's review of similar cases and discussions with the patient and family could be considered a patient-centered approach. Making a decision based on the committee's own values would be value based. A decision based on an analysis of the specific ethical principles involved would be principle based. Basing the decision on *a priori* rules could be described as a deontological approach. Care-based ethical decision-making would emphasize relationships among key participants and focus on providing care. (DeGrazia and Beauchamp 2001) *Answer 3.42: B*

3.43

The leader of a national society of psychiatrists advocates for people living with mental disorders characterized by cognitive decline and intermittent psychotic symptoms to receive the COVID-19 vaccine ahead of non-ill, age-matched individuals in the general population. The psychiatrist leader, in making her argument, states that "individuals with cognitive decline and intermittent psychotic symptoms are more likely than healthy individuals to be economically disadvantaged and to encounter greater barriers to health care."

The reasoning offered by the psychiatrist leader is primarily based on which ethical principle?

A.   Autonomy.
B.   Beneficence.
C.   Confidentiality.
D.   Nonmaleficence.
E.   Justice.

Although the psychiatrist leader's argument involves the ethical principles of beneficence (doing good) and nonmaleficence (doing no

harm), the argument is primarily based on the ethical principle of justice, or fairness. Vaccine distribution during a pandemic involves the principle of *distributive justice*, which refers to the fair distribution of resources and burdens through society. (Williams and Dawson 2020)
Answer 3.43: E

CHAPTER 4

ETHICS AND PROFESSIONALISM IN CLINICAL CARE

4.1

A 17-year-old male college freshman presents to a psychiatrist in private practice, complaining of a 2-week history of anxiety attacks. After asking her for an assurance of confidentiality, the patient explains that his anxiety is the result of being recently beaten by college fraternity members during a secret initiation ritual. Although the patient is terrified that he will be beaten again, he believes that he will suffer a worse fate if he tries to quit the fraternity. He asks for medication to control his fear until the initiation period is over in 1 week. The psychiatrist asks for details of the assault and is convinced that it posed a significant risk of permanent physical injury or death. The psychiatrist urges the patient to inform the authorities of the assault, but he adamantly refuses and reminds the psychiatrist of her pledge of confidentiality.

What is the best course of action for the psychiatrist to take?

- A. Do not inform the authorities and attempt to forge a therapeutic alliance by providing antianxiety medication.
- B. Do not inform the authorities but refuse to facilitate the abusive situation by providing antianxiety medication.
- C. Inform the patient that she is obligated to report the assault and do so immediately.
- D. Inform the patient that she is obligated to report the assault but will wait several days to give him time to tell the authorities himself.
- E. Inform the patient that she will keep his confidence but later anonymously report her patient's physical abuse to the authorities.

Doctor-patient confidentiality is one of the most important ethical aspects of clinical care, and it holds a special place in psychiatry, in which patients share the most intimate aspects of their lives. This said, confidentiality is a privilege (not a right, per se) that has certain limitations within the tradition of clinical care and mandated by law. A psychiatrist can never in advance and under all circumstances guarantee the absolute privacy of a patient's personal material. For instance, when a dependent elder or a child may be experiencing significant neglect or any form of abuse, or when a seriously ill and violent individual threatens to kill a named individual, the clinician must report the risky or dangerous situation to appropriate authorities. Physicians are justified in not maintaining the privilege of confidentiality when doing so is necessary to ensure the patient's safety or that of others. In this case, the psychiatrist has a duty to report her concerns to prevent further physical injury to her patient as well as to others who may be pledging the same fraternity. Because this patient is only 17 years of age, the psychiatrist may also be mandated by state law to report the assault as an instance of child abuse.

In some situations, the therapeutic relationship may be preserved if the psychiatrist can convince the patient to step forward himself. However, waiting several days for the patient to change his mind is unwise when the abuse is ongoing and probably involves other victims. Recklessly or unthinkingly breaching confidentiality violates the principle of truth telling, can undermine the therapeutic relationship, and can erode the image of psychiatrists generally as worthy of trust. Most dilemmas of this sort may be prevented by informing patients in advance that clinical information will be kept confidential unless doing so could result in harm. (American Psychiatric Association 2010; Group for the Advancement of Psychiatry 1990; Roberts 2002a) *Answer 4.1: C*

4.2

Involuntary treatment for a suicidal individual at risk for immediate harm is permitted in most states based on which of the following principles?

    A.   Autonomy.
    B.   Confidentiality.
    C.   Fidelity.
    D.   Nonmaleficence.
    E.   Veracity.

Involuntary treatment is a clear example of conflicting ethical principles: the obligation to respect patient autonomy and the obligation of nonmaleficence (do no harm). Choosing not to override a patient's treatment refusal is an expression of respect for patient autonomy, but blind adherence to a patient's wishes about treatment may not be ethically justifiable and may cause harm. Two principles are used to justify the legality of involuntary treatment. *Parens patriae*, literally the "father of the people," is the ideal that mental, medical, and legal professionals act out of compassion to commit patients against their will to protect their well-being. Underlying this theory is an assumption that severely psychotic, addicted, or suicidal patients are often not truly decisionally capable and that involuntarily hospitalizing such patients enables their autonomy to be restored. Police power is a legal warrant that states that immediate, foreseeable, and preventable danger to self or others justifies curtailing the liberty of patients. (Appelbaum and Gutheil 2020; Byatt et al. 2007; Menninger 2001) *Answer 4.2: D*

4.3

A 45-year-old married father of four children is brought to the emergency department of a university hospital with internal bleeding from injuries sustained in a motor vehicle crash. The patient has been stabilized but will require a blood transfusion to replace blood lost and prepare for exploratory surgery. When approached to consent for the transfusion, the patient refuses, stating that it is forbidden by his religion. The attending physician calls for a psychiatric consult. The psychiatry fellow on call proceeds to the emergency room.

Which of the following is the most appropriate first step in evaluating this patient?

A. Assess the patient's decisional capacity to refuse the transfusion.
B. Call the patient's wife to find out if she agrees with his decision to refuse the transfusion.
C. Obtain a complete psychiatric history, using collateral sources as needed.
D. Order the transfusion against the patient's wishes.
E. Talk to the patient about blood substitutes and ask him if he would consider accepting one.

The first step in approaching this case should be to assess the patient's decision-making capacity, because without this clinical information, no determinations about the appropriate course of action can be made. Depending on the results of the bedside capacity evaluation, it may be suitable to call the patient's wife so that she might act as a surrogate, to obtain further psychiatric history, or to explore other treatment options. Ordering the transfusion against the patient's wishes not only would be a violation of clinical protocol but also would go against legal and ethical precedent to respect the autonomy of patients and to consult with surrogates except in a true emergency. Although the medical situation is urgent, it does not require such a drastic action. (Gutheil and Appelbaum 2019; Roberts 2016) *Answer 4.3: A*

4.4

Match the following statements with the most appropriate term.

    A.   Physician orders for life-sustaining treatment (POLST).
    B.   Do-not-resuscitate/do-not-intubate (DNR/DNI) orders.
    C.   Living will.

    _____ A written document that provides guidance regarding the health care wishes of a decisionally capable individual
    _____ A medical order entered into a patient's health record
    _____ A standardized one-page form that provides information to responders regarding interventions in urgent situations when the patient cannot provide consent and there is no time to reach a usual provider or decision-maker

A living will is a document written by a decisionally capable individual that specifies the health care wishes of the individual should he or she become unable to make decisions for himself or herself due to illness or incapacity. DNR/DNI orders are entered into a patient's health record and are followed only if the patient lacks decisional capacity to give the order in real time (Braun 2017). POLST is a pragmatic, one-page standardized form that specifies a patient's preferences regarding emergency treatments and end-of-life care and defines how a physician should respond in urgent situations in which a patient cannot provide consent and there is no time to reach a usual provider or decision-maker. In a POLST, the patient's preferences are recorded as medical orders. A physician (or, depending on the state, a nurse practitioner or other independently licensed practitioner) must sign the POLST form. (Hickman et al. 2009) *Answers 4.4: C, B, A*

4.5

A woman who was recently raped seeks help from a therapist who specializes in posttraumatic stress disorder treatment. The patient says she has read about eye movement desensitization and reprocessing (EMDR) and asks the therapist to use this specific intervention. The therapist is not trained to use EMDR and is skeptical about its efficacy.

What is the therapist's most ethical course of action?

A. Inform the patient that the therapist is not trained to use EMDR and offer a referral.

B. Inform the patient that the therapist is not trained to use EMDR and that it is a controversial treatment. Offer to refer the patient or to treat her using another therapy.

C. Inform the patient that the therapist is not trained to use EMDR, discuss its weaknesses, and dissuade her from pursuing it.

D. Learn as much as possible about EMDR and initiate treatment.

E. To encourage a therapeutic alliance, agree to treat the patient with any modality she believes may be helpful.

When considering the use of a new or controversial treatment, the need for collaboration in the patient-physician relationship becomes particularly important. In such circumstances, it is important for patient care to be guided by sound theoretical reasoning, the best available research, and mainstream clinical experience. The clinical use of novel or nonstandard interventions should be grounded in a robust informed consent process, shared decision-making, and the patient's clear understanding of the alternatives, risks, and benefits of treatment. In this case, the best option is the one that provides the patient with the most options and the most information—including information about controversy surrounding the patient's preferred treatment. (American Psychiatric Association 2010) *Answer 4.5: B*

4.6

A 26-year-old woman with major depression is hospitalized because she is suicidal. Three days after admission, her psychiatrist documents in the progress notes that the woman, although still depressed, is no longer suicidal. The insurance reviewer notifies the psychiatrist that the patient will need to be discharged to outpatient treatment. The woman has little support outside the hospital, and the psychiatrist does not feel that she is stable enough for discharge. The patient is struggling financially and cannot afford to pay out of pocket for continued hospitalization.

Which of the following is the most ethical course of action?

A. Discharge the patient as requested by the insurance reviewer and arrange for outpatient follow-up.

B. Continue the hospitalization even though the patient may have to pay the bill.

C. To gain insurance coverage for more hospital days, document in the medical record that the patient is again suicidal.

D. Suggest that the patient call her insurance company and tell them that she may hurt herself if she doesn't have coverage for more hospital days.

E. Phone the insurance reviewer to explain the need for continued hospitalization without implying that the patient is suicidal.

Psychiatrists who would never consider lying for their own benefit may nonetheless be tempted to do so on behalf of their patients. Surveys indicate that a substantial minority of physicians will alter or even falsify a diagnosis, prognosis, or recommended treatment to obtain a procedure or medication they feel is necessary or important to a patient. Such deception is most common regarding reporting to insurance companies. Physicians may rationalize lying to insurers or managed care companies because they feel that the companies are motivated only by profits, are medically uninformed, or force physicians to practice substandard medicine.

Even if these are legitimate concerns, they do not justify falsification of records. Documenting that a patient is suicidal when she is not is a failure to honor the ethical duty of veracity, or truth telling, which requires the positive obligation to convey information and impressions accurately as well as the negative obligation not to mislead or deceive through omissions or alterations of the truth. Deceiving insurance companies may create some short-term benefit for patients (and save physicians time by avoiding the need to make appeals), but it may also have far-reaching deleterious consequences, including the loss of the clinician's credibility, criminal charges of fraud against the clinician or the facility where he or she works, sanctions against the physician by the state medical board, or cancellation of the patient's insurance coverage. Although it may seem that a patient would be grateful for the physician's attempts to game the system on his or her behalf and that the therapeutic relationship would thereby be strengthened, it may be more likely that a patient would question the doctor's integrity and begin to mistrust his or her other decisions.

In this case, suggesting that the patient directly request further hospitalization unfairly burdens her with the physician's responsibility; encouraging her to overdramatize her symptoms is blatantly unethical. Making an appeal to the insurance company for further consideration of the patient's clinical needs and circumstances is the optimal course of action. If the request is denied, as it may well be, the physician and patient should work together to create the best treatment plan possible given the limitations. (Roberts 2016; Werner et al. 2004) *Answer 4.6: E*

4.7

Standards for involuntary commitment of individuals with mental disorders typically include which of the following?

    A.   Dangerousness toward self or others.
    B.   Definite or provisional diagnosis of mental disorder directly linked to need for intervention.
    C.   Inability to provide adequate self-care.
    D.   Proposed intervention is less restrictive than other alternatives.
    E.   All of the above.

In addition to evidence of dangerousness toward self or others, standards for involuntary commitment of individuals with mental disorders typically include a rationale based in the diagnosis of a mental disorder, evidence of a patient's inability to provide adequate self-care, and a determination that involuntary commitment would be less restrictive than other alternatives. (Testa and West 2010) *Answer 4.7: E*

4.8

A psychiatrist searches public postings on the internet to learn more about a new patient prior to their first appointment. The psychiatrist is intrigued by what is revealed by the search, and before he knows it, he has spent nearly an hour on the search, finding more and more interesting tidbits.

Which of the following descriptions best describes a professional risk in this situation?

    A.   No professional risk because the psychiatrist is being thorough in preparing for a new patient visit.

B.   No professional risk because the psychiatrist is engaged in a usual and accepted clinical practice.

C.   Some professional risk because the patient did not provide consent for the search.

D.   Some professional risk because the psychiatrist is serving his own gratification rather than the patient's needs.

E.   Serious professional risk because the psychiatrist meets the definition of "stalking" the patient.

Although googling a patient is not, in itself, unethical, the psychiatrist's motivations are ethically problematic. Clinicians must be critical of their reasons for conducting an internet search: Is the search in the best interest of the patient? Why is the clinician not seeking information from the patient directly? Conducting an internet search to gratify personal curiosity or voyeurism represents a professional risk. (Sabin and Harland 2017) *Answer 4.8: D*

4.9

A psychologist is treating a 21-year-old woman for complicated grief related to the death of her parents in an automobile crash. The psychologist lost his own parents when he was a teenager, and he identifies strongly with this patient. The psychologist often sees her after regular clinical hours and has canceled other appointments to see her on short notice.

Which ethical pitfall is the psychologist in danger of committing?

A.   Abandonment of the therapeutic alliance.

B.   Breach of confidentiality.

C.   Divided loyalties as a dual agent.

D.   Erosion of professional boundaries.

E.   Practicing outside his scope of clinical competence.

This clinical scenario involves a patient who can be considered difficult because she resembles the clinician in a way that threatens his ability to maintain professional boundaries. The concept of difficult patients encompasses a broad spectrum, ranging from the type of patient in this vignette to hostile, aggressive, or unlikable personalities who evoke strong negative reactions. The psychologist's habit of seeing this patient after hours and canceling other appointments to see her suggests therapeutic boundaries are being threatened.

Abandonment of the therapeutic alliance describes a situation in which a clinician may pay less attention to a patient, subtly encourage the patient to leave treatment, or simply stop seeing the patient. Confidentiality breaches occur when clinicians share information about patients with others inappropriately. Divided loyalties as a dual agent refer to a therapist's simultaneous allegiance to more than one party. Scope of clinical competence pertains to the psychologist's ability to recognize his areas of expertise as well as his limitations as a treatment provider. (Roberts 2016) *Answer 4.9: D*

4.10

Young children cannot make fully informed and autonomous decisions regarding their own health care. In addition to what is believed to be in the best interests of a child, which of the following standards are given consideration in decisions related to the child's health care?

    A.   Burden and discomfort of care plan.
    B.   Parental wishes.
    C.   Physician recommendations.
    D.   Preferences of the child.
    E.   All of the above.

When making decisions related to the health care of a young child, the burden and discomfort of the care plan, parental wishes, physician recommendations, and the preferences of the child are given consideration, in addition to what is believed to be in the best interests of the child. The values and opinions of multiple stakeholders are weighed in decisions related to a child's health care. (Grootens-Wiegers et al. 2017) *Answer 4.10: E*

4.11

A patient asks his psychiatrist for a disability evaluation. He has been depressed since the death of his wife 3 months ago, and now he does not wish to ever return to work. His psychiatrist has been supportive, assisting him through the grieving process and helping him plan for a return to work. The psychiatrist believes a short course of therapy will return the patient to his previous occupational functioning. The psychiatrist fears that confronting the patient about returning to work may lead to regression and a longer course of treatment.

Which of the following is the best option for the psychiatrist?

A. Conduct the evaluation and, no matter what the findings, advocate for the patient's request.
B. Conduct the evaluation and discuss all findings, positive and negative, with the patient before submitting them to the employer.
C. Conduct the evaluation and divulge the findings only to the employer.
D. Conduct the evaluation without referring to the patient's current treatment.
E. Refer the patient to a colleague with forensic expertise to conduct the evaluation.

Clinical psychiatrists who take on a forensic role with their patients may find that both their therapeutic work and their forensic objectivity are undermined by the different requirements of the two roles. Forensic evaluations generally require reviewing corroborating materials, exposing private information to public scrutiny, and subjecting evaluees to potential sanctions. These requirements may all undermine a therapeutic alliance. At the same time, the credibility and objectivity of the forensic evaluation may be undermined by the clinician's interest in advocating for the patient. Recent scholarship is identifying a place for compassion or patient advocacy in forensic evaluations, but this has not yet supplanted the ideal of separating the two roles whenever possible. It is consequently safest to avoid acting as a forensic expert for one's own patients.

In situations in which this dual role is unavoidable, as in workers' compensation, civil commitment, or guardianship proceedings, identifying the conflict for the patient and the court, describing the sources of information completely, and remaining sensitive to the differences in role are important methods of managing the dual roles. (American Academy of Psychiatry and the Law 2005; Knoll 2018; Strasburger et al. 1997) *Answer 4.11: E*

4.12

An adolescent with nonspecific abdominal pain and evidence of bruising and scars is accompanied by an adult for medical treatment in an emergency room. The adolescent seems frightened and shy and often looks to the adult before responding to questions from the health care provider. After offering initial reassurance to the adolescent, what is the most important next step in the evaluation by the emergency room physician?

A. Calling the police for suspected trafficking of the adolescent.
B. Consulting with the hospital administrator.
C. Giving the adolescent a sandwich.
D. Requesting that a psychiatrist see the adolescent.
E. Speaking with the adolescent separately from the accompanying adult.

If a child or adolescent seems wary of an accompanying adult, speaking with the child or adolescent separately, without the adult present, is clinically indicated. Physicians, nurses, and other health care workers are mandated by law to report child maltreatment to child protective services. A report must be made if a physician suspects or has reason to believe that a child has been abused or neglected. The physician is not required to provide proof that abuse or neglect occurred. (Children's Bureau 2019) *Answer 4.12: E*

4.13

HIV testing has been introduced in many clinics as a routine test that patients must opt out of, rather than directly request. Which of the following statements is correct about the relative weighting of ethically important ideas underlying the public health efforts in support of such a practice?

A. Individual autonomy of patients over interests of the public.
B. Benefit to individuals over interests of health providers.
C. Confidentiality of patients over financial interests of patients.
D. Interests of health providers over financial interests of patients.
E. Interests of the public over individual autonomy.

HIV represents a persistent public health crisis. In the United States, nearly 38,000 people are newly infected with HIV each year, and 14% of those living with HIV are unaware of their HIV-positive status (HIV.gov 2020). The opt out approach to HIV testing was devised to make testing more normative. The opt out approach has been effective in reducing stigma surrounding HIV testing and increasing testing rates compared with an "opt in" approach (Young et al. 2009). Opt out testing places the interests of the public over individual autonomy—an HIV test will be conducted unless an individual explicitly declines to be tested. *Answer 4.13: E*

4.14

A first-year psychiatry resident rotating through a busy outpatient pediatrics clinic is assigned to see a 16-year-old girl for a new patient evaluation. The patient was registered at the front desk by her mother, who then left. The patient reports that she is "relieved" to come to the doctor's office because she gets "stressed out sometimes." Relevant state law indicates that adolescents must have parental consent for medical evaluation and treatment, except in relation to sexual health and mental health.
Which of the following is the resident's best option?

A. Contact a legal representative regarding the appointment of a guardian for the patient.
B. Contact the state child protective services to report that the patient was left at the clinic without parental supervision.
C. Tell the patient that the visit must be rescheduled for a time when her mother can be present.
D. Assign a staff member to act as the patient's guardian during the evaluation.
E. If the patient agrees, start the evaluation even though the mother is not present.

Laws regarding adolescent medical and mental health care and parental consent vary from state to state. In many localities, advising adolescents about specific topics such as contraception and sexually transmitted diseases does not require parental consent for evaluation and treatment. When parental consent for treatment is needed, it may be demonstrated in a number of ways: if the parent participates in the medical visit, sends the teen with written permission for treatment, or gives consent by telephone. In this case, by registering the patient and leaving her in the waiting room, the mother's action may be viewed as giving implied consent for the visit to proceed without the mother's presence. The patient can also give assent to the visit: a 16-year-old can be expected to say whether he or she prefers to wait for the parent to return and to be able to give a relevant and adequate medical history. (American Psychiatric Association 2010; Beauchamp and Childress 2001) *Answer 4.14: E*

4.15

The parents of a healthy 12-year-old boy ask a child psychiatrist to test the boy for a genetic predisposition to Alzheimer's disease. Although there is no family history of the disease, the parents express their belief that "knowledge is power" and say that they intend to have the boy tested for the genetic predisposition to all common disorders as the technology becomes feasible. The psychiatrist is aware that genetic testing is clinically available.

What is the psychiatrist's best course of action, based on ethical guidelines concerning susceptibility genetic testing?

A. Order the test if the parents give written consent.
B. Order the test if the parents and the son give written consent.
C. Order the test if the parents and the son give written consent and if the parents agree to undergo testing themselves.
D. Explore the reasons for the request at this time and clarify whether additional therapeutic support for the family is indicated.
E. Disclose the psychiatrist's own family history of Alzheimer's disease and personal decision regarding undergoing susceptibility genetic testing.

Genetic tests to predict an asymptomatic person's future risk of illness raise several ethical concerns. The psychiatrist's positive ethical duty is to understand the concerns that may lead to the request for genetic susceptibility testing and to determine whether additional psychiatric support is necessary for the patient and family. In this case, the request is on behalf of a child, which introduces complexity regarding informed consent and the psychological distress of disclosure of results. The potential harms of genetic susceptibility testing in the absence of disease are many in number, including opening the door to future insurance or employment discrimination. In certain circumstances, these risks are outweighed by the test's benefits—for example, if a positive test result leads to an effective intervention to prevent or ameliorate the disease (i.e., newborn screening for phenylketonuria) or if the test result can assist individuals in life planning (i.e., predictive testing for Huntington's disease). In this case, there is no clear medical benefit to the child knowing his genetic susceptibility status at this age, and by testing the child now based on the parents' wishes, the child is deprived of the right to make the decision for himself in the future. (Burke et al. 2001; Post et al. 1997; Roberts and Uhlmann 2013; Ross and Moon 2000) *Answer 4.15: D*

4.16

A second-year psychiatry resident is performing an intake evaluation in the outpatient clinic. The new patient, who is 36 years old, recounts a history of repeated sexual molestation by several male relatives during her childhood and teenage years. She indicates that she is no longer at risk for assault because she resides "halfway across the country" from her family of origin. She requests that the resident not document her abuse because she is ashamed of what happened and is concerned that clerical staff in the clinic will find out about her past. The patient will be seen in the clinic for pharmacotherapy only.

What should the resident tell the patient?

A.   Documenting the abuse is part of the patient's recovery.
B.   No other clinic employees will have access to the medical chart.
C.   The resident must document the abuse in detail as part of her assessment.
D.   The resident will document only that there is a history of abuse without extensive details.
E.   The resident will not document the history of abuse.

Balancing the need for accuracy in the medical record with protecting patient privacy is an important skill for psychiatrists to master. Psychiatrists should not assure patients that their records are completely confidential because in modern medical practice this may be virtually impossible to maintain. In the age of third-party payers, quality assurance reviewers, and electronic medical records, the principle of confidentiality has become a much more limited and partial protection than in the days of Hippocrates. It is especially important to inform patients during the initial intake evaluation of the limitations of confidentiality. Although health care facilities must take every precaution to prevent unauthorized access to medical records, it is probable that many eyes other than the physician's will see the record.

Probity may seem to call for recording absolutely nothing about the childhood trauma because it may not seem material to the patient's treatment with pharmacotherapy. However, even if the patient does not receive formal psychotherapy at the clinic, supportive therapy will likely be part of her medication management. Therapeutic mistakes could occur if future treating clinicians are unaware of her history of abuse. However, this type of chart does not require detailed accounts of the circumstances or emotions surrounding the abuse, which the patient would probably consider highly private and stigmatizing. (Carman and Britten 1995; Dewald and Clark 2001; Siegler 1982) *Answer 4.16: D*

4.17

A psychiatry resident misses an appointment with a pharmacotherapy patient because her car breaks down. When she explains this to the patient, he offers to give her "a really great buy" on a car from his brother's car dealership. The resident urgently needs to buy a new car, and she has limited financial resources.

Which of the following is correct?

A. It is ethical to accept the offer, because the patient made it without coercion.

B. It is ethical to accept the offer, because the patient will not directly gain financial benefit from the transaction.

C. It is ethical to accept the offer, because the patient is being treated with pharmacotherapy only, not psychotherapy.

D. It is unethical to accept the offer, because such an arrangement may be a trick by the patient.

E. It is unethical to accept the offer, because such an arrangement may exploit the patient and may impair the resident's clinical judgment.

The ethical precept that a psychiatrist does not accept gifts of significant monetary value is founded on the principle that the inherent inequality of the psychotherapeutic relationship makes the patient vulnerable to exploitation. For this reason alone, the offer of "a really great buy" on a car represents a gift that is too significant to be accepted ethically. The patient may also assume that the resident is entering into a quid pro quo arrangement and that he will receive preferential treatment from her in return for the deal he has arranged. Even if this is not his assumption, the resident may feel indebted to the patient, and this may subtly influence her case management. Her clinical judgment and objectivity may be diminished or distorted because of this business transaction. (American Psychiatric Association 2001a; Backlar and Cutler 2002; Roberts 2006) *Answer 4.17: E*

4.18

A psychiatrist is flying aboard a commercial airplane when a male passenger begins having a generalized tonic-clonic seizure in the aisle. The psychiatrist identifies himself to the flight crew as a doctor. The ill man's wife tells the psychiatrist that her husband stopped drinking recently and that he has a history of withdrawal seizures. The flight attendant produces the medical kit, which contains a syringe of lorazepam. The psychiatrist quickly thinks about the potential ramifications of administering the benzodiazepine to the patient, who continues to seize, and subsequently gives the lorazepam. The seizure stops, to everyone's great relief. This type of professional action is ethically acceptable, even though the intervention does not involve formal informed consent, because it deals with a situation involving which of the following?

A. A therapeutic privilege between provider and patient.
B. An emergency situation in which immediate treatment is necessary to prevent serious harm.
C. The wife's implied waiver of the patient's need to be informed.
D. Treatment by a physician who does not have an established relationship with the patient.
E. Treatment of an incompetent individual.

There are several exceptions to the usual requirement that a patient provide informed consent for his treatment. One is the granting of consent to treatment by a surrogate decision-maker for a patient who lacks the capacity to make the decision. Another exception is therapeutic privilege, rarely invoked today, in which a provider determines that the patient's welfare would not be served by his granting informed consent. In many jurisdictions Good Samaritan statutes immunize health care professionals from untoward sequela from aid rendered. The provision of needed emergency medical services to an unconscious patient is an example of the emergency exception to the informed consent rule. (Berg et al. 2001; Roberts 2016) *Answer 4.18: B*

4.19

The obligation of a physician to assess clinically a patient who arrives unconscious in the psychiatric emergency room is based on which of the following duties?

A. Duty to autonomy.
B. Duty of care.
C. Duty of confidentiality.
D. Duty to be truthful.
E. Duty to warn.

Duty of care loosely equates with the principle of beneficence. A physician has a duty to care for any patient, conscious or unconscious, and provide a thorough clinical assessment (Samartzis and Talias 2019). Medical negligence represents a failure to fulfill the duty of care. *Answer 4.19: B*

4.20

Which of the following is the concept that an individual can have the decision-making capacity to consent to less risky procedures with a more certain benefit, yet at the same time lack the capacity to consent to a more risky procedure with less certain benefit?

A. Autonomy.
B. Coercion.
C. Paternalism.
D. Sliding scale of competency.
E. Transparency in informed consent.

Sliding scale of competency is the concept that the standard for consent becomes more stringent as the risks associated with the medical decision increase. For example, a patient with mild dementia may have adequate capacity to consent to receiving intravenous hydration but may not have adequate capacity to consent to a risky surgical procedure with uncertain benefit. A surrogate decision-maker may be required in the latter case but not in the former. (Drane 1984; Roberts 2016) *Answer 4.20: D*

4.21

A medic sends a 19-year-old army private to a field hospital because the private had an anxiety reaction that paralyzed him during battle. The private reports a history of panic attacks, which have become worse under the stress of deployment. The psychologist diagnoses panic disorder, and the acute symptoms respond well to a sedative medication. The private asks that the psychologist not record the panic disorder diagnosis because he wants to rejoin his company immediately and hopes to stay in the military to earn college benefits. Instead, the private suggests that the psychologist document an allergic reaction. This case raises which of the following ethical issues?

A. Confidentiality, dual agency, and scope of practice.
B. Confidentiality, dual agency, and veracity.
C. Confidentiality, justice, and respect for persons.
D. Confidentiality, nonmaleficence, and respect for autonomy.
E. Confidentiality, respect for persons, and scope of practice.

Mental health professionals in the military are similar to occupational physicians in that they have different, and often conflicting, sets of obligations when compared with a civilian clinician. These obligations are sometimes referred to as *dual agency situations*. Confidentiality would obligate the clinician in a nonmilitary practice not to disclose the details of the patient's diagnosis to his employer or any third party without the patient's permission or being required by law. However, a military practitioner also has a professional responsibility to promote the effectiveness and cohesion of the fighting force. Sending a soldier with diagnosed panic disorder—one who has already become immobilized in battle—back to the theater would endanger other soldiers and the overall mission of the military. By documenting that the patient had an allergic reaction, the psychologist would fail to fulfill his duties to the military and would also fail to uphold the ethical principle of veracity, or truth telling. (Howe 1981; Schneider and Bradley 2018) *Answer 4.21: B*

4.22

The obligation of a physician to inform child protective services if a child appears to be physically abused is based on which of the following duties?

A. Duty to autonomy.
B. Duty of care.
C. Duty to report.
D. Duty to warn.
E. Duty to be truthful.

Physicians, nurses, and other health care workers are mandated by law to report child maltreatment to child protective services. A report must be made if a physician suspects or has reason to believe that a child has been abused or neglected. The physician must report the facts or circumstances that led to the suspicion that the child has been abused or neglected. The physician is not required to provide proof that abuse or neglect occurred. (Children's Bureau 2019) *Answer 4.22: C*

4.23

A 64-year-old divorced woman who had been in brief psychotherapy with a psychiatrist returns a year after leaving therapy. The patient informs her psychiatrist that she has just been diagnosed with metastatic ovarian cancer. The patient has spoken with an attorney about advanced directives and talked with a niece, her only living relative, about her will. The patient appears vulnerable and slightly tearful at the end of the session. The psychiatrist gives the patient a gentle pat on the shoulder before she goes out the door.

Which of the following is the most appropriate description of the psychiatrist's choice to touch the psychotherapy patient on the shoulder?

- A. The behavior is a boundary violation likely to jeopardize treatment.
- B. The behavior is inappropriate because it exploits the patient.
- C. The behavior may have been appropriate under these particular circumstances.
- D. The behavior should be a standard response to such vulnerable and sad patients.
- E. The behavior should be reported to the state medical ethics board.

In general, physical contact with patients should not be standard practice for a variety of reasons (such as unequal power relationships, transference, the need to maintain therapeutic neutrality), and therapists are trained to avoid such behavior. However, there may be circumstances in which nonsexual touching is an empathic and compassionate gesture. Assuming the therapist does not exhibit such behavior in a standard fashion, this may have been an appropriate response. In this context, the action is not necessarily a damaging, exploitative, or reportable offense. (Epstein and Simon 1990; Gabbard and Nadelson 1995) *Answer 4.23: C*

4.24

A psychologist forms the impression that his therapy patient has been physically abusive to his children, ages 6 and 7, who live with the patient and his physically disabled mother. The psychologist has never seen the children, and the children are not his patients.

Which of the following is the psychologist's best course of action?

- A. Do not report the impression of abuse, because it may harm the therapeutic relationship with the father.
- B. Do not report the impression of abuse, because he has never seen the children.

C.   Require the patient to bring in his children for an evaluation be-
     fore deciding whether or not to report the impression of abuse.
D.   Report the impression of abuse to the proper child protection
     authorities or encourage the patient to do so with the psycholo-
     gist's support.
E.   Report the impression of abuse to the proper child protection
     authorities and also report suspected abuse to elder protection
     authorities because of the likelihood that the patient is abusive to
     his mother if he is abusive to the children.

In this situation, the best course of action is to inform the patient of
the health professional's requirement to report suspected abuse. If possible, it is ideal to encourage the patient to participate in the reporting
process and to provide emotional support and, if necessary, to use intervention and community resources as the report is investigated. The reporting process thus may be included in the therapeutic process, rather
than being seen as an act of "disloyalty" in the treatment relationship.
Failure to report suspected abuse of children is a serious breach of professional and legal responsibilities for psychologists or psychologists in
training, physicians, including advanced physicians in training, and physicians who work on multidisciplinary treatment teams. In the absence
of a clear impression of potential abuse of the physically disabled mother,
however, it would be a breach of patient confidentiality to report the patient to the elder protective services authority. (American Psychiatric
Association 2001a; Roberts 2016; Simon 1992) *Answer 4.24: D*

4.25

Sometimes patients wish to leave the hospital before they are medically
ready. When the treatment team permits this type of discharge, it may
be called leaving "against medical advice," or an "AMA" discharge.
    Which of the patients described below is most appropriate to be dis-
charged against medical advice?

A.   A clear-thinking patient with a history of cocaine abuse who is
     being worked up for a possible gastrointestinal bleed but de-
     clines to stay for an endoscopy.
B.   A febrile patient recently diagnosed with treatment-resistant
     tuberculosis (TB) who wants to see his girlfriend.
C.   A patient in the intensive care unit after a suicide attempt by an-
     tidepressant overdose who insists he has to "finish the job."

D.   A patient with moderate dementia and pneumonia who gets on the elevator thinking he is catching a bus.

E.   A patient with postsurgical delirium who begins pulling out her intravenous lines and demanding to leave.

When a patient asks to leave before he or she is medically ready, clinicians must conduct a careful assessment of decision-making capacity. A patient who possesses decision-making capacity is free to refuse any treatment, including hospitalization, even if such a refusal results in serious morbidity or mortality. In the vignettes presented, it is highly probable that the demented and delirious patients portrayed are incapable of making informed decisions about leaving the hospital. The suicidal patient is still dangerous to himself and is likely impaired by a mental illness. The patient with TB may very well be decisionally capable, but public health considerations preclude discharging him because his communicable disease presents a danger to the community. The fact that he has a fever suggests that there may be an unresolved medical issue as well; this alone would not be sufficient to keep him in the hospital, but the overall clinical picture warrants caution.

Although the patient with the possible gastrointestinal bleed may be withdrawing from or craving cocaine, he appears to be the most capable of making the decision to leave the hospital. In such a case, the clinician should assess whether the patient understands that the gastrointestinal bleed is potentially life threatening, has reasoned through the risks of leaving, appreciates the effects of the situation on him, and is communicating a stable, authentic choice. If the patient chooses to leave, he should be discharged with documentation that he is decisionally capable, that he has declined further medical evaluation, and that he has been warned that this is an unwise decision. Because clinicians may be happy to see difficult patients leave the hospital, even if against medical advice, they should be mindful of their own reactions to the patient and ensure that they are not subtly influencing the decision to leave. (Gostin 2002; Stern et al. 2018) *Answer 4.25: A*

4.26

A very traditional Asian family asks their grandmother's physician not to inform her of the severity of her illness. They prefer to tell her as a group once family members are gathered at their home. The physician believes the disclosure must be made soon because the standard treatment for the woman's condition will work best only if begun quickly.

Which of the following is the physician's most appropriate next step?

A. Ask the patient to clarify her wishes regarding the disclosure of her diagnosis.
B. Conduct a decision-making capacity assessment of the patient.
C. Consult with hospital attorneys to clarify the physician's legal obligations.
D. Identify a surrogate decision-maker for the woman.
E. Withdraw from the case to avoid being forced by the family to behave unethically.

Informed consent in the United States is driven by individualistic notions of autonomy and decision-making. Patients are expected to collaborate with physicians as equal partners despite feelings of vulnerability and imperfect medical knowledge. In some communities, however, decision-making is familial, and this places different requirements on the informed consent process.

The physician in this case may consequently be torn between his or her training on informed consent and the family's needs and preferences. Tensions in ethics similarly arise between commentators who try to identify fundamental similarities between cultures (i.e., the importance of providing relevant information) and those who honor the specific cultural requirements of the community (i.e., hiding information about terminal illness). An ethically justifiable response in such cases is to ask the patient her preferences for information disclosure, thus honoring her autonomy and cultural preferences at the same time. (Fan and Tao 2004; Macklin 1998; Ozdemir et al. 2019) *Answer 4.26: A*

4.27

The obligation of a physician providing an expert opinion in an involuntary hospitalization hearing is based on which of the following duties?

A. Duty of care.
B. Duty to report.
C. Duty to serve.
D. Duty to be truthful.
E. Duty to warn.

Upholding the moral ideal of veracity involves being truthful in one's statements as well as not telling lies and avoiding misimpressions. A physician providing an expert opinion is obligated to provide a truthful account of his or her reason for recommending, or not recommending, an involuntary hospitalization. (Holder et al. 2018) *Answer 4.27: D*

4.28

Caring for individuals with mental disorders can expose clinicians to occupational risks. Which of the following represents recognized best practices for hospitals and clinics in managing such risks?

A. Acknowledge the fears of clinicians.
B. Create a safe and secure clinical environment to the extent possible.
C. Engage in training to help reduce risks, for example, in dealing with patients with altered mental status.
D. Provide care and support to clinicians who are injured by patients in health care settings.
E. All of the above.

In managing occupational risks, hospitals and clinicians should acknowledge the fears of clinicians, create a safe and secure clinical environment to the extent possible, engage in training to help reduce risks, and provide care and support to clinicians who are injured by patients in health care settings. *Answer 4.28: E*

4.29

A 6-year-old child is brought to a psychiatrist for individual psychotherapy. The child states that he does not want to see the psychiatrist, that he does not want to be in therapy, and that he is coming only so that he will not "get into trouble" with his parents. The psychiatrist continues the psychotherapy.

What is the best ethical justification for the psychiatrist's continuation of treatment despite the patient's lack of agreement?

A. The child is not being physically forced to come.
B. The child is unlikely to be developmentally capable of free and autonomous informed consent.
C. The child's oppositional behavior demonstrates the need for therapy.

D. The psychiatrist has specialized knowledge about what is best for the child.

E. There is no ethical justification for the treatment of this child.

It is always important to respect children who are patients and to attempt to obtain their assent for treatment. However, the capacity to make treatment decisions in a truly free and autonomous manner is tied to the developmental stage of the child. At age 6 years, a child does not have the cognitive capability for his consent to be informed. The cognitive capacities grow through the developmental trajectory, and the importance of obtaining a child's assent and eventual consent become more and more important. The same statements about therapy made by a 16-year-old should be given much greater weight. (Hurley and Underwood 2002; Nurcombe 2002) *Answer 4.29: B*

4.30

Psychiatrists may often be in stressful and unsafe situations and may feel uncomfortable caring for certain "difficult" patients. Which of the following is accurate regarding professional expectations of psychiatrists?

A. Psychiatrists are obligated to provide emergency care under all circumstances.

B. Psychiatrists are obligated to provide care to established patients indefinitely.

C. Psychiatrists are obligated to see all patients irrespective of their ability to pay.

D. Psychiatrists are obligated to perform clinical duties even if the duties violate their sincere religious or moral beliefs.

E. None of the above.

Psychiatrists are *not* obligated to provide emergency care under all circumstances (e.g., in the care of patients with religious beliefs that override the obligation or in the care of patients who have provided informed refusal for treatment). Psychiatrists, moreover, are not obligated to provide care indefinitely, to see all patients irrespective of their ability to pay, or to perform duties that violate their sustained, sincere moral beliefs. According to accepted ethical standards in medicine, physicians are generally "free to choose whom to serve" (American Psychiatric Association 2010). Once an ongoing doctor-patient relationship has been established, however, the physician may not abandon the patient (e.g., due to lack of payment). Transferring a patient's care to another physician is not considered patient abandonment if the treating psychiatrist is unable to provide necessary care and when the situation is not an emergency. *Answer 4.30: E*

4.31

A patient in psychotherapy for a mild anxiety disorder applies for life insurance. He signs a consent form for the release of his medical records to his insurance company, and the company subsequently requests a copy of his entire clinical record from the therapist.

Which of the following is the most appropriate action for the therapist to take?

- A. Advise the patient of the need for confidentiality of treatment records.
- B. Ask the insurance company if a treatment summary would suffice.
- C. Comply with the request and send a copy of the entire record.
- D. Explain to the insurance company the need for confidentiality of psychotherapy records.
- E. Refuse to send the records, citing doctor-patient confidentiality.

Often insurance companies do not require complete psychotherapy records to determine coverage and are satisfied with a treatment summary including diagnosis, dates of treatment, and prognosis. Although patients have the right to waive confidentiality, they are not always cognizant of the full implication of the release-of-information forms they sign. When releasing confidential patient information for any reason, physicians should release only the minimum amount of information required for the particular situation. In addition to checking with the insurance company, it is also useful to discuss with the patient the implications of the waiver of confidentiality. (Roberts 2016; U.S. Department of Health and Human Services 1996) *Answer 4.31: B*

4.32

For each of the following descriptions, choose the most appropriate term related to the principle of informed consent. Each answer option may be used once, more than once, or not at all.

A. Durable power of attorney for health care.
B. Power of attorney.
C. Presumed consent.
D. Psychiatric advance directive.
E. Psychiatric research advance directive.

_____ A person with bipolar disorder specifies his preferences for disenrollment and/or medication treatment if he develops severe symptoms and becomes decisionally incapable during a washout period of a research protocol in which he is enrolled.

_____ An unconscious person is treated at an emergency department after being struck in a hit-and-run accident.

_____ A terminally ill individual specifies whom he wishes to make medical decisions for him once he has become decisionally incapable.

_____ A seriously ill individual specifies whom he wishes to represent him at a real estate closing in another state because he cannot travel.

_____ A person with a family history of Alzheimer's disease specifies whom she wishes to make medical decisions for her if she becomes decisionally incapable.

Power of attorney refers to any transfer of legal authority to another person, usually for the purpose of conveniently completing a contract. Durable power of attorney for health care refers to the appointment of a state-sanctioned health care agent who may make medical decisions for a person who lacks decisional capacity. A psychiatric advance directive is a document that records a psychiatric patient's wishes regarding treatment should he lose decisional capacity. A psychiatric research advance directive records the wishes of a psychiatric research subject regarding participation in research should he become nondecisional. Informed consent is typically required for medical procedures, but presumed consent is sufficient in emergent cases in which life-threatening problems require immediate medical intervention for patients who are nondecisional (e.g., unconscious). (Roberts 2016; Simon 1992) *Answers 4.32: E, C, A, B, A*

4.33

A medical student is asked to evaluate a patient with opiate dependency who presented to the emergency department with abdominal pain and probable pancreatitis. The patient is well known to the medical and surgical services, and the chart states in several places that she is "med-seeking." When approached for a physical examination, the patient yells, "Bring me some morphine!" The student notes that the patient appears uncomfortable, is tachycardic, and has dilated pupils. The student believes that the patient's pain is not being treated adequately, probably because she is tolerant to the level of opiate medication that is being administered. She quickly asks her supervising resident to write an order for more pain medication.

Which of the following is the ethical principle most clearly illustrated by the medical student's clinical care recommendation?

A. Autonomy.
B. Compassion.
C. Fidelity.
D. Scope of practice.
E. Veracity.

The medical student in this scenario is appropriately treating this patient with compassion, as she would treat any other suffering human being in need of medical help. Patients who deservedly or not receive the reputation of being difficult present special challenges for physicians that may lead to substandard care. A physician's responsibility is to alleviate suffering, even in those patients who may not be grateful for the care they receive or who may have exacerbated their problems by self-injurious behavior or the use of alcohol or drugs. (Jonsen et al. 2002; Roberts 2016) *Answer 4.33: B*

4.34

An elderly man with chronic paranoid schizophrenia has received care for many years at a community mental health center. One day before the Christmas holidays, he brings his psychiatrist and case manager a cake that he has baked in appreciation for their help.

What is the most appropriate response to this gift from this patient?

A. Accept the cake as a gesture of gratitude.
B. Accept the cake but only after thoroughly discussing the meaning of the gift and transference with the patient.
C. Decline the cake because it is a minor ethical breach to accept any gift from a patient.

D. Decline the cake because it is a serious ethical breach to accept any gift from a patient.
E. Request an ethics consultation to help make an appropriate decision.

Accepting expensive or significant gifts from patients is unwise for ethical and clinical reasons. Transference feelings and the unequal power relationship between doctors and patients make some patients vulnerable to financial exploitation, and it may therefore be difficult to determine whether a patient's offer of an expensive gift is truly voluntary. In addition, expensive gifts may carry multiple meanings, including disguised hostility or negative feelings that the patient might wish to keep out of the therapeutic relationship.

The ethical implications of accepting a token, inexpensive gift from a patient depend on the context. In this case, offering a gift of food during the holiday season appears to be a positive development in someone with a paranoid psychosis. If the treatment providers were to refuse the cake, the patient's feelings might be hurt and he might no longer feel safe and accepted at the mental health center. The relationship of this seriously mentally ill patient to the clinic staff is very different from that of a neurotic person to a therapist providing dynamic psychotherapy. In the latter situation, the clinician should analyze the underlying meaning involved in the token gift and then decide to accept it or not, depending on the result of that analysis. (American Psychiatric Association 2001a; Backlar and Cutler 2002; Gabbard 1999) *Answer 4.34: A*

4.35

After the death of a patient, at what time, if ever, does the psychiatrist's duty of confidentiality end?

A. Ends at the time of the patient's death.
B. Ends 2 years after the patient's death.
C. Ends 100 years after the patient's death.
D. Lasts indefinitely except under proper legal compulsions.
E. Lasts indefinitely except with regard to the deceased patient's immediate family.

A psychiatrist is obligated to keep a patient's confidences even after the patient's death and even if immediate family members request information about the deceased person. Exceptions to the physician's ob-

ligation for confidentiality include abiding by legal requirements and protecting others from imminent harm. (Roberts 2005; Roberts 2016)
Answer 4.35: D

4.36

A 36-year-old patient with chronic paranoid schizophrenia and type 2 diabetes stops receiving his monthly depot injections of antipsychotic medications and stops taking his diabetes medications. Over the next 2 months, the patient is brought to the hospital three times with diabetic ketoacidosis, each time requiring hospitalization. The treatment teams have not been able to convince the patient to restart either his diabetes or antipsychotic drugs. He tells them that he does not have diabetes but was infected by drinking bottled water. On the fourth hospitalization, an attending consultation-liaison psychiatrist transfers the patient to the psychiatric unit and places him on a medical hold. He tells the staff this hold is on the basis of *parens patriae*.

In this case, which of the following is the most appropriate description of the concept of acting with *parens patriae*?

    A.   Acting as a parent to protect the patient from harming himself.
    B.   Acting clinically to provide better treatment for the patient.
    C.   Acting institutionally to protect the hospital from an adverse event.
    D.   Acting medicolegally to protect the psychiatrist from a lawsuit.
    E.   Acting with police powers to protect the community from harm.

Parens patriae is a Latin phrase meaning literally "the state as parent." The concept derives from Anglo-American law in which kings, as the fathers of their country, would protect their subjects when they were incapable of protecting themselves. Since colonial times, *parens patriae* has been used as a justification for involuntary commitment of the mentally ill. For psychiatrists, the ethical foundation of the concept is in beneficence theory: the psychiatrist acts out of beneficence to hospitalize the patient whose delusions prevent him from taking lifesaving medications. Without hospitalization, the patient may die. The treatment and policy goal is to provide treatment that restores the patient's capacity to care for himself.

There is no evidence that the patient in this case is a likely danger to the community, and the parental role is not an example of the police powers invoked when a patient is a threat to others. Acting to prevent a lawsuit or an adverse event is not consonant with the beneficent foundation of *parens patriae* or with the collaborative nature of the doctor-patient relationship. And although the physician behaves clinically, the clinical intervention also serves an underlying social policy. (Gutheil and Appelbaum 2019; Roberts 2016) *Answer 4.36: A*

4.37

Which of the following statements about accidental deaths due to overdose is correct?

   A.   Most are due to acetaminophen.
   B.   Most are due to amphetamines.
   C.   Most are due to cannabis.
   D.   Most are due to opioids.
   E.   Most are due to tricyclic antidepressants.

   Most accidental overdose deaths are due to opioids. (Wilson et al. 2020) *Answer 4.37: D*

4.38

Which of the following is an accurate statement regarding how employers may use genetic information in adherence with the 2008 federal Genetic Information Nondiscrimination Act?

   A.   Employers are permitted to use genetic information to determine eligibility for employee promotions.
   B.   Employers are permitted to use genetic information to determine eligibility for job reassignments.
   C.   Employers are permitted to use genetic information to evaluate retirement benefits for employees.
   D.   Employers are permitted to use genetic information to evaluate job applicants.
   E.   None of the above.

   The 2008 Genetic Information Nondiscrimination Act (National Institutes of Health 2008) prohibits employers from requiring genetic information or using genetic information in employment decisions. Genetic information may not be used to determine eligibility for promotions or reassignments, may not be used to evaluate retirement benefits, and may not be used to evaluate job applicants. *Answer 4.38: E*

4.39

A delirious Hispanic man is admitted to a hospital with pneumonia. Soon after admission, he requests to leave, even though the medical workup is incomplete. He is determined to lack decisional capacity. The medical team discusses with the patient and his family the risk of leaving. The family reports that the patient is a proud man who has always been fairly stoic, but he now seems to be "talking crazy."

Which of the following is the most appropriate next course of action for the medical team?

A. Consult with an expert in Hispanic culture to understand the cultural context of his refusal to accept treatment.
B. Discharge him immediately against medical advice, honoring the man's autonomy.
C. Identify the appropriate surrogate decision-maker and discuss the case with that individual.
D. Transfer the man to the psychiatric service because staff there will be better at handling him.
E. Try to convince the patient to stay by informing him that the police will be called if he leaves.

Refusal of treatment does not, by itself, demonstrate a lack of decision-making capacity. In this case, however, it has already been determined that the patient is delirious. It would be negligent to discharge the patient in such a condition. Although staff on the inpatient psychiatric unit may have experience working with confused and uncooperative patients, delirium is a medical urgency and requires acute medical stabilization. Coercion with a threat may be controversial and could be an abuse of power. The best option would be to identify the surrogate decision-maker and educate this person about risks, benefits, and options so that he or she can make an informed decision on behalf of the patient. It would also be helpful to ask the family to help encourage the patient to stay, because confused patients sometimes are more willing to listen to their loved ones than to the medical team. (Beauchamp and Childress 2001; Roberts 2016) *Answer 4.39: C*

4.40

What is the most common cause of substance-related aggressive behavior?

A. Alcohol.
B. Cannabis.
C. Cocaine.
D. Hallucinogens.
E. Opioids.

Alcohol intoxication and withdrawal are associated with aggressive behavior. Cocaine and hallucinogens are associated with impulsive or disorganized behavior and sensory disruption. Cannabis and opioids are least likely to result in aggressive behavior of the substances noted here. *Answer 4.40: A*

4.41

A psychiatrist is conducting her initial meeting with a 25-year-old inpatient who was brought to the emergency room the previous night. Congruent with state law, the patient had been placed on a 72-hour hold because he is considered a danger to others. The patient was known to have assaulted a neighbor the preceding evening, claiming that the neighbor was spying on him. The patient has no known previous psychiatric history. The patient is suspicious of the psychiatrist, is relatively noncommunicative, and repeatedly asks when he will be allowed to leave. The psychiatrist suggests to the patient that he will probably be able to leave in a day or two if he consents to taking medication.

What ethical problem is suggested by the psychiatrist's statement?

A. The psychiatrist fails to demonstrate beneficence by not immediately ordering an injection of an antipsychotic medication.
B. The psychiatrist is wrong to imply that the patient has the capacity to consent to medications because the patient is obviously psychotic.
C. The psychiatrist may be coercive in linking the patient's consent to medication to a rapid discharge.
D. The psychiatrist violates the neighbor's right to protection by discussing discharge without the neighbor's involvement.
E. The psychiatrist violates the patient's autonomy by taking away his right to decide when he is ready for discharge.

Because the psychiatrist is seeing the patient for the first time and because the patient has no previous psychiatric history, it is unlikely that the psychiatrist has sufficient knowledge (such as an accurate diagnosis) to be able to predict the patient's response to medication. Therefore, the statement linking medication consent to a rapid discharge is not a factually based clinical judgment. It is more likely that the psychiatrist was instead attempting to use the patient's wish to leave as leverage to obtain consent to medication. The implication is that refusal to consent to medication will lead to prolonged hospitalization. Such consent would therefore be coerced rather than autonomous. The process of informed consent requires disclosure, voluntariness, and decision-making capacity. The psychiatrist's use of coercion in this case hinders the informed consent process by impairing the patient's ability to make a voluntary choice. (American Psychiatric Association 1996; Nurcombe 2002; Roberts 2016) *Answer 4.41: C*

4.42

Boundary crossings are behaviors within the therapeutic relationship that push the limits of acceptable professional conduct but may serve to advance the treatment. Boundary violations, on the other hand, are behaviors that do go beyond the parameters of appropriate professional behavior and have the clear potential for exploiting the patient.

Which of the following is a boundary crossing as opposed to a more serious boundary violation?

    A.   Accepting a hand-painted dish towel from a withdrawn patient.
    B.   Accepting expensive jewelry from a wealthy patient.
    C.   Giving one's favorite patients a small handmade gift on their birthdays.
    D.   Going out on a date with a former psychotherapy patient.
    E.   Hiring a patient who is a landscaper to work on one's yard.

Boundary crossings and violations are the subject of increasing scrutiny in psychiatric ethics, and although experts may debate the nuances of specific situations, the essence of each type of therapeutic disturbance is clear. Boundary crossings are situations that may or may not be justified by contextual features, particularly if they occur on an infrequent basis. Accepting a gift that is inexpensive but that a withdrawn patient has made meaningful through embellishment may serve to advance the treatment by making the patient feel more relaxed and accepted in the treatment setting. However, if the clinician makes a habit of accepting (or giving) token gifts, then the tenor of the relationship begins to change from doctor-patient to friendship, even if this is not a conscious intention of the therapist or an explicit understanding of the patient. Boundary crossings may thus be harbingers of a moral slippery slope in which the bounds of an ethical therapeutic relationship become looser and more unclear, and they therefore may not infrequently lead to true boundary violations.

Boundary violations are actions that are completely outside the scope of acceptable professional practice. Examples of boundary violations include going out on a date with a patient or former patient or accepting expensive jewelry from a patient. Hiring a patient to work on one's yard is an obvious boundary violation because it creates a business relationship alongside the therapeutic one. (Dewald and Clark 2001; Gutheil and Gabbard 1998; Roberts 2016) *Answer 4.42: A*

4.43

Which of the following is an accurate statement regarding the 2008 Genetic Information Nondiscrimination Act (GINA)?

A. Insurers are permitted to use genetic information to set health premiums for an individual.
B. Insurers are permitted to use genetic information to determine eligibility for an individual's health insurance.
C. Insurers are permitted to use genetic information of family members to determine eligibility of an individual for health insurance.
D. Insurers are permitted to use genetic information to determine eligibility for an individual's life insurance.
E. All of the above.

GINA prohibits the discriminatory use of genetic information in health insurance and employment. GINA does not extend to long-term care insurance, disability insurance, or life insurance. (National Institutes of Health 2008) *Answer 4.43: D*

4.44

A 26-year-old woman is admitted to an inpatient psychiatric unit after a suicide attempt. To protect her from further self-harm, the patient is dressed in pajamas and given a bed in the hallway near the nurses' station. When a male nursing assistant attempts to take her vital signs, she becomes agitated, screams, and pushes him away. The inpatient psychiatrist is called.

Which of the following is the most appropriate first step for the psychiatrist?

A. Ask the patient what has upset her.
B. Assign only female care providers to this patient.
C. Instruct the nursing assistant to persist in checking vital signs.
D. Prescribe sedative medication.
E. Request a consultation from an expert in cultural psychiatry.

A patient's unusual or difficult behavior is a clinical sign that requires inquiry and interpretation. Once the underlying reasons for unusual behavior are understood, it is possible to respond therapeutically instead of precipitously reacting.

The possibility that culture is influencing behavior should always be considered. This woman may believe that an unmarried woman who is not properly dressed should not be seen by unrelated men. If this is the case, the male nursing assistant's good intentions may mean little in the face of the patient's concern. To jump to a conclusion that her behavior is the result of her psychiatric illness could result in inappropriate treatment, such as restraint or sedation, when her distress would appear normal to those who share her values and social expectations. Uncritical cultural assumptions are equally dangerous. To assume the patient's unusual behavior has a cultural basis could result in undertreatment of her mental illness.

If inquiry reveals that her distress is based on her cultural values, thoughtful attention to those values will minimize inadvertent psychological trauma and inform the progress of her psychiatric treatment. Specific steps might be to assign only female staff to care for the patient and to move her out of the hallway as soon as it is safe to do so. Other helpful steps would be to see if there are mental health professionals or advocates from her culture who could help advise the treatment team and educate and reassure the patient. (Backlar and Cutler 2002; Roberts and Dyer 2004) *Answer 4.44: A*

4.45

Which of the following statements about violence and mental illness is most accurate?

A. Individuals with mental illness frequently engage in violent behavior.
B. Individuals experiencing first-episode psychosis are most likely to engage in violent behavior.
C. Individuals with mental illness engage in violent behavior less frequently than members of the general population.
D. Individuals with mental illness are most likely to engage in violent behavior.
E. Individuals with mental illness engage in violent behavior more than do individuals with substance disorders.

Individuals with mental illness do not frequently engage in violent behavior. Individuals with substance-related conditions overall are more likely to engage in violent behavior than individuals with mental illness alone. Among individuals with mental illness, those who are experiencing first-episode psychosis are most likely to engage in violent behavior. (Swanson et al. 2015) *Answer 4.45: B*

4.46

An elderly man with moderate dementia has refused amputation of his gangrenous foot because he believes that it is merely discolored by soot or dirt. After meeting with the patient to thoroughly inform him about his illness and the risks and benefits of treatment options, the vascular surgeon calls for a psychiatry consultant to determine the patient's decisional capacity. After evaluating the patient, the consultant determines that he lacks the capacity to decline the amputation.

Which of the following is the most salient rationale for determining that this patient lacks the capacity to make this medical decision?

A. He cannot communicate a choice.
B. He does not understand and appreciate his medical situation.
C. He has a diagnosis of moderate dementia.
D. He has not been informed of the benefits and risks of the proposed therapeutic procedure.
E. His decision is not consistent with his values and goals.

Clinical standards for medical decision-making capacity include a genuine appreciation of the medical situation, the nature of the recommended care, and potential alternative courses for care along with the benefits, risks, and consequences of each alternative. In addition, the individual should have the ability to communicate a choice and to understand the information relevant to the medical situation. Decisions need to be arrived at through reasoning and must be consistent with the patient's values and goals.

In this case, the patient is able to clearly communicate a choice but appears incapable of recognizing the facts of his own medical situation. He does not acknowledge the reality that he has a gangrenous foot. As a result, he does not recognize and cannot appreciate the potential consequences of his medical situation.

It is important to note that a patient does not need to choose what most people would consider reasonable to possess decision-making capacity. For example, if the patient had said that he understood his medical condition but nonetheless preferred death to amputation, he might be considered capable of making that decision under certain circumstances. (Appelbaum and Grisso 1988; Lo 2020b; Roberts 2016) *Answer 4.46: B*

4.47

A psychology intern has been seeing a patient for psychodynamic psychotherapy for the last 4 months. The patient is a 45-year-old man with narcissistic personality disorder and associated depression. During the last month, the patient has been leaving angry messages with the department secretary, sending the intern critical letters, and insulting her during sessions. She has repeatedly tried to work constructively with the patient's negative feelings under the guidance of an experienced supervisor. She and her supervisor suspect that the patient's anger is directed toward women in general and that he might do better with a male therapist. At this point, the intern believes that her countertransference toward the patient is so strong that she cannot work with him therapeutically. She discusses her situation with her supervisor.

What would be the most appropriate response of the supervisor?

A. Assist the intern in transferring the patient to another therapist.
B. Inform the intern that termination in this context, by definition, is patient abandonment.
C. Inform the intern that she must work through her countertransference and continue treating this patient.
D. Notify security that the patient is harassing the intern.
E. Suggest the intern refer the patient to group psychotherapy.

The goal of a therapeutic alliance is a mutually respectful partnership in which positive change can occur. It would seem that this is no longer possible in the scenario described. Despite adequate supervision and a reasonable period of time, the intern has been unable to achieve a therapeutic alliance, perhaps because of her sex. Trainees, and even experienced clinicians, are often afraid that terminating any treatment relationship is equivalent to abandoning the patient and may result in serious professional and legal repercussions, but patients are not abandoned when they are referred to other appropriate treaters. In this case, it is likely that referral to another therapist may give the patient a chance to develop a relationship in which he can accomplish therapeutic goals. By contrast, referring the patient for group therapy might constitute abandonment because this form of treatment is not specifically indicated. It is not clear that the patient's behavior reaches the level of harassment requiring the supervisor to contact security, which would certainly be a viable option if the patient's behavior escalated. (American Psychiatric Association 2001a; Gutheil and Appelbaum 2019) *Answer 4.47: A*

4.48

Patient information that is faxed or emailed between health care providers in the United States is governed by which legal statute?

A. The Consolidated Omnibus Budget Reconciliation Act.
B. The Employee Retirement Income Security Act.
C. The Health Insurance Portability and Accountability Act (HIPAA).
D. The Privacy Act and Patriot Act.
E. The Protected Health Information Act.

HIPAA has many features, one of which deals with the protection of privileged information disclosed in the health care setting. According to HIPAA, information provided to a health care provider (including nurses, physicians, psychologists, and social workers) is disclosed in confidence and should not be disseminated without the permission of the patient, unless it is related to the emergency treatment of that patient, to reportable offenses such as suspected child abuse, and to other specific exceptions. (U.S. Department of Health and Human Services 1996) *Answer 4.48: C*

4.49

In cases of terminal illness, caregivers, family members, and patients may all have different perspectives on how to approach end-of-life treatment decisions. If the patient or family and health care providers have different views about the appropriateness of life-sustaining or invasive interventions, which of the following options should be the physician's first step toward resolving the disagreement?

A. Call an ethics committee consultation.
B. Consult a legal expert.
C. Make an independent decision about medical treatment that is grounded in evidence-based practice.
D. Meet with the patient (or proxy decision-maker), family, and health care team.
E. Transfer the patient to another provider.

End-of-life care may require trade-offs of quality of life for longevity that involve painful personal choices. Such decisions are not purely medical or scientific but are informed by personal values, local customs and traditions, and cultural beliefs. Ideally, respectful and open discussions among patients, proxy decision-makers, family members, and physicians can help patients and surrogates explore the values that inform their choices and can provide a venue for assessing decision-making capacity if the patient becomes impaired. This process-based approach to making end-of-life treatment decisions can avoid adversarial court proceedings and unilateral, paternalistic decision-making. If there is an impasse between treatment providers and the patient or surrogate, involving an ethics committee or transferring the patient may well become necessary, but such steps should not occur before the physician begins a respectful discussion that involves deliberation, exploration of values, and negotiation. (American Medical Association, Council on Ethical and Judicial Affairs 1999; Candilis et al. 2004) *Answer 4.49: D*

4.50

Which of the following is an accurate statement regarding the ethical concerns associated with artificial intelligence and its applications in precision medicine?

A. Artificial intelligence algorithms may be trained on nonrepresentative populations.
B. Artificial intelligence algorithms may have biased assumptions.
C. Artificial intelligence algorithms may not be applicable in many clinical situations.
D. Artificial intelligence algorithm standards for validation are not transparent.
E. Artificial intelligence algorithm use may widen health disparities in many clinical situations.
F. All of the above.

A number of concerns are being raised with respect to artificial intelligence (Vayena et al. 2018). Algorithms trained on nonrepresentative populations have been shown to provide suboptimal results when applied to populations not represented in the training data. Moreover, because many algorithms are disproportionately trained on people who can access novel technology, they risk widening existing health disparities. Furthermore, the conscious and unconscious biases of algorithms' designers tend to inhere in the algorithms themselves and could reinforce existing harmful biases that result in suboptimal care. Algorithms' underlying code is not legible outside a specialist community, and most contemporary classes of algorithm, such as deep learning, proceed mostly in black boxes, hidden even to their creators. It is uncertain whether artificial intelligence algorithms are applicable to real clinical settings, where decisions are made in real time by physicians who take in many subtle kinds of information. *Answer 4.50: F*

4.51

Approximately what proportion of firearm fatalities are suicides?

A. 10%.
B. 25%.
C. 60%.
D. 75%.
E. 90%.

Suicides account for 6 out of every 10 firearm fatalities in the United States according to the Centers for Disease Control and Prevention (2020). *Answer 4.51: C*

4.52

A 22-year-old college student presents to the student health center after taking an intentional overdose of "a handful of pills." She is being treated for depression and reports that she took the pills while in acute distress because her boyfriend is leaving for combat duty. Medically stable, she regrets taking the overdose and has no prior history of suicide gestures or attempts, psychosis, or substance abuse. The patient is offered psychiatric hospitalization but declines because she wants to spend time with her boyfriend before he leaves. She is accompanied by her parents, who plan to stay the weekend and provide support. The patient denies any current suicidal ideation and agrees to return to see the psychologist on Monday morning. The psychologist feels that parental supervision and clinical follow-up are appropriate.

Which of the following is the best explanation of why this psychologist's plan fulfills the concept of the "least restrictive alternative"?

A. Because depressed patients should be given psychotherapy before medications are tried.

B. Because effective treatments that do not limit liberty should be used before those that do restrict individual freedom, such as psychiatric hospitalization.

C. Because persons who have made a suicide attempt should not be treated as outpatients.

D. Because psychiatric admission should be to a community facility rather than to a university hospital.

E. Because when suicidal patients have family who can watch them, hospitalization is not required.

The least restrictive alternative concept emerged from several legal cases in which courts ruled that if there are several equally effective treatment options, the alternative that least limits the patient's freedom and rights must be used first. In this case, the patient impulsively made a suicide attempt. She regrets the attempt, and her parents are able to monitor her condition. In addition, she refuses hospitalization and is no longer suicidal. She has agreed to return for close outpatient follow-up. These facts would suggest that involuntary hospitalization is not warranted and is an overly restrictive option. Many patients who make first suicide attempts do require involuntary hospitalization, and some patients would be too suicidal to be allowed to return home even if family were available. Both psychotherapy and medication intervention are appropriate for treatment of depression, and the choice of one over the other or of a combination of treatments is a clinical decision. There is no ethical reason why a community hospital would be preferable to one at a university, except perhaps confidentiality, but this is not related to the concept of least restrictive alternative. (Chiles et al. 2019; Gutheil and Appelbaum 2019; Roberts 2016) *Answer 4.52: B*

4.53

A child psychiatry fellow has been providing weekly psychotherapy for an 8-year-old boy for 1 year. The treatment began shortly after the death of the boy's mother and is going well. During a meeting with the boy's father to discuss his progress, she feels a strong sexual attraction to the widower. A week later, the boy's father telephones to ask her on a date. She would like to accept but wonders if it would be ethical to do so.

Which of the following is the best course of action?

A. Agree to date the father but immediately transfer the son's care to another child psychiatry fellow.
B. Agree to date the father, continue to treat the child, and encourage the child to express his feelings about the adults' relationship.
C. Agree to date the father, continue to treat the child, but keep the adults' relationship a secret from the child.
D. Explain to the father the need to maintain a professional relationship with him to meet the therapeutic needs of the son.
E. Seek formal, written permission from the training director to enter into a dating relationship with the parent of a patient.

A psychiatrist has an ethical obligation to refrain from sexual or romantic relationships not only with current and former patients, but also with key third parties to the doctor-patient dyad, such as the parent, spouse, or guardian of a patient. In all these cases, romantic involvement may severely compromise the physician's primary obligation to the therapeutic relationship. In this scenario, the fellow's best option is to decline the offer to date the father and perhaps seek supervision to understand how her feelings about the father may affect the treatment of the son. Abruptly transferring the son's care could be devastating to a child whose mother has recently died, and doing so simply to gratify the psychiatrist's own needs would call into question her professionalism. Finally, even if a training director were inclined to give written permission to trainees to engage in questionable relationships, such a document would not relieve the fellow of her ethical obligations to her patient. (American Psychiatric Association 2001a, 2010) *Answer 4.53: D*

4.54

Identify whether the statement is not supported or supported by existing evidence regarding differential health risks and health disparities.

    A. Not supported.
    B. Supported.

    ____ LGBTQ+ individuals are at risk for poor mental health outcomes and substance use disorders.
    ____ Sexual minority youth are more likely to experience suicidal ideation than nonsexual minority youth.
    ____ Peer victimization (bullying) is a significant psychological health risk for sexual minority youth.
    ____ LGBTQ+ individuals encounter significant stigma in health care settings, which may contribute to an inadequate standard of care and avoidance of care-seeking.

Lesbian, gay, bisexual, transgender, queer, intersex, asexual, and other sexual or gender minority (LGBTQ+) individuals are at greater risk for poor mental health outcomes, substance use disorders, and suicidal ideation than cisgender heterosexual individuals. Discrimination, victimization, bias, poor self-esteem due to internalized homophobia and transphobia, and a perceived inability to live an open life may contribute to these health disparities (Drescher et al. 2019; Yarbrough 2018). In one study, 23% of transgender and gender diverse respondents reported that they did not seek needed health care the prior year because of a fear of mistreatment, and 33% reported at least one negative experience with a health care provider related to their identity (James et al. 2016). In another study, one-third of LGBTQ respondents reported having somewhat or very difficult access to care, and 15% reported having a negative experience in health care because of their identity (Macapagal et al. 2016). *Answers 4.54: B, B, B, B*

4.55

Identify whether the statement is not supported or is supported by existing evidence regarding violence and suicide and mental disorders.

A.   Not supported.

B.   Supported.

_____   Men are more at risk for violent behavior than women.

_____   Mentally ill individuals are responsible for most violence in society.

_____   Men are more at risk for suicide with a firearm than women.

_____   Living with a child under age 18 years is a protective factor against suicide.

_____   After discharge from an inpatient unit, risk for suicide is heightened in the first week.

_____   Men are more likely to attempt suicide than women.

_____   A positive therapeutic alliance between therapist and patient is a protective factor against suicide.

_____   Suicide risk assessment is highly accurate in predicting who will commit suicide.

_____   Suicide risk assessment is highly accurate in predicting who will not commit suicide.

_____   Violent threats or behaviors toward others are suicide risk factors.

_____   Individuals with mental illness who attempt suicide are more impulsive than individuals in the general population.

_____   Certain sleep disorders elevate risk for violent behavior.

_____   Certain personality disorders elevate risk for violent behavior.

Suicide risk assessment tools are inaccurate in predicting who will or will not commit suicide. Suicidality is relatively widespread, with suicidal ideation (i.e., thoughts of killing oneself) being most common, attempted suicide being slightly less common, and completed suicide being least common. Data suggest that men and boys are more likely to die by suicide, whereas women and girls are more likely to attempt suicide. Men are also more likely to commit suicide by using a firearm (Chiles et al. 2019). Protective factors for suicide include living with children under 18 and having a positive therapeutic alliance. Risk factors for suicide include having been recently discharged from an inpatient unit and having impulsive or aggressive behaviors (Dumais et al. 2005; McGirr et al. 2008). Studies show that people with mental illness comprise only a small proportion of those who commit acts of violence overall. In fact, individuals with mental illness are more likely to be a victim of violence than a perpetrator of violence (Beeber 2018). Certain sleep disorders and certain personality disorders may elevate risk for violent behavior (Gallegos et al. 2019; Winsper et al. 2013; Yu et al. 2012). Most violent crimes are committed by men rather than women. *Answers 4.55: B, A, B, B, B, A, B, A, A, B, B, B, B*

4.56

A 50-year-old man with chronic obstructive pulmonary disease (COPD) and schizoaffective disorder lives independently and takes his medication as prescribed, but is unable to work due to hallucinations that are distracting and upsetting to him. At a routine visit to his psychiatrist, he is offered an appointment to receive the COVID-19 vaccine. The patient declines, stating that he is concerned about taking the vaccine away from other people who "need it more." After talking further with his psychiatrist, he confides that he also is worried about being poisoned. Which of the following is the best next step for the psychiatrist?

A. Clarify whether the patient's family members have received the vaccine.

B. Explore the patient's concerns further.

C. Increase the patient's antipsychotic medication.

D. Inquire about the patient's political beliefs.

E. Schedule a vaccine appointment for the patient.

By offering the patient an appointment for the COVID-19 vaccine, the psychiatrist is taking steps to ensure that an individual who is a member of a vulnerable population has access to an important intervention to help prevent very serious health outcomes, such as acute respiratory distress, cardiac complications, or even death. Recent evidence has shown, moreover, that COVID-19 is associated with inflammatory neurological conditions with chronic sequelae. Individuals living with schizophrenia, early in the pandemic, were shown to have twice the mortality rate associated with COVID-19 infection as age-matched peers (Nemani et al. 2021). In this case, the therapeutic relationship between the patient and the psychiatrist appears strong, given the fact that the patient confided his concern about being poisoned. The psychiatrist's first obligation is to explore the degree to which the patient's thinking is affected by his mental disorder. The psychiatrist's second, and closely linked obligation, is to provide accurate information to the patient, setting the stage for informed consent for the vaccine. Informed consent relies on information, voluntarism, and decisional capacity. In this case, the patient's statement that others "need the vaccine more" may be in tune with his personal values, but it may also reflect a lack of appreciation for his own medical situation, which puts him at risk for severe illness associated with COVID-19. A patient does not need to choose what most people would consider reasonable to possess decision-making capacity, and this patient is free to decline to be vaccinated; however, a fear of being poisoned may be associated with this patient's mental disorder or may reflect a lack of information about the nature and safety of the vaccine itself and its potential benefits for an older person living with COPD. Exploring the patient's concerns further allows the psychiatrist to support the patient in making an informed decision about the vaccine. (Nemani et al. 2021; Roberts 2016; Sallam et al. 2021; Shen and Dubey 2019) *Answer 4.56: B*

CHAPTER 5

ETHICS AND PROFESSIONALISM IN MEDICAL RESEARCH

5.1

Which of the following is the set of three ethics principles identified in the *Belmont Report* as constituting the foundation of ethically sound human research?

    A. Autonomy, beneficence, compassion.
    B. Beneficence, confidentiality, respect for persons.
    C. Beneficence, justice, respect for persons.
    D. Beneficence, nonmaleficence, respect for persons.
    E. Justice, nonmaleficence, respect for persons.

The *Belmont Report*, published by the National Commission for the Protection of Human Subjects of Biomedical and Behavioral Research in 1979, stands as one of the most important documents outlining the ethical duties of medical researchers. The three ethical principles identified in the report as the foundation for ethically sound human subjects research are respect for persons, beneficence, and justice. (Brody 1998; National Commission for the Protection of Human Subjects of Biomedical and Behavioral Research 1979; Roberts 2002a) *Answer 5.1: C*

5.2

Which of the following terms best characterizes each situation described?

    A. Research misconduct.
    B. Not research misconduct.

_____ An academic psychiatrist oversees the analysis of data from a recent small research project for which she serves as the principal investigator. The data do not support the original hypothesis of the study. The academic psychiatrist decides to abandon the project.

_____ An academic psychiatrist oversees the analysis of data from a recent small research project for which she serves as the principal investigator. The data do not support the original hypothesis of the study. The academic psychiatrist decides to try to publish the findings of the project.

_____ An academic psychiatrist oversees the analysis of data from a recent small research project for which she serves as the principal investigator. The data do not support the original hypothesis of the study. The academic psychiatrist continues the project to see if data from additional participants lead to a different result.

Research misconduct includes fabricating (recording or reporting made-up data or results), falsifying (manipulating any part of the research process or altering data or results so that the research is not accurately represented in the research record), or plagiarizing (using another's ideas, processes, results, or words without credit) during any part of the research process (Office of Science and Technology Policy 2000; see also Caplan and Redman 2018). The principal investigator of a research project has the authority and accountability to decide when or if to discontinue a project. The principal investigator may also decide whether or not to recruit participants. *Answers 5.2: B, B, B*

5.3

A research volunteer describes her motivation for entering a minimal risk study as "wanting to help other people." Her mother has died of the disease being studied, and she is willing and decisionally capable. Which of the following best describes her motivation?

A. Altruistic.
B. Coerced.
C. Induced.
D. Involuntary.
E. Unreasonable.

The desire to help others through research participation is a form of altruism. Individuals offer many reasons for choosing to participate in research protocols. Assessing self-reported motivations is an important part of the research informed consent process. The authenticity and consistency of reasons offered by prospective study volunteers are important to consider. Whether a volunteer's motivations are reasonable is a value-laden judgment that may simply ignore the prospective participants' values or disguise the wishes or values of investigators. Consequently, it is not seen by many as an acceptable standard for assessing motivation or decision-making capacity. (Appelbaum and Roth 1982; Kaminsky et al. 2003; Roberts et al. 2000b) *Answer 5.3: A*

5.4

A medication in a blinded foil packet is inadvertently given to the wrong patient in a clinical research protocol. One hour later, the study nurse discovers the error and is able to reach the study participant, who returns the unopened packet. The study nurse fills out an error report. The principal investigator later removes the error report from the protocol records and destroys it, stating, "No harm was done."

Which of the following ethics principles is most compromised in this decision?

A. Beneficence.
B. Integrity.
C. Justice.
D. Nonmaleficence.
E. Respect for persons.

Researchers are responsible for providing sufficient information about the conduct of their research to allow for an adequate judgment of scientific merit. Attention to detail and taking (and retaining) accurate notes facilitates disclosure of methodological issues as they arise. Excellence in such administrative matters demonstrates the integrity of the research project and of the investigators themselves. (Brody 1998; Coverdale et al. 2006; Roberts 1999; Roberts 2016) *Answer 5.4: B*

5.5

Which of the following terms best characterizes each situation described?

A. Ethical.
B. Unethical.

_____ Accidental misinterpretation of data
_____ Falsification of data
_____ Imputation of missing data by standard methods
_____ Suppression of data that does not support hypothesis
_____ Intentional misinterpretation of data
_____ Plagiarism
_____ Reporting a research-related error to the institutional review board

Research misconduct includes fabricating (recording or reporting made-up data or results), falsifying (manipulating any part of the research process or altering data or results so that the research is not accurately represented in the research record), or plagiarizing (using another's ideas, processes, results, or words without credit) during any part of the research process. Honest error is not considered research misconduct. (Office of Science and Technology Policy 2000; see also Caplan and Redman 2018) *Answers 5.5: A, B, A, B, B, B, A*

5.6

The conduct of human research is founded on several bioethics principles. Which of the following bioethics principles is reflected in the idea that vulnerable, disadvantaged, or minority groups should neither be overrepresented in dangerous research studies nor should they be underrepresented in research trials of promising new therapies?

    A.   Autonomy.
    B.   Beneficence.
    C.   Justice.
    D.   Nonmaleficence.
    E.   Veracity.

Justice is the principle that benefits and burdens should be equitably distributed in society. In human subjects research, the potential risks and advantages of protocol participation should not be assigned inappropriately or disproportionately to certain groups. (Beauchamp and Childress 2001; Lo 2020b; Roberts 1999) *Answer 5.6: C*

5.7

A psychiatric nurse at a university hospital is assigned to care for an inpatient with severe obsessive-compulsive disorder (OCD). The patient is enrolled in a research study being conducted by a member of the faculty to determine the efficacy of a new medication for OCD. The patient reports to the nurse that he has had diarrhea since starting the medication. The patient states that when he informed the study investigator about the problem, he was told that he would receive extra compensation and that he should not stop taking the experimental medication. The nurse is unable to contact the investigator or a member of the research team to talk about this issue.

Which of the following can provide the most helpful guidance to the nurse?

    A. The hospital attorney's office.
    B. The hospital institutional review board.
    C. The hospital risk management office.
    D. The hospital utilization review committee.
    E. The state medical board.

Learning to obtain appropriate consultation is a key skill for all health professionals. This skill is especially important for psychiatric professionals who deal routinely with cases involving medical, legal, and institutional matters as well as ethical uncertainties, ambiguities, and complexities. In this scenario, it is reasonable for the nurse to be concerned about the patient/participant being told he would receive extra compensation rather than having the study medication discontinued or receiving a medical treatment for the apparent side effect. Because the study investigator and his team cannot be contacted, the nurse's best option is to discuss the matter with a member of the hospital's institutional review board, which is charged with the protection of human subjects in medical research. Although the other entities listed, such as the hospital's risk management office, ethics committee, and attorney, may provide helpful counsel and assistance about ethical matters, they are not as appropriate for initial consultation in the scenario presented. (Pincus et al. 1999; U.S. Department of Health and Human Services 2018) *Answer 5.7: B*

5.8

Research involving animals is ethically controversial. Which of the following combination of principles is used to guide ethical practices related to animal research?

    A. Caution, containment, and constraint.
    B. Definition, diminishment, and determination.

C.   Generosity, guardianship, and guarantee.
D.   Replacement, reduction, and refinement.
E.   Respect, repetition, and return.

The three principles of replacement, reduction, and refinement (3Rs) are standard in animal research. The 3Rs were introduced in 1959 by William Russell and Rex Burch in "The Principles of Humane Experimental Technique." In research involving animals, every effort should be made to *replace* animals with alternatives, to *reduce* the number of animals used, and to *refine* experiments to minimize pain and distress to animals. (Flecknell 2002) *Answer 5.8: D*

5.9

A researcher systematically recruits recent immigrants with few financial resources to participate in a 12-week study of an atypical antipsychotic medication in the treatment of mild anxiety. The participants are asked to remain at a research center in a rural site during the course of the project to facilitate study adherence. This practice represents a violation of which of the following concepts underlying ethically sound research?

A.   Enhance voluntarism of participants.
B.   Include the least vulnerable population necessary to test the scientific hypothesis.
C.   Minimize coercive pressures on participants.
D.   Minimize risk to participants.
E.   All of the above.

From an ethical perspective, this study's design and its procedures are highly problematic. Its scientific purpose and value are unclear, and the overall beneficent aim of the study is not apparent. Therefore, the appropriateness of the risks to which participants are exposed is doubtful. The tactic of recruiting potentially vulnerable immigrants with multiple disadvantages when other clinically relevant populations exist and the practice of intentionally isolating study participants in a rural site for an extended period of time are violations of the principles of justice and respect for persons, respectively. This study, as described, is ethically unacceptable. (American Psychiatric Association, Task Force on Research Ethics 2006; Emanuel et al. 2000; National Commission for the Protection of Human Subjects of Biomedical and Behavioral Research 1979; Roberts 1999; Roberts and Heinrich 2005) *Answer 5.9: E*

5.10

It is widely accepted that some individuals with severe mental illness may experience periods of compromised decisional capacity. A number of safeguards to support and ensure the autonomy of participants in psychiatric protocols have been developed.

Which of the following statements is correct about these safeguards?

A. All individuals with mental illness require a surrogate decision-maker prior to entering a protocol that poses greater than minimal risk.
B. All individuals with mental illness are required to undergo a decisional capacity evaluation prior to enrolling in any protocol.
C. All individuals with mental illness are required to have a family member cosign the consent form at the time of entering a protocol that poses greater than minimal risk.
D. All individuals with mental illness are required to have a complete psychiatric evaluation prior to enrolling in any protocol.
E. Special safeguards are implemented for patients with certain symptoms, such as severe psychosis, rather than for all patients with mental illness.

The protective measures outlined in items A–D above are not usual or customary in research protocols and are inappropriate because they arguably diminish (not enhance) the autonomy of mentally ill research participants. Research advance directives (i.e., a document in which the study volunteer outlines in advance his preferences for decision-making across the course of research participation) represent one important example of a research safeguard that supports individual autonomy by providing a roadmap or plan for decision-making that honors the preferences and values of the study volunteer. Safeguards that automatically build in requirements for cosigners, evaluations (e.g., of symptoms, of decisional capacity), and surrogate decision-makers may be stigmatizing, paternalistic, and unnecessary to adequately ensure the safety and well-being of participants, simply on the basis of the diagnosis of mental illness. Better alternatives are, for instance, evaluations that are triggered by certain illness features, such as the presence of severe psychotic symptoms, or a more rigorous institutional review board review triggered by certain protocol features, such as studies that are high risk with no prospect of benefit for individual volunteers. (Brody 1998; Levine et al. 2004; Oldham et al. 1999; Roberts 2016) *Answer 5.10: E*

5.11

Conflicts of interest raise which concerns in the conduct of research?

A. The potential for bias in data collection.
B. The potential for bias in data analysis.
C. The potential for adverse effects on the credibility of research results.
D. The potential for improper behaviors on the part of investigators, such as insider information stock trading based on study findings.
E. All of the above.

The mere existence of a conflict of interest, be it actual or potential, need not prohibit research. However, investigators should recognize the multiple concerns that conflicts of interest may raise about the quality of the data and the behavior of the researchers. Investigators should acknowledge the conflict (or potential for conflict) to key stakeholders in the research enterprise, such as participants, the public, institutional review boards, and funding agencies. Researchers should also take appropriate steps to manage the conflict, for example, by clearly defining and separating the clinical and research roles. (Hilty et al. 2006; Roberts 2016; West et al. 1995) *Answer 5.11: E*

5.12

A healthy college student enters a research study that offers $250 for her participation. She meets all legal and ethical requirements for capacity to consent. During the consent process she tells the investigator, "I wouldn't do this if the money weren't right."

In this context, which of the following best describes the $250 compensation?

A. Bribery.
B. Coercion.
C. Incentive.
D. Reimbursement.
E. Undue inducement.

A key feature of the informed consent process for medical research is that potential subjects must be capable of making a voluntary decision about participation, free from coercive influences. Research volunteers often receive payment for their participation in clinical research, and this payment is considered noncoercive so long as it is reasonably commensurate with the participants' time and effort. Payment may become an undue inducement or influence if volunteers are financially desperate and are motivated by the study compensation to take on risks they might not otherwise assume. Payment for study participation is also considered more problematic when offered to persons who are seriously ill or in severe pain rather than to healthy volunteers. (Dunn and Gordon 2005; Grady 2005) *Answer 5.12: C*

5.13

Trademarks embody which of the following characteristics that allow the owner to identify and distinguish some concept, service, or product from those of a competitor?

    A.   Picture(s).
    B.   Sound(s).
    C.   Writing(s).
    D.   Device(s) or object(s).
    E.   All of the above.

Trademarks can embody any distinguishing characteristic in a concept, service, or product. Trademarks are a form of intellectual property, like patents, registered designs, and copyrights, but, unlike other forms of intellectual property, trademarks exist indefinitely, provided registration is renewed. Trademarks are registered with the U.S. Patent and Trademark Office and are protected by intellectual property laws. (Blackett 2016) *Answer 5.13: E*

5.14

For each of the following scenarios, choose the most appropriate term. Each answer option may be used once, more than once, or not at all.

    A.   Anonymous method for data collection.
    B.   Confidential method for data collection.

    ____   A faculty member invites residents by email to participate in a written survey of preferences for learning and assessment in the residency program. He encourages the residents to print out the survey and return it without any identifying information. He discards any surveys that are returned electronically or have identifiable data on them.

_____ A faculty member recruits volunteers for a protocol from a psychiatric inpatient unit; the protocol involves a written survey that has a randomly selected code on each page of the survey. The faculty member maintains a list with participant names and the assigned code number in a locked file cabinet in a different building.

An anonymous survey is one in which no one anywhere can link the data provided by a participant with his or her name. Therefore, the first scenario represents an anonymous survey method. The second scenario does offer some privacy protections for participants, but their anonymity is not absolutely ensured because a list is maintained—even if it is off-site. For this reason, the second study involves a confidential data collection method. (Roberts 2016; U.S. Department of Health and Human Services 2018) *Answers 5.14: A, B*

5.15

In the 1970s and 1990s, the National Cancer Institute experienced difficulty in recruiting sufficient participants for its comparison of mastectomy and lumpectomy in the treatment of breast cancer. Some investigators felt significant discomfort offering interventions when they were uncertain about which option was best. Others already favored one intervention over the other. In both studies, the participants themselves had clear ideas of which intervention they preferred, influencing their willingness to participate.

Which ethically important precondition for the research process appears to have been lacking in this situation?

A. Adequacy of safeguards.
B. Informed consent.
C. Scientific equipoise.
D. Therapeutic misconception.
E. Weighing research risks.

For a clinical trial to be ethically justifiable, there must be true uncertainty regarding the efficacy of the intervention being studied. Otherwise, research subjects are exposed to risk without good cause. The condition in which the opinions of researchers and clinicians balance "on the knife's edge" of certainty is called *equipoise*. Commentators have suggested that the National Cancer Institute's accrual difficulties were the result of a lack of equipoise on the part of investigators and subjects. When researchers and subjects have established views of which treatment is best, the requirement of uncertainty justifying a clinical trial cannot exist. The need for a research study to determine which treatment is superior may consequently require both professional consensus and community agreement. (Freedman 1987; Karlawish and Lantos 1997) *Answer 5.15: C*

5.16

For each of the following scenarios, indicate whether the activity meets criteria for human subjects research in the U.S. Department of Health and Human Services regulations. Each answer option may be used once, more than once, or not at all.

A.   Does not meet criteria for human subjects research.
B.   Meets criteria for human subjects research.

_____   Systematic examination of obituaries published in the local newspaper for documented cause of death that may be related to mental illness.
_____   Systematic examination of pathology reports in the university hospital morgue for documented cause of death that may be related to mental illness.
_____   Written survey distributed anonymously in the medical school cafeteria regarding nutritional preferences of students for use in planning cafeteria menus.
_____   Written survey distributed anonymously in the medical school mailroom regarding personal mental health care needs of medical students and residents for use in planning clinical service programs in the affiliated department of psychiatry.
_____   Systematic examination of clinical charts comparing HIV status, related diagnoses, and lab test use in a psychiatric inpatient unit and medical inpatient unit at the university hospital to facilitate quality assurance processes.
_____   Prescription of a psychotropic medication for an off-label use by an individual practitioner in caring for an individual patient with a severe and treatment-resistant mental illness.

A human subject is defined as a "living individual about whom an investigator (whether professional or student) conducting research: (1) Obtains information or biospecimens through intervention or interaction with the individual and uses, studies, or analyzes the information or biospecimens; or (2) Obtains, uses, studies, analyzes, or generates identifiable private information or identifiable biospecimens" (Code of Federal Regulations, Title 45, Part 46, Section 102.e). The first two scenarios involve deceased persons. Furthermore, in the first scenario, all information obtained is public, and in the second and third, there is no identifiable information. Finally, although the final four scenarios involve human subjects, they do not qualify as research because they are being conducted for quality assurance or treatment purposes and not to contribute to generalizable knowledge (i.e., the original purpose is not to publish the results). Thus, none of the scenarios meet the U.S. Department of Health and Human Services criteria for human subjects research. (Amdur and Bankert 2002; Brody 1998; Hilty et al. 2006; U.S. Department of Health and Human Services 2018) *Answers 5.16: A, A, A, A, A, A*

5.17

Copyrights protect which of the following?

    A.   Representation of an idea.
    B.   An idea.
    C.   A concept.
    D.   A methodology.
    E.   None of the above.

Copyright law protects original works of authorship that are "fixed in any tangible medium of expression…from which they can be perceived, reproduced, or otherwise communicated" (U.S. Copyright Office 2020). Examples include literary works, artistic works, musical works, architectural works, and computer software (Joyce et al. 2016). Copyright protection does not extend to any idea or concept. In the United States, copyright protection generally expires 70 years after the death of the author of the work. Creative Commons offers copyright licenses that allow works to be shared and reused by others (Creative Commons 2020). Works in the public domain are not protected by copyright. *Answer 5.17: A*

5.18

A psychiatrist in private practice receives an invitation from a pharmaceutical company to participate in an investigative trial in which she is asked to treat depressed patients with a new antidepressant. She will receive an honorarium of $500 for each patient she enrolls and an additional $500 for each patient who completes the trial. At the end of the study period, she will be asked to make an informal report on her patients' responses.

Which of the following is the most important initial action for the psychiatrist to take to fulfill her ethical obligations?

A. Agree to participate only if she can split the honoraria with the patients she enrolls.
B. Contact the appropriate human investigations committee for study approval.
C. Obtain written, informed consent from patients before enrolling them in the study.
D. Question the methodology and purpose of this study.
E. Recruit patients for the study only if she believes they are likely to benefit from the new drug.

Clinical research must be scientifically rigorous to be of value. This protocol, in which the physician is paid to make an informal report on the results of prescribing the company's medication, appears to be of dubious scientific value. Physicians are already expected to report adverse reactions to medication to the U.S. Food and Drug Administration. A physician receiving such payments has a clear financial conflict of interest, because she makes money from the drug company if her patients take the new medication and stay on it for a given period of time, yet the doctor is already receiving payment for services from the patient or from the patient's insurance company. Accepting these payments from the drug company could be construed not as medical research but as receiving a kickback for prescribing a particular medication. (Roberts 1999; Studdert et al. 2004) *Answer 5.18: D*

5.19

For which of the following populations do special human subjects regulations exist in the United States in 2020?

A. 18-year-old adults in good health.
B. 38-year-old adults diagnosed with mental illness.
C. 30-year-old adults who are incarcerated.
D. 32-year-old adults who are employed.
E. 75-year-old adults in poor health.

Pregnant women, human fetuses, and neonates; children; and prisoners all require additional protections in research according to federal regulations. Incarceration may affect prisoners' ability to make a voluntary, uncoerced decision about whether to participate in research, and thus additional safeguards are required (45 CFR 46, Subpart C). Other populations not specified in federal regulations may be potentially vulnerable to coercion or manipulation in the research situation. Some individuals may have multiple sources of vulnerability. Authentic voluntarism involves: "1) developmental factors, 2) illness-related considerations, 3) psychological issues and cultural and religious values, and 4) contextual factors" (Roberts 2016, p. 245).

Concerns about the potential vulnerability of psychiatrically ill research subjects and the risks of further stigmatizing the mentally ill by developing policies and practices in the absence of empirical research on these issues has thus fueled numerous endeavors to examine specific, ethically relevant issues in psychiatric research (Dunn and Roberts 2005; Dunn et al. 2006a). These studies, taken as a whole, have affirmed that patients with serious neuropsychiatric disorders are generally able to provide adequate informed consent for research, that enhancements to consent procedures result in improved understanding of research consent, and that participants' motivations for enrolling in psychiatric research are very similar to those of people with medical illnesses. *Answer 5.19: C*

5.20

For each of the following vignettes, choose the best manuscript designation from the list below. Each answer option may be used once, more than once, or not at all.

A. First author.
B. Second or subsequent author.
C. Acknowledged.
D. Not acknowledged.

_____ A medical student spends 2 months with a psychiatric research group. He attends team meetings, listens to research discussions, and enters psychiatric research data into a spreadsheet. Two years later, after the data are analyzed, a manuscript is generated. The student's role is _____.

_____ A resident comes up with an idea for a scholarly project based on a medical chart review. Because the resident has never done any research, she asks a senior faculty member for assistance. With the faculty member guiding each step of the process, the resident refines her idea and writes the first draft of the scholarly proposal and the institutional review board application. The faculty member provides detailed and specific advice on the interpretation of the findings and closely edits the resulting manuscript for style and content. The role of the faculty member should be reflected on the manuscript as _____.

____ The chairman of a psychiatry department is extremely supportive of the scholarly efforts of young faculty. He helps augment their budgets and he is happy to talk about research ideas in a general way. However, he is too busy for direct involvement. A faculty member sends him multiple drafts of a manuscript, but he returns only one—with the addition of a comma. His role in this manuscript is _____.

Ideally, authorship issues should be discussed among collaborators and coworkers early in a project, long before a manuscript is ready for submission to a publication. In the first scenario, the student's role does not meet authorship criteria. He did not contribute to the design, the data analysis, or the writing or review of the manuscript. The student is, however, embarking on a professional career, and his role in the project might have sparked his interest in research or might be significant to others in the profession. His work should be acknowledged in the manuscript. The faculty member in the second scenario meets criteria for authorship in that he made substantial contributions to the resident's concept and to the interpretation of data. He helped to critically revise the manuscript, and it should have his approval before it is published. In the third scenario, the department chairman is not entitled to authorship for this particular manuscript. Acknowledging his sustentative support would be correct. (International Committee of Medical Journal Editors 2006; Smith and Master 2017) *Answers 5.20: C, B, C*

5.21

The parents of a 14-year-old girl want her included in a research study that is investigating a new medication that may or may not offer a modest benefit for diabetes and that involves numerous blood draws. The parents sign the informed consent form. The girl, however, does not wish to participate in the study.

What should the researchers do?

A. Enroll the girl because she is a minor and legally unable to provide informed consent.
B. Enroll the girl because the legal guardians consented to her participation.
C. Enroll the girl without informing her of her participation.
D. Not enroll the girl because she did not provide her assent to participate.
E. Not enroll the girl because she is decisionally impaired.

Guidelines from the U.S. Department of Health and Human Services stipulate that in addition to receiving parental permission for a minor child to participate in research, investigators must obtain the assent of the child before he or she can be included in the research protocol. Information about the research needs to be presented to children in a manner that is congruent to their age and level of cognitive development. Assent must be communicated in the form of an affirmative agreement; children can therefore veto their own participation. (Arnold et al. 1995; Office for Human Research Protections 2005; Rosato 2000) *Answer 5.21: D*

5.22

For which of the following populations do special human subjects regulations exist that emphasize potential for personal benefit in evaluating whether a greater than minimal risk protocol can enroll subjects?

A. 14-year-olds who are in good health.
B. 38-year-olds who are diagnosed with mental illness.
C. 30-year-olds who are incarcerated.
D. 32-year-olds who are employed.
E. 75-year-olds who are in good health.

In the United States, adults are individuals 18 years of age or older. Children and adolescents participate in research involving greater than minimal risk if the benefits are greater than the risks. The benefit must be at least equal to the potential benefit of other available treatments or approaches. Parents or guardians must grant permission and the child must assent (Roberts 2016). Research with children may involve greater than minimal risk and not offer direct benefit to the participant if the study will generate essential knowledge for children with the participant's same disorder and the risks are not greater than a minor increase over minimal risk (i.e., will not exceed the discomfort of a medical, dental, psychological, social, or educational situation) (Roberts 2016). Children may participate in research not involving minimal risk if parents or guardians grant permission and the child assents (45 CFR 46, Subpart D). *Answer 5.22: A*

5.23

Match the information element with its status as protected health information, or not, under Health Insurance Portability and Accountability Act (HIPAA) regulations.

    A.   Protected health information.
    B.   Not protected health information.

    _____ Name
    _____ Social Security number
    _____ Date of birth
    _____ Implanted medical device serial number
    _____ Phone number
    _____ Cousin's name
    _____ Employer's name
    _____ Full face photograph
    _____ Medical record number
    _____ Fax number
    _____ Sister-in-law's name

HIPAA protects individually identifiable health information in any form or media. This information is called protected health information. Protected health information includes any information that identifies an individual or could be used to identify an individual, including common identifiers such as name, address, and birth date. (Office for Civil Rights 2013) *Answers 5.23: A, A, A, A, A, B, A, A, A, A, B*

5.24

For each of the following scenarios, select the single best term from the list below. Each answer option may be used once, more than once, or not at all.

    A.   Honest mistakes.
    B.   Research errors.
    C.   Research misconduct.

____ Research mistakes resulting from negligence, such as those related to haste.

____ Research undertaken using accepted methods that are later discovered to be flawed and, as a result, yield flawed data.

____ Errors that involve deception, such as fabrication of results, falsification, and plagiarism.

Science and scientists are inherently imperfect. Not only do human beings make mistakes, but the very nature of science is iterative and provisional, allowing for the possibility of mistake making along the journey of scientific inquiry. The sorts of scientific errors for which one is not ethically at fault include what might loosely be called *honest mistakes*. If an investigator is using accepted methods that later turn out to be flawed, the researcher is not ethically at fault. Errors resulting from negligence are sometimes blameworthy. Errors that involve deception are clearly unethical and can carry harsh punishments. (Friedman 1992; Lafollette 1992) *Answers 5.24: B, A, C*

5.25

Gene editing is ethically controversial because of the potential for irreparable and unforeseeable harm in which of the following applications?

A. Modification of the genetic code of human embryos.

B. Modification of the genetic code of certain insects, such as disease-carrying mosquitoes.

C. Modification of the genetic code of certain plants, such as nutrition-rich plants.

D. Modification of the genetic code of microorganisms.

E. All of the above.

CRISPR-Cas9 gene-editing technology has already led to the modification of the genetic code of human embryos, crops, livestock, microorganisms, and insects (Rossant 2018). Gene-editing technology could allow for improved crop and livestock breeding, new antimicrobial and antivirals, and control over disease-carrying insects (Barrangou and Doudna 2016), but all of these applications are ethically controversial. The ability to edit human embryos is especially controversial, given the potential for "designer babies" (Cavaliere 2019; "Germline Gene-Editing Research Needs Rules" 2019). Many ethical arguments have been made for and against human genome editing (see Cavaliere 2019). *Answer 5.25: E*

5.26

A medical student must complete a required scholarly project and chooses to interview residents at a nearby nursing home to explore their mental health care experiences. She gets the idea for her project when she visits her aunt, who is a nursing home resident herself. The medical student asks her faculty preceptor whether she has to obtain approval from the institutional review board (IRB) before presenting the information in a scientific poster session. The faculty member's response should be which of the following?

A. No, because this is a minimal risk interview study.
B. No, because this is a student project for a personal learning experience.
C. No, because this is a student project that involves collecting information from consenting adults.
D. Yes, because this is a project that involves collecting identifiable information from living human volunteers.
E. Yes, because this is a project that involves collecting identifiable information from living human volunteers about sensitive topics and the intention is to contribute to generalizable knowledge.

According to the U.S. Department of Health and Human Services guidelines, this project meets criteria for human research, and it involves gathering identifiable data for a potentially vulnerable population. Because the student intends to present the data in a scientific poster session, there is no question that it is a project with the intent to contribute to generalizable knowledge. The student's project thus meets the definition for human research and must therefore receive prospective IRB approval. (Brody 1998; Roberts 2016; U.S. Department of Health and Human Services 2018) *Answer 5.26: E*

5.27

Methods for safeguarding against conflicts of interest of researchers include which of the following?

A. Disclosure of financial interests.
B. Financial limits.
C. Oversight of research-related activities.

    D.   Role separation.
    E.   All of the above.

Conflicts of interest refer to competing roles, relationships, or interests that threaten an investigator's integrity, distort an investigator's judgment, or compromise an investigator's ability to act according to the moral requirements of his or her role. Such situations may naturally occur in clinical care and research, and they are not inherently unethical, but must be recognized and managed. Conflicts of interest might include large monetary incentives for enrolling participants in protocols, large financial investments in entities sponsoring protocols, and even interests in obtaining a promotion or national recognition through experiments. (Roberts 2016) *Answer 5.27: E*

5.28

Which of the following descriptions best characterizes each situation described?

    A.   Violates professionalism expectations.
    B.   Conforms to professionalism expectations.

    _____   In authoring a manuscript on a related topic, a scientific reviewer uses unpublished figures that he has encountered in a recent grant proposal.
    _____   In authoring a manuscript on a related topic, a scientific reviewer cites published figures that he has encountered in a recent grant proposal.

Peer reviewers have an obligation to "respect the confidentiality of the peer review process and refrain from using information obtained during the peer review process for [their] own…advantage" (Committee on Publication Ethics 2017). Using another's ideas, processes, results, words, or figures without credit is clear plagiarism. Plagiarism is a form of research misconduct. If an author wishes to reproduce a figure from a published article or book, the author must obtain permissions from the copyright holder. *Answers 5.28: A, B*

5.29

For each of the following scenarios, select the correct description from the list below of how the activity should be dealt with by institutional review boards (IRBs) as defined in U.S. Department of Health and Human Services regulations for human subjects research. Each answer option may be used once, more than once, or not at all.

A. Requires full IRB committee review.
B. May be eligible for expedited IRB review.
C. May be deemed exempt from IRB oversight.
D. Not appropriate for IRB review.

_____ Systematic examination of obituaries published in the local newspaper for documented cause of death.

_____ Written survey distributed anonymously in a medical school cafeteria regarding nutritional preferences of students for use in planning cafeteria menus.

_____ Written survey distributed anonymously in a medical school mailroom regarding personal mental health care needs of medical students and residents for use in planning critical service programs in the affiliated department of psychiatry.

_____ Written survey distributed anonymously via mailboxes to medical students and residents regarding personal mental health care needs to serve as the basis of an empirical manuscript in a peer-reviewed journal.

_____ Systematic examination of clinical charts comparing HIV status, related diagnoses, and lab test use in a psychiatric inpatient unit and medical inpatient unit at the university hospital to serve as the basis of an empirical manuscript in a peer-reviewed journal.

_____ Systematic examination of clinical charts comparing HIV status, related diagnoses, and lab test use in a psychiatric inpatient unit and medical inpatient unit at the university hospital to facilitate quality assurance processes.

_____ Prescription of a psychotropic medication for an off-label use by an individual practitioner in caring for an individual patient.

IRBs prospectively review animal and human research occurring in an institution and have the following two major purposes: to ensure scientific merit and to ensure that study participants are treated ethically and that their rights and welfare are protected. In the first three scenarios, IRB approval would not be required because they are not scientific studies with intention to disseminate or publish results. The first scenario describes a review of already publicized data; the following two describe quality improvement projects. The fourth scenario does involve research (a survey) with intent to publish the results and therefore would require

IRB approval; however, because the study design is simple and keeps the participants anonymous, it may be eligible for being reviewed in an expeditious fashion. Many IRBs have this capability. In the fifth scenario, the study is a bit more complex and describes plans for publication and therefore would require IRB approval. The sixth scenario again involves a quality assurance project, and as long as it will not be used for dissemination, IRB approval would not be required. The final scenario involves clinical prescribing practice, does not involve research, and therefore would not require IRB approval. (Roberts 2016) *Answers 5.29: D, D, D, B, A, D, D*

5.30

For each of the following descriptions, select the most relevant term in institutional review board (IRB) oversight of human research protocols. Each answer option may be used once, more than once, or not at all.

    A.   Adverse event.
    B.   Amendment.
    C.   Audit.
    D.   Assent.
    E.   Serious adverse event.

_____ Performing experimental procedure on the wrong arm of a study participant.

_____ Seeking prospective approval for a change in a protocol.

_____ Hospitalizing a study participant who experiences unexpected severe side effects of an experimental medication.

_____ Seeking affirmative agreement by a potential research subject to participate in a study.

_____ Reviewing research records, activities, personnel, or facilities to ensure compliance with professional standards.

_____ Reporting mild dizziness of an otherwise healthy participant who remains in a research study.

_____ Discovering evidence of significant bone marrow suppression in a research subject who has been exposed to a placebo administered in a protocol.

_____ Hospitalizing a schizophrenia study participant who experiences severe psychotic symptoms during a washout phase of a clinical trial.

_____ Examining documentation of policies and procedures after a participant has made a complaint about the conduct of a protocol by a researcher.

Potential research subjects assent to participate in a study by providing informed consent. An adverse event is any untoward occurrence in a subject, or any unfavorable or unintended sign, symptom, or disease in a subject, that is temporarily associated with the use of an investigational product, although this occurrence may not have a causal relationship with the product (ICH 2016). An adverse event that leads to a serious outcome, such as death, substantial risk of death, inpatient hospitalization or extension of existing hospitalization, disability or permanent damage, or congenital anomaly or birth defect, is a serious adverse event (21 CFR 312). Adverse events must be reported to the IRB if they represent unanticipated problems that may place subjects at greater risk than what was previously recognized (Office for Human Research Protections 2016).

If investigators wish to change any part of an approved study, they must submit an amendment to the IRB. The IRB must review and approve the amendment before the change is implemented. Protocol violations or deviations must be reported to the IRB. Protocol violations or deviations are considered noncompliance.

An audit is an independent examination of trial-related activities and document. An audit is conducted to verify data integrity and ensure that all protocol, regulatory requirements, and standard operating procedures are being followed. (ICH 2016) *Answers 5.30: E, B, E, D, C, A, E, E, C*

5.31

According to U.S. Department of Health and Human Services regulations, institutional review boards (IRBs) are required to include unaffiliated members as well as individuals with expertise, individuals who represent affiliate institutions, and others. This is to help ensure that community values are considered when evaluating the merit, safety, and safeguards related to human studies.

Which of the following individuals is best suited to serve as an unaffiliated representative on a medical school IRB?

A. The daughter of the chairman of the psychiatry department.
B. The husband of the medical school hospital chief executive officer.
C. The neighbor of an employee of the cancer center.
D. The owner of a sandwich shop that caters many medical school events.
E. The sister of the administrator for the surgery department.

All of the individuals listed have some kind of relationship with the medical school or its affiliated institutions, facilities, and offices. Of the individuals listed, the neighbor of the employee has the most remote connection and most properly may represent community perspectives. The neighbor does not appear to be dependent for his or her livelihood on the medical school, but this should be clarified before an appointment is made. Some kind of connection with the medical school is acceptable; however, the nature of the relationship must be evaluated to ensure that the community participation role may be fulfilled. (U.S. Department of Health and Human Services 2018) *Answer 5.31: C*

5.32

What principles, known as the 3Rs, guide the ethical conduct of animal research?

    A.   Ramifications, rationalization, recognition.
    B.   Recruiting, refining, remedying.
    C.   Replacing, reducing, refining.
    D.   Rejection, resolution, responsibility.
    E.   Renouncing, replacing, restricting.

Perspectives on animal research have evolved in recent years, and three main ethical principles currently pertain to scientific research using animals. First, *replacing* refers to finding alternative methods to using animals in research, such as computer models and tissue experiments. *Reducing* focuses on minimizing the use of animals in research by pursuing other avenues of experimental design. *Refining*, the third guideline, encompasses the improvement of research techniques to alleviate potential harm in experiments that do involve animals. (Mandal and Parija 2013) *Answer 5.32: C*

5.33

For each of the following research scenarios, select the Belmont principle that most substantively informs the research design.

    A.   Respect for persons.
    B.   Beneficence.
    C.   Justice.

_____ Studying a problem associated with healthy aging by engaging with a population of elders living independently in the community rather than in a residential program for cognitively impaired elders.

_____ Informing and seeking sound and voluntary decisions to participate in a research project rather than failing to inform and pressuring people to participate in a research project.

_____ Optimizing the knowledge and potentially helpful impact that derive from a research project.

Respect for persons is a broad concept that encompasses respect for autonomy plus a deep regard for the worth and dignity of all human beings. The protection of potentially vulnerable groups of people represents a key aspect of respect for persons and is embodied in specific ethical guidelines.

Beneficence refers to the belief that individuals should try to do good and to seek benefit for others. Beneficence encompasses the notion of *utility*, the duty to act in a way that provides the greatest positive consequences and the least negative consequences.

Justice is a moral principle that relates to treating people fairly and, in modern society, without prejudice. Justice addresses principles of fairness in recruitment and in distribution of knowledge gained in research. *Distributive justice* refers to equitable distribution of benefits and burdens among members of society. (National Commission for the Protection of Human Subjects of Biomedical and Behavioral Research 1979)
Answers 5.33: C, A, B

5.34

Which of the following describes a "minimal risk" benchmark as defined in U.S. human subjects regulations, such as the Common Rule?

A. A risk that is greater than those encountered in daily life activities.

B. A risk that is greater than those encountered in having knee replacement surgery.

C. A risk that is not greater than the risk of a mastectomy for a patient with breast cancer.

D. A risk that is not greater than the risk of having a broken bone set in a cast.

E. A risk that is not greater than the risk of routine medical or psychological tests or exams.

The Common Rule defines minimal risk as a risk that is not greater than "those ordinarily encountered in daily life or during the performance of routine physical or psychological examinations or tests." (45 CFR 46.102) *Answer 5.34: E*

5.35

For each of the following descriptions, select the correct term. Each answer option may be used once, more than once, or not at all.

- A. Data safety and monitoring board.
- B. Data use agreement.
- C. De-identification.
- D. Double-blinding.
- E. Randomization.
- F. Negligence.

_____ An agreement between institutions that allows for the sharing of research data.

_____ A committee that monitors data from human subjects in a protocol to protect the subjects from harm.

_____ A process to prevent human research subjects and researchers from discovering who is receiving an experimental treatment versus another treatment, such as a placebo.

_____ A committee that may recommend the discontinuation or alteration of a protocol based on concerns about participant welfare.

_____ A process to remove information, such as name or medical record number, which makes it possible to learn who provided data or a biological sample.

_____ A failure to follow appropriate standards in the conduct of research and resulting in direct harm.

Data safety monitoring boards represent an additional review activity to help ensure the safety of research participants. Data safety monitoring boards can prospectively or retrospectively evaluate trial procedures and data to determine whether participants are exposed to unexpected risks (Roberts 2016).

A data use agreement establishes the requirements and permitted uses for a limited data set shared between institutions. A limited data set is protected health information, and thus a data use agreement is required under the HIPAA Privacy Rule before data can be shared. De-identified data are no longer considered protected health information, as individual identifiers are removed, and thus their use is not restricted by the Privacy Rule. The Privacy Rule specifies two appropriate methods for deidentification. The first method is expert determination, under which an expert applies statistical and scientific principles to render the information nonidentifiable. The second method is safe harbor, under which 18 types of identifiers are removed, including all geographic information smaller than a state and all elements of dates except year, and there is no actual knowledge that the information could be used to identify an individual (Office for Civil Rights 2015).

A study is double-blind if neither the participants nor the researchers know who is receiving an experimental treatment and who is receiving another treatment. The blind may be broken in a medical emergency if it is necessary to identify the treatment that a participant is receiving to determine the appropriate medical response.

Negligence in the research situation refers to a failure to follow appropriate standards, resulting in direct harm to individual participants.
Answers 5.35: B, A, D, A, C, F

5.36

Human subjects regulations, referred to as the Common Rule, were recently updated. Which of the following was changed in the updated rules?

A.   Guidelines related to the definition of human research.
B.   Guidelines related to institutional review of education research.
C.   Guidelines related to nonliving persons.
D.   Guidelines related to research involving public records or media reports.
E.   Guidelines related to who may deem human research exempt.

The revisions to the Common Rule allow for education research to be handled differently in some circumstances than under the prior regulations (see 45 CFR 46.104[d][2] of the revised Common Rule). All of the other elements of the Common Rule listed here are substantively the same. The Common Rule and the revised Common Rule did not change the definition of human research. An institutional review board is allowed to deem human research exempt—this responsibility does not reside with other agents, such as investigators, in the process. Research related to nonliving persons, public records, and media reports do not meet the definition of human research and do not fall under the Common Rule regulations 45.CFR.46. (Office for Human Research Protections 2018) *Answer 5.36: B*

CHAPTER 6

ETHICS AND PROFESSIONALISM IN INTERACTIONS WITH COLLEAGUES AND TRAINEES

6.1

A psychologist working in a large medical center approaches a psychiatric colleague and asks for a prescription for something to help her sleep for a few weeks. She explains that she has been going through a tough divorce and repeatedly waking up very early in the morning, unable to return to sleep. She says that sleep deprivation is causing her to have problems concentrating and is making her irritable.

Which of the following is the most appropriate course of action for the psychiatrist?

A. Explain that a full evaluation would be best and offer a referral to a trusted colleague.

B. Offer sympathy but do not respond to the request for a prescription.

C. Offer to make an appointment to see her for medication management.

D. Prescribe a sedative-hypnotic to the psychologist for 2 weeks for situational insomnia.

E. Prescribe a 2-week supply of a sedative-hypnotic and refer her to a trusted colleague for therapy.

Every clinician will at some time encounter a situation similar to the one described in the vignette. The prevalence of this practice does not, however, mean that it is wise or ethical. A host of difficulties accompany treating colleagues, including the failure to conduct a full assessment and to make a reasonable diagnosis as well as the lack of adequate follow-up. This is especially true in mental health treatment because the personal, sensitive health information that is essential to diagnosis and treatment is less likely to be exchanged in the context of an overlapping relationship. Treating those too like us can also lead to overidentification with the patient-colleague, which impairs the clinical objectivity needed to provide good care. The safest and most responsible approach in these situations is to arrange a referral to a clinician not professionally or personally involved with the colleague. In the setting of a large medical center, making such a referral should not be difficult. (American Psychiatric Association 2001a; American Psychoanalytic Association 2008) *Answer 6.1: A*

6.2

Psychiatrists may be asked to help intervene with physician colleagues who have become impaired. Which of the following reasons to intervene is the most representative of the ethical foundation of a profession?

A. To avoid personal legal liability.
B. To defend the reputation of medical doctors.
C. To enhance the role of psychiatry in medical practice.
D. To protect patients from harm.
E. To strengthen the physician workforce.

An impaired clinician is defined as one whose condition may result in ineffective interventions and/or harm toward a patient (American Psychological Association 2006). Extreme stress may be a primary cause of distress and impairment in the health professions (Belitz 2020). Intervening when a physician colleague becomes impaired follows the ethical principle of nonmaleficence, protecting patients against harm that may result from the physician working with an impairment. *Answer 6.2: D*

6.3

On a busy night of call, a psychiatry intern rotating on a neurology service is asked by his senior resident to perform a lumbar puncture on a patient being worked up for meningitis. The intern's previous attempts at a lumbar puncture have been either unsuccessful or required multiple punctures. When the intern talks with the patient about the risks, benefits, and alternatives for the procedure, he describes his level of expertise and explains that the senior neurology resident will be present during the lumbar puncture to provide direction and take over if necessary.

Which of the following describes the intern's disclosure of his level of expertise?

A. Appropriate, because the patient has a right to be informed about the qualifications and experience of treatment providers.
B. Inappropriate, because it gives the patient an opportunity to refuse the procedure.
C. Inappropriate, because it is likely to increase the patient's anxiety about the procedure.
D. Inappropriate, because it may undermine the senior resident's authority in assigning the lumbar puncture to the intern.
E. Unnecessary, because patients in teaching hospitals should know that they will be treated by trainees.

The imperative for trainees to learn the art of medicine may conflict with their duty of beneficence and nonmaleficence toward their patients. At times, it may be in a patient's best interests to have a more capable individual perform a procedure rather than an inexperienced trainee. In such cases, the issue should be addressed openly with the patient as a demonstration of respect for the patient's autonomy.

In obtaining informed consent for the procedure, the trainee's level of expertise should be discussed with the patient. Procedural safeguards, such as the presence of a more senior clinician to direct and observe the trainee, should also be described. Many patients take pleasure in being helpful and in participating in the education of future doctors and specialists, and they may willingly consent. If a patient declines, a more senior resident should perform the lumbar puncture if possible. The mere fact that the patient has been admitted to a teaching facility does not mean that the patient has given up the right to be fully informed about the circumstances of treatment. (American Medical Association, Council on Ethical and Judicial Affairs 2002; Dubois et al. 2004; Hoop 2004; Lo 2020b; Santen et al. 2005) *Answer 6.3: A*

6.4

A junior faculty member in an academic department of psychiatry and behavioral medicine is told by a resident supervisee that a senior member of the faculty has been behaving erratically. The resident says that she suspects that the senior clinician has been abusing alcohol and that she believes his clinical judgment has been adversely affected. The faculty member has had little contact with his senior colleague, but he has no reason to question the resident's judgment. He encourages the resident to speak to her training director about her concerns. She refuses, saying that she fears retribution. Which of the following is the junior faculty member's next best course of action?

A. Discuss the matter with the senior colleague and then report it to the department chairman.
B. Do nothing for now, but plan to take action if another resident complains.
C. Encourage the resident to be more assertive in her professional interactions.
D. Inform the training director that the residents are having problems with the senior colleague.
E. Leave an anonymous note in the senior colleague's mailbox informing him that his abuse of alcohol has become a matter of public discussion and urging him to seek appropriate help.

Determining when and how to report suspected impairment in a colleague is often extremely difficult for physicians, and it becomes especially tricky if the colleague is in a position of power over the person who believes that impairment may be an issue. In this case, because the resident believes the senior colleague's clinical judgment is affected, the safety of patients is at stake and immediate action must be taken. By speaking to the senior colleague directly about the concern and then reporting it to the department chairman, the junior faculty member will fulfill his ethical duties to expose impaired colleagues and to deal honestly with other doctors. (Belitz 2020) *Answer 6.4: A*

6.5

A psychiatrist serves as an associate dean of a medical school and is asked by the dean to provide an impression of the mental health of a faculty member based on interactions in a recent committee meeting.

Which of the following responses is the most appropriate next step for the associate dean to take?

A. Decline to offer a psychiatric opinion but try to clarify the dean's concern.

B. Give a psychiatric impression based on the limited observation at the recent meeting.
C. Offer to assess the colleague more closely at an upcoming committee meeting.
D. Refer the faculty member to a psychiatrist for an evaluation.
E. State the relevant DSM criteria for the dean to draw his own conclusion.

A psychiatrist should not evaluate someone outside of a physician-patient relationship. If a physician-patient relationship exists, the psychiatrist should not disclose any information about the patient unless obligated to do so by law or unless the patient has given prior authorization. The APA's *Principles of Medical Ethics With Annotations Especially Applicable to Psychiatry* state that "A physician shall respect the rights of patients, colleagues, and other health professionals, and shall safeguard patient confidences and privacy within the constraints of the law" (American Psychiatric Association 2010, p. 6). In the case of an impaired or unethical colleague, the psychiatrist has an obligation to intervene (Belitz 2020). Misconduct must be reported in adherence with local laws and institutional and professional codes of conduct. *Answer 6.5: A*

6.6

For each of the following statements, select the most appropriate term. Each answer option may be used once, more than once, or not at all.

A. Disclosure of conflicting interests.
B. Committee oversight of professionals with potential conflicting interests.
C. Rules to protect against large financial conflicts of interest.
D. Separation of conflicting roles to protect patient interests.

_____ An institution does not permit its employed physicians from accepting paid consulting roles with outside commercial entities.
_____ An institution allows its employed physicians to accept paid consulting roles with outside commercial entities so long as the total amount of pay received is less than $15,000.
_____ An institution allows its employed physicians to accept paid consulting roles with outside commercial entities so long as the consultation does not relate to patient care activities.

Physicians have an obligation to place the welfare of their patients above their obligations to others (Roberts 2016). To protect patients' interests, institutions may prohibit physicians from occupying conflicting roles with industry. A paid consulting role with an outside commercial entity represents a conflict of interest that may negatively impact patient care. Relationships with industry can alter physicians' behavior (Appelbaum and Gold 2010) and safeguards are essential to protect the integrity of individuals and their institutions. (Roberts 2016) *Answers 6.6: D, C, D*

6.7

Which of the following should third-year medical student Angela Jones be introduced as by her attending psychiatrist to patients?

    A.   Angela.
    B.   Clinical Clerk Jones.
    C.   Doctor Jones.
    D.   Medical student Jones.
    E.   Student-psychiatrist Jones.

Patients are entitled to know the identity of those who provide care to them, and so medical students should be introduced accurately. Misrepresenting the role of a health care provider undermines trust and may lead to a patient feeling betrayed. In addition, informed consent requires physicians to disclose pertinent information to patients, and the qualifications of personnel who provide care is pertinent to a patient's decisions. Unfamiliar titles such as "clinical clerk," although factually accurate, should be avoided, because they are not meaningful to most patients. The titles "student doctor" and "student physician" are clearly preferable to "doctor" but are considered by some to be less appropriate than the more common label of "medical student." Students, faculty, and administrators routinely describe individuals at this level of training as medical students when talking among themselves. Using a different descriptor only when introducing students to patients is unnecessary and may mislead patients into thinking that the student is at a more advanced level of training. (Lo 2020b) *Answer 6.7: D*

6.8

A first-year psychiatric resident has received above-average clinical evaluations and has scored in the ninetieth percentile on his in-house training examination. However, two administrative assistants inform the training director that the resident has been rude and demanding in his dealings with them.

Which of the following is the most appropriate response for the training director?

A.   Ask the chief resident to tell all the residents to behave cordially with staff.

B.   Do not act on the comments, because the resident's strong academic and clinical performance should outweigh minor problems with staff.

C.   Meet with the resident to discuss the administrative staff's concerns.

D.   Reprimand the resident for his inappropriate behavior.

E.   Tell the administrative assistants that they should not have unrealistic expectations about the behavior of hard-working trainees.

As a matter of professionalism, residents must be capable of maintaining good working relationships, and not only with attending physicians and patients. The quality of a resident's interactions with staff and with peers also demonstrates his or her professionalism, communication, and interpersonal skills. For this reason, the Accreditation Council for Graduate Medical Education expects residents to be evaluated for competency in these areas by someone other than their supervising attending physicians. Training directors should therefore take seriously any concerns expressed by staff about residents. The appropriate first step is to discuss the situation with the resident. Reprimands should be reserved for continued egregious behavior. (Accreditation Council for Graduate Medical Education 2020) *Answer 6.8: C*

6.9

For each of the following dual roles, select the most appropriate description. Each answer option may be used once, more than once, or not at all.

A.   No inherent ethical conflicts; no special or additional safeguards necessary to protect patient interests because of the dual role.

B.   Some inherent ethical conflicts possible; special or additional safeguards may be necessary to protect patient interests because of the dual role.

C. Some inherent ethical conflicts very likely; special and additional safeguards may be necessary to protect patient interests because of the dual role.

D. Always inherent ethical conflicts; special and additional safeguards always necessary to protect patient interests because of the dual role.

_____ Providing care as a psychiatrist and also volunteering at the local pet shelter.

_____ Providing care as a psychiatrist and splitting fees with the psychotherapist to whom patients are referred.

_____ Providing care as a psychiatrist and living in the community with a patient.

_____ Providing care as a psychiatrist and owning a significant stake in the local mental health clinic where patients receive care.

_____ Providing care as a psychiatrist and taking a weekly Zumba class at the local YMCA with patients.

_____ Providing care as a psychiatrist and purchasing fuel with a "friends and family" discount from a patient who owns the local gas station.

_____ Providing care as a psychiatrist and going out on a date with the patient.

_____ Providing care as a psychiatrist and serving as an unpaid advisor for medical students at a university hospital in another state.

_____ Providing care as a psychiatrist and promoting the sale of a new herbal remedy made by a company owned by the psychiatrist.

_____ Providing care as a psychiatrist and fundraising for a national mental health charity.

Mental health professionals inhabit multiple roles professionally and within the community. "The intense, intimate, and asymmetrical nature of the psychotherapeutic relationship renders patients vulnerable to exploitation and, for this reason, psychiatrists must act with strictest professionalism to assure that patient well-being is placed above all other interests that may exist in psychiatrist-patient interactions" (Roberts 2006, p. 772).

Volunteering at a local pet shelter, attending a weekly Zumba class, and living in the community do not represent inherent ethical conflicts. Serving as an unpaid advisor for medical students also does not represent an inherent ethical conflict. Owning a stake in the local mental health clinic or fundraising for a national mental health charity may require

additional safeguards, as these roles could impact patient care or conflict with patient interests depending on the situation. Fee splitting, promoting the sale of a product made by one's company, and accepting a
discount from a patient on a personal service represent obvious ethical
conflicts, as the mental health professional's financial interests conflict
with the interests of patients. Dating a patient is also an obvious ethical
conflict. As stated in the APA's *Principles of Medical Ethics With Annotations Especially Applicable to Psychiatry*, "the necessary intensity of the
treatment relationship may tend to activate sexual and other needs and
fantasies on the part of both patient and psychiatrist, while weakening
the objectivity necessary for control" (American Psychiatric Association
2010, p. 4). Mental health professionals must uphold the standards of professionalism and act accordingly. *Answers 6.9: A, D, A, C, A, D, D, A, D, C*

6.10

A patient with new-onset schizophrenia is hospitalized at an academic
center. After noticing that the patient has unusual facial features, nasal
speech, and an abnormal blood calcium level, the psychiatrist orders a
chromosome analysis for 22q deletion syndrome (velocardiofacial syndrome). Although the patient and family consent to testing, the patient's
nurse refuses to draw blood for the order, saying that it is unethical to
participate in the genetic testing of psychiatric patients.

Which of the following is the appropriate next step for the psychiatrist
to handle the conflict with the nurse in an ethically sensitive manner?

A. Ask the patient's family to assure the nurse that they want testing.
B. Discontinue the order after reconsidering the ethical implications
   of genetic testing.
C. Meet with the nurse to hear her concerns and to explain why ge-
   netic testing is beneficial in this case.
D. Order the test on a day when the nurse is not present.
E. Recommend that the nurse be reprimanded for failing in her
   ethical duty to follow the physician's orders.

Nurses, like physicians, have professional duties to their patients. Genetic testing is highly controversial in psychiatry, and the nurse's opinion
in this case is not uncommon. However, because 22q deletion syndrome
may be associated with treatable cardiac and endocrine defects, this diagnostic test is potentially therapeutically beneficial and likely carries few
risks. Unlike predictive or susceptibility testing, diagnostic genetic testing

in a patient already known to have a chronic and potentially disabling condition, such as schizophrenia, may be less likely to increase the risk of insurance or employment discrimination. Patients and families may still suffer psychological distress as a result of the genetic testing, however, and this must be recognized and addressed. A reasonable first step toward resolving the conflict with the nurse would be to meet with the nurse to hear her concerns and to explain the physician's reasoning about the risks and benefits to the patient. (American Nurses Association, Center for Ethics and Human Rights 2015; Burke et al. 2001) *Answer 6.10: C*

6.11

An attending psychiatrist has been working closely with a third-year resident on a clinical service for the past month. The attending psychiatrist has begun to feel a sexual attraction to the resident but has not acted on it. After a particularly busy day, the resident flirtatiously asks the attending psychiatrist to go out for drinks and dinner. The prospect of spending the evening in the resident's company is extremely appealing to the attending psychiatrist.

Which of the following is the attending psychiatrist's most appropriate response to this situation?

A. Accept the invitation without ethical concerns because the interest is clearly mutual and between consenting adults.
B. Accept the invitation and limit professional boundary issues by informing the resident that they must not talk about patients during their evening together.
C. Accept the invitation and limit the appearance of impropriety by informing the resident that the encounter must be kept secret from other residents and faculty.
D. Decline the invitation.
E. Decline the invitation and immediately report the resident's unprofessional behavior to the program director.

Residents and faculty are human beings who, on occasion, may find themselves attracted to one another. However, the relationship between a student or resident and a supervisor is an asymmetrical one, in which the supervisor has power over the trainee. In such relationships, issues of trust, transference, and countertransference arise that are not unlike, although not precisely duplicating, those in a doctor-patient relationship. Nonprofessional relationships between trainees and supervisors may cause numerous problems. Other trainees may feel that the peer in the relationship with a supervisor receives preferential treatment. The supervisor may find it difficult to assess the work of the trainee objectively. If the relationship ends, the trainee may feel subjected to a hostile work environment. For all these reasons, such relationships are best avoided entirely or at least pursued after the supervisor-trainee relationship has terminated. If the attraction is strong and interferes with the professional relationship, the faculty member should consider seeking consultation and supervision. Although the resident in this case attempted to initiate the relationship, the faculty member is still responsible for maintaining professional roles because of his position of power and authority. (American Medical Association 2016; American Psychiatric Association 2010) *Answer 6.11: D*

6.12

A psychiatry resident on a consultation-liaison rotation is asked to determine who should be the proper alternative decision-maker for a patient who has sustained a massive stroke and is on life support. The patient did not leave an advance directive designating a substitute decision-maker. There are two adult children involved, and each has a different set of end-of-life preferences for their father.

Which of the following professionals should the resident consult with first about this difficult case?

A. The chairman of the hospital ethics committee.
B. The chairman of the institutional review board.
C. The hospital attorney.
D. The hospital risk manager.
E. The supervisor/attending psychiatrist.

Trainees should consult with their attending supervisors frequently, especially in ethically problematic or high-risk situations such as this one. Because the attending psychiatrist has the responsibility of oversight on clinical cases, the resident has a duty to keep him or her informed and to be open and truthful about the circumstances of the case, even though it may lead to disagreements about appropriate care. Factors the resident and attending psychiatrist should consider when making a recommendation for an alternative decision-maker in this case include the maturity of the two adult children and the familiarity of each with their father's likely wishes regarding medical care. (Roberts 2016) *Answer 6.12: E*

6.13

A medical student applying for residency training waived his right to review his letters of recommendation from medical school faculty members. After he was accepted into a hospital residency training program, the training director placed all the application materials, including the letters of recommendation, into the new resident's permanent file. A year later, the resident requests to examine his permanent file.

Which of the following best describes what actions the training director should take?

    A. Explain to the resident that he is not allowed to see certain parts of the file.
    B. Permit the resident to examine the entire file.
    C. Photocopy the file for the resident, but do not include the letters.
    D. Remove any letters of recommendation before showing the resident the file.
    E. Require that the files be viewed with staff present.

A student's waiver of the right to review a letter of recommendation is designed to protect the confidentiality of the letter writer, so that the writer can freely describe the applicant's weaknesses as well as strengths. To fully protect the letter writers, once the letters have served their purpose (i.e., helped determine whether a student should gain admittance to a training program), the letters should be destroyed. By law, an accepted resident has the right to review his entire training file, and the training director thus may not restrict access to it. (Association of American Medical Colleges 2015) *Answer 6.13: B*

6.14

For each of the following scenarios, select the most appropriate ethical characterization based on standards of professionalism and management of the competing obligations of dual roles. Each answer option may be used once, more than once, or not at all.

    A. Ethically acceptable.
    B. Ethically problematic.
    C. Ethically unacceptable.

_____ A residency program director participating in a local community drive to register voters.

_____ A residency program director participating in a local community drive to register voters sponsored by his synagogue or church.

_____ A residency program director requiring his trainees to participate in a local community drive to register voters sponsored by his church or synagogue to fulfill a "community engagement" obligation prior to graduating residency.

_____ A residency program director serving on a graduate medical education accreditation committee that evaluates programs at a competing medical school in the same geographical area.

_____ A residency program director providing psychiatric care to his own trainees in the context of a large mental health clinic with many clinical providers.

_____ A residency program director becoming close personal friends with one of his trainees.

_____ A residency program director becoming close personal friends with one of his former trainees.

Participating in a local community drive does not represent an unethical conflict of interest, but it would be unethical to require trainees to participate. The resident must respect the rights of trainees, especially given the unequal nature of the relationship (American Psychiatric Association 2010). Whereas it is acceptable to become close personal friends with a former trainee, developing a similar relationship with a current trainee is ethically unacceptable. A residency program director providing psychiatric care to his own trainees represents a serious conflict of interest and is ethically unacceptable when many clinical providers are available to provide psychiatric care. These same obligations extend to psychologists. According to the American Psychological Association's *Ethical Principles of Psychologists and Code of Conduct*, a multiple relationship or dual role is considered unethical if it "could reasonably be expected to impair the psychologist's objectivity, competence, or effectiveness in performing his or her functions as a psychologist, or otherwise risks exploitation or harm to the person with whom the professional relationship exists" (American Psychological Association 2017, Section 3.05). *Answers 6.14: A, A, C, B, C, C, A*

6.15

A psychiatry faculty member notices that a psychiatric intern is moving slowly and not talking very much. During a private moment, the attending psychiatrist expresses concern to the intern, and the intern says that he is extremely depressed but that he has seen a physician and has started taking antidepressants. Over the next few weeks the intern shows no sign of improvement, and when the faculty member inquires again, the intern says he is beginning to feel suicidal, but he hasn't told his treating physician. The faculty member urges him to notify his physician. The intern refuses.

What is the psychiatrist's best course of action?

A. Ask the other interns to offer the ill colleague their emotional support.
B. Call the state board of medical examiners and report the intern as an impaired physician.
C. Encourage the intern to talk with the residency training director about the problem, and accompany the intern to the residency training director's office.
D. Find the name of the intern's physician in his medical records and notify the physician that the intern is becoming suicidal.
E. Suggest the intern increase his antidepressant dosage.

It appears that the faculty member has done everything reasonable to encourage the intern to disclose the very serious nature of his symptoms to his physician. Because the intern cannot bring himself to disclose his suicidality and he is getting worse, the faculty member is ethically obligated to act on his behalf. Of the options presented, encouraging him to talk with the training director is most respectful of the intern's privacy, and it allows the faculty member to avoid overstepping his role as the intern's colleague while getting the information to someone with the authority to discreetly intervene. *Answer 6.15: C*

6.16

Several psychiatry residents want to organize a mental health educational fair for medical students, but they have no funds for the project. A pharmaceutical company offers to fully sponsor the fair if it is allowed to advertise its medications by distributing sales literature and hanging banners.

Which of the following is the residents' most ethically conservative course of action?

A. Accept the offer only if other pharmaceutical companies are also allowed to advertise.

B.   Accept the offer only if the pharmaceutical company agrees not to distribute the sales literature.
C.   Accept the offer only if the pharmaceutical company agrees not to hang the banners.
D.   Refuse the offer and negotiate better terms with another pharmaceutical company.
E.   Refuse the offer and have a bake sale to fund the fair.

The appropriate role of the pharmaceutical industry in sponsoring medical education events is a matter of intense contemporary ethical debate. In this case, the most ethically conservative response would be to give the pharmaceutical company no part in the fair and to identify other means of generating funds that do not carry the same possibility of a conflict of interest. A much less conservative view would be to argue that it would be acceptable to have industry funding and product advertising if other companies were also allowed to advertise, but many academic psychiatrists would see this option as merely greater commercialization of the event. A more pragmatic, middle-ground approach would be to allow the company to provide an unrestricted educational grant to fund the event without allowing advertising of specific products. (American Medical Association, Council on Ethical and Judicial Affairs 2005; Snyder Sulmasy et al. 2019) *Answer 6.16: E*

6.17

A psychiatrist working in a university mental health clinic has been treating a 45-year-old used car salesman for bipolar disorder and cocaine dependence. The patient presents for follow-up reporting excruciating new-onset back pain and difficulty walking. The psychiatrist refers him to the university's urgent primary care clinic. The patient returns to the psychiatrist's office 4 hours later, saying that the primary care physician treated him skeptically after he told her of his history of drug abuse. The doctor refused to prescribe pain medications or to order an X-ray or MRI of his back and suggested he should just "tough it out."
   Which of the following is the psychiatrist's most appropriate ethical course of action?

A.   Advise the patient of his right to sue the physician for malpractice.
B.   Call the chief of staff and report the physician for unethical behavior.
C.   Call the hospital ethics committee for an emergency consult.

D. Call the primary care physician and request further medical work-up.

E. Treat the back injury to the best of the psychiatrist's ability.

Psychiatrists have an important role to play in educating their medical colleagues about the appropriate treatment of so-called difficult or stigmatized patients, whose clinical needs are often dismissed more readily than those of other patients. Advising the patient to sue the colleague is unprofessional and distracts from the immediate goal of providing for the clinical needs of the patient. The psychiatrist should not treat the patient's back pain himself, because this most likely departs from his scope of practice and could place the patient at risk for substandard care. Calling the urgent care physician and explaining the reasons for requesting a medical work-up, and in the process providing education about addiction, may accomplish both the goal of getting good care for the patient and the goal of helping the physician rethink her attitude toward such patients. (American Medical Association, Council on Ethical and Judicial Affairs 2005) *Answer 6.17: D*

6.18

For each of the following scenarios, select the most appropriate ethical characterization based on standards of professionalism and management of the competing obligations of dual roles. Each answer option may be used once, more than once, or not at all.

A. Ethically acceptable.
B. Ethically problematic.
C. Ethically unacceptable.

_____ A fellowship program director recommending personal psychotherapy to his trainees with therapists in the community.

_____ A fellowship program director referring his trainees for personal psychotherapy in his own private practice clinic in the community.

_____ A fellowship program director requiring his trainees engage in personal psychotherapy with his wife who is a therapist in the community.

_____ A fellowship program director providing expertise in the development of institutional policies related to physician wellness at the training institution.

_____ A fellowship program director providing expertise in the development of institutional programs related to physician wellness at the training institution.

_____ A fellowship program director providing clinical care to trainees outside of his department in the context of an institutional physician well-being program.

_____ A fellowship program director providing clinical care to trainees from his department in the context of a large institutional physician well-being program with multiple providers.

A training program director may recommend treatment and may, in some circumstances (e.g., suspected or demonstrated impairment or mental health or substance-related condition placing the trainee at risk for impairment), require treatment. The training program director should not make referrals that result in personal financial gain. The training program director should not provide psychiatric or mental health treatment to individuals in the training program because of overlapping role problems. A training program director may offer expertise to assist in the development or ongoing implementation of a mental health program. These same concepts apply to psychologists. The American Psychological Association's *Ethical Principles of Psychologists and Code of Conduct* state, "When individual or group therapy is a program or course requirement, psychologists responsible for that program [must] allow students in undergraduate and graduate programs the option of selecting such therapy from practitioners unaffiliated with the program" and, furthermore, "faculty who are or are likely to be responsible for evaluating students' academic performance [must] not themselves provide that therapy" (American Psychological Association 2017, Standard 7.05). See 6.14. *Answers 6.18: A, C, C, A, A, B, C*

6.19

A psychiatry resident working with a highly critical psychotherapy supervisor begins fabricating his psychotherapy process notes. The resident feels guilty but believes the only way to obtain an acceptable evaluation from the supervisor is to pretend that the resident is an astute therapist who rarely makes mistakes.

Which ethical principle does the resident's action violate?

A. Confidentiality.
B. Fidelity.

   C.   Justice.
   D.   Respect for autonomy.
   E.   Veracity.

Residents who fabricate process notes have been reported in the psychiatric literature, and this practice may not be a rare occurrence. Deceiving a difficult supervisor may give an embattled resident a feeling of control or an insecure resident a means to avoid shameful feelings of inadequacy. As an ethical matter, the practice is a grievous violation of the principle of veracity, or truth telling. Physicians have a professional obligation to tell the truth not just to patients but also to supervisors, colleagues, insurance companies, administrators, and all other professional contacts. By lying to his supervisor, the resident directly harms his supervisor, who may be the attending physician of record on the case and who needs accurate information to fulfill his duty in that role. The deception also harms the patient by preventing the individual from receiving care that is informed by the experience of the more senior colleague. (Hantoot 2000; Hoop 2004) *Answer 6.19: E*

6.20

A resident with deficiencies in his clinical performance contemplates transferring to another residency program. The resident asks a faculty member for a letter of recommendation to the training director of the other program. The faculty member has been a mentor of the resident, and he is well aware of the resident's performance difficulties. Which of the following is the faculty member's most ethically rigorous action?

   A.   Agree to write the letter and do not include any negative information.
   B.   Agree to write the letter and do not include any negative information, but communicate that information to the residency director off the record.
   C.   Agree to write the letter, but first talk to the resident about the negative information the letter would contain.
   D.   Decline to write the letter, saying that it is against the faculty member's general policy to write letters of recommendation.
   E.   Decline to write the letter without giving a reason.

Physicians are often reluctant to divulge information to third parties that may be harmful to a colleague's career. However, the medical profession's social contract includes the requirement for self-regulation, and thus there is an obligation to communicate accurately about trainees and colleagues. A useful recommendation letter would describe the resident's weaknesses as well as strengths. To fulfill the ethical duty of veracity, the faculty member should inform the resident of his assessment before writing the letter. This demonstrates the faculty member's commitment to honesty, facilitates the resident's self-perception, and gives the resident an opportunity to withdraw the request for the letter. (Layde and Roberts 2020) *Answer 6.20: C*

6.21

A faculty member invites a medical student to participate in writing an invited review paper. The student researches the material and writes several drafts. The faculty member reviews the student's final version, makes a few minor grammatical and formatting changes, and submits the paper for publication. The faculty member informs the student that because he was asked to write the paper, the faculty member will be the first author.

Which of the following best describes this situation?

A. The faculty member is correct in placing his name first because faculty members are ultimately responsible for the integrity of their publications.

B. The faculty member is correct in placing his name first because it is standard for an invited paper to name the invited author first.

C. The student has an ethical duty to insist on first authorship.

D. The student should consider herself fortunate to be included on a paper in any authorship category.

E. The student should receive first author credit.

Honesty about the significance of the contribution is the principle governing the order of authorship. The first author of a publication is expected to have made a significant contribution to the paper, and in this case, the medical student's contribution far overshadows that of the faculty member. In addition, it is part of the faculty member's fiduciary relationship as a teacher and mentor not to exploit his position of power over residents and students. Given the asymmetrical relationship with faculty, it is often not realistic to expect students and residents to make demands or even advocate for rightful recognition. (Committee on Publication Ethics 2019; Roberts 2017) *Answer 6.21: E*

6.22

A psychologist has been treating a female patient for depression. During the course of psychotherapy, the patient reveals that she had sexual relations with a prior therapist. Which of the following is the psychologist's most appropriate immediate response to this revelation?

    A.   Allow the patient to continue to tell her story without pressuring her to act.

    B.   Encourage the patient to report the incident to a professional ethics committee.

    C.   Encourage the patient to report the incident to the state licensing board.

    D.   Offer to contact the prior therapist and confront him on the patient's behalf.

    E.   Question the patient gently but firmly to establish the identity of the prior therapist.

As a member of a profession charged with self-regulation, the psychologist has a duty to help identify colleagues who behave unethically. However, in this case, that duty does not outweigh the responsibility to be clinically helpful to this patient. At some point, it may be therapeutic for this patient to take action, such as reporting her prior therapist to the state licensing board or professional ethics committee. However, the psychologist should not push the patient to do anything before the patient is prepared to do so. In addition, taking matters into the psychologist's own hands may also have detrimental effects on the patient. When and if the patient is ready to proceed, options for reporting should be explained. Some states have criminalized therapists' sexual relationships with patients and have codified the response that subsequent treating therapists should follow. (American Psychiatric Association 2010) *Answer 6.22: A*

6.23

For each of the following scenarios, select the most appropriate ethical characterization based on standards of professionalism. Each answer option may be used once, more than once, or not at all.

    A.   Ethically acceptable.

    B.   Ethically problematic.

    C.   Ethically unacceptable.

____ A department chair setting compensation higher for faculty members with multiple dependents.

____ A department chair setting compensation higher for faculty members with additional professional duties that have accumulated with more years of service in the department.

____ A department chair setting compensation higher for faculty members with additional subspecialty fellowship training.

____ A department chair setting compensation higher for faculty members in whom he has the greatest confidence that they will "do a great job."

Salary equity refers to the ability of employees to "earn and be paid similar compensation for comparable work, given shared qualifications— regardless of differences in individual characteristics such as gender, race, age, sexual orientation, religion, and disability" (Association of American Medical Colleges 2019, p. 6). Pay raises may be based on productivity, performance reviews, length of time at an institution, or negotiations (Association of American Medical Colleges 2019). Salary equity is a moral imperative. *Answers 6.23: C, A, A, B*

6.24

A patient is brought to the emergency department after being injured when his tractor toppled over in a rocky farm field. The patient, although weak, is lucid and rational. He refuses a transfusion, stating that he is a Jehovah's Witness. The hospital chaplain confirms that the patient's refusal of the transfusion is consistent with the religious beliefs of his denomination. The psychiatry fellow is consulted to assess the patient's decisional capacity. He informs the emergency medicine attending physician that the patient is capable of making the decision to refuse the transfusion and that the patient accepts the risk that he may die as a result. The emergency medicine attending physician understands but states that he will proceed with the transfusion because his own values do not permit him to allow the patient to die needlessly.

Which of the following is the psychiatry fellow's most appropriate ethical response?

A. Call an elder of the Jehovah's Witness church to talk to the attending physician about his religion's values and beliefs.

B. Call security to keep the attending physician from performing the transfusion.

C. Call the chief of emergency medicine to ask him to overrule the attending physician.

D.   Call the hospital attorney to ask about the hospital's liability in the situation.

E.   Call the hospital ethics committee for an emergency consultation.

Ethics committees are available in almost every hospital precisely to help resolve ethical dilemmas such as that described in this case. Conflicts among staff members about the care of a patient are one of the primary problems ethics committee members are trained to resolve. Calling security would likely cause a tense situation to become even more conflictual. Consulting the hospital attorney might be somewhat useful, but it is not as likely to provide a mediated resolution as would consulting the ethics committee. Representatives from a distinct religious community are often willing to come to a hospital to provide emergency counseling and education, but it is unlikely that this would persuade this attending physician because the hospital chaplain has already been involved. The chief of emergency medicine would likely transfer the patient to another physician willing to respect the patient's wishes, yet this still is a unilateral solution. The optimal approach is to contact the ethics committee members on call to educate the attending about the issue of treatment refusal and to work out a solution that balances the need to respect a competent patient's preferences regarding medical care with the physician's mandate to preserve life. The understanding that surgery will proceed without transfusion or with the use of a blood substitute might offer such a balance. (Gutheil and Appelbaum 2019; Roberts 2016) *Answer 6.24: E*

6.25

Which of the following should third-year psychiatry resident Bob Smith be introduced as to patients?

A.   Doctor Smith.
B.   Mister Smith.
C.   Psychiatrist Smith.
D.   Student doctor Smith.
E.   Student-psychiatrist Smith.

Bob Smith has completed medical school and is a licensed physician, so he can correctly be introduced as Dr. Smith. To be clear about their roles, the attending physician may also wish to specify that Dr. Smith is in his third year of specialty training in psychiatry. For patients to be fully informed about their treatment, they need to be informed about the level of training of their clinicians. Because many patients are unfamiliar with the medical education process, terms such as *resident* and *intern* may not have a precise meaning to patients and should be explained. (Santen et al. 2004) *Answer 6.25: A*

6.26

The senior resident on an inpatient psychiatry unit asks a third-year medical student if he would mind picking up the resident's laundry. The resident apologizes for making the request and explains that because he is on call he will not be able to get his laundry before the dry cleaner closes for the weekend. The medical student cheerfully says, "Your wish is my command, sir!" and embarks on the errand.

Which of the following describes this request of the medical student?

A. Acceptable because the student is obviously willing to help out this way.
B. Acceptable if the resident offers to mention the "team spirit" shown by the student when writing an evaluation.
C. An inappropriate use of power by the resident.
D. An inappropriate use of power only if the medical student voices a complaint.
E. Unconventional but acceptable given the resident's demanding work schedule.

This request is not an appropriate use of the medical student's time. The resident is failing to fulfill his duties as a teacher and exploiting his position as a supervisor. By sending the student off the unit to perform a personal errand, the resident prevents the medical student from learning psychiatry through clinical work, but the primary ethical problem is that he asks the medical student to perform the resident's personal bidding outside the bounds of professional duty. Offering to mention the medical student's team spirit when writing the evaluation is a subtle form of coercion, because the medical student is likely dependent on the resident for an evaluation as well as for the quality of his day-to-day life on the rotation. The fact that the medical student cheerfully agrees to the request does not mean that the medical student does not feel coerced, and it does not make the resident's behavior more acceptable. (Plaut and Baker 2011) *Answer 6.26: C*

6.27

For each of the following scenarios, select the most appropriate ethical characterization based on standards of professionalism and management of the competing obligations of dual roles. Each answer option may be used once, more than once, or not at all.

    A.   Ethically acceptable.
    B.   Ethically problematic.
    C.   Ethically unacceptable.

    ____   A faculty member serving as a peer reviewer on a manuscript submission by an author whose work is unknown to her but falls within the reviewer's scope of expertise.

    ____   A faculty member serving as a peer reviewer on a manuscript submission by an author whose work is well known to her and falls within the reviewer's scope of expertise.

    ____   A faculty member serving as a peer reviewer on a manuscript submission by an author who is a close personal friend and whose work falls outside the reviewer's scope of expertise.

The integrity of the peer reviewer process relies on the ethical participation of expert reviewers. The Committee on Publication Ethics has clear guidance regarding ethical peer review (Committee on Publication Ethics 2017). Simply put, peer reviewers should not agree to review manuscripts when they do not have sufficient expertise or for which they have a clear conflict of interest. Peer reviewers should notify the journal if a competing interest arises or is discovered that may prevent the completion of an unbiased review. Peer reviewers should not review manuscripts for which they lack the appropriate expertise. Peer reviewers should not agree to review manuscripts authored by "recent (e.g., within the past 3 years) mentors, mentees, close collaborators or joint grant holders" or by authors employed at the reviewer's same institution (Committee on Publication Ethics 2017, p. 3). Peer reviewers should also not agree to review manuscripts that are similar to the reviewer's own unpublished works in preparation. *Answers 6.27: A, A, C*

6.28

For each of the following descriptions, select the most appropriate term. Each answer option may be used once, more than once, or not at all.

A. Bias.
B. Discrimination.
C. Harassment.
D. Inequity.

____ Lack of fairness or justice
____ Inclination or prejudice for or against some thing
____ Unjust or prejudicial treatment of one category of person
____ Aggression, intimidation, or pressure
____ Men paid more than women for equal work
____ A man paid more than a woman for equal work in the same setting at the same institution
____ Implicit or explicit view that a white medical student is more qualified than medical students of other racial backgrounds
____ Implicit or explicit view that female medical students are less qualified than male medical students
____ Male residents being offered more professional opportunities than female residents because of concern that female residents will have more parenting responsibilities and lose time away from work

Discrimination is defined as the intentional unjust treatment of individuals on the basis of some actual or perceived characteristic. *Bias* is defined as an inclination or prejudice for or against something (see Chapman et al. 2013; Sue et al. 2007). *Harassment* is unwelcome conduct on the basis of some characteristic that may create an intimidating, hostile, or abusive work environment (U.S. Equal Employment Opportunity Commission 2020a). *Inequity* is a lack of fairness or justice. *Answers 6.28: D, A, B, C, D, B, A, A, B*

6.29

For each of the following scenarios, indicate whether the situation represents an ethically justifiable use of confidential information in the educational/academic setting. Each answer option may be used once, more than once, or not at all.

A. Justifiable.
B. Not justifiable.

____ Without obtaining the patient's consent, a senior psychiatry resident publishes a psychotherapy case report that includes identifiable details about the patient.

_____ A psychiatric resident discusses a case with her supervisor without disguising identifying details about the patient.

_____ A faculty psychologist shows a carefully edited videotape of a former patient at a small, closed professional meeting after having obtained written informed consent from the patient.

_____ A well-known academic psychiatrist asks a long-term and highly dependent psychotherapy patient to make media appearances to help promote the psychiatrist's new book.

An ethical tension exists between the duty to protect patient confidentiality and the need to discuss cases with other psychiatrists in academic settings. If such a discussion occurs in the context of obtaining supervision or consultation to provide a patient with better care, it is clearly ethically justifiable. The situation is less straightforward if a patient's confidentiality is breached because a physician writes or speaks publicly about a case to advance the field of psychiatry and/or his or her own career. Clear and uniform ethical guidelines for the scientific publication of patient material have not been established. At a minimum, patients should be given the opportunity to consent or to refuse, and ideally the identifying details of the case should be thoroughly disguised. Voluntariness, one of the requisite features of informed consent, may not be possible in some cases—such as in the example of a highly dependent therapy patient who is asked to surrender privacy to help promote the psychiatrist's career. (Roberts 2016; U.S. Department of Health and Human Services 2013) *Answers 6.29: B, A, A, B*

6.30

The sister of the chairman of internal medicine at an academic medical center requires inpatient psychiatric hospitalization. After she has been in the hospital for 2 days, the chairman of internal medicine pages the psychiatric resident in charge of the case and angrily asks why he was not informed that his sister had been hospitalized. He demands to be told about her clinical condition. The patient is catatonic and cannot give consent to allow the resident to speak to others about her medical situation.

Consulting with which of the following individuals is the most appropriate first step for the resident to take?

A. The attending psychiatrist.
B. The chairman of the department of internal medicine.
C. The chairman of the department of psychiatry.

D.   The hospital attorney.

E.   The psychiatry residency program director.

Because of the power discrepancy between a resident and a faculty member or chairman (even one from a different department) and because of the added pressures of caring for a VIP patient, it is important for a resident to consult with the attending psychiatrist for assistance in identifying the ethical issues involved in the case and working toward a reasoned solution. Even though caring for this patient may pose special challenges for the resident, the resident must still uphold his or her duty to preserve the patient's confidentiality and should therefore discuss the case only with individuals who have a legitimate need to know. Describing the situation to numerous high-ranking members of the medical school may make the resident feel supported, but it would be an unnecessary violation of the patient's privacy. (Roberts 2016; Stoudemire and Rhoads 1983) *Answer 6.30: A*

6.31

A psychology intern is struggling to complete her dissertation while also finishing her clinical internship in a large university hospital. She confides to one of her fellow interns that the data for her dissertation did not come out as she expected and that she had to "massage the numbers quite a bit" to make them fit her hypothesis. Which of the following is the peer intern's most appropriate first response?

A.   Do nothing because it is not appropriate for one intern to criticize another.

B.   Call the other interns together to decide as a group how to handle the situation.

C.   Educate the intern about the ethical implications of falsifying her data and encourage her to talk to her advisor about how to handle the problems with her dissertation.

D.   Immediately report the intern's unethical behavior to the supervisor of the internship.

E.   Write an anonymous letter to the intern's dissertation advisor, reporting the intern's unethical behavior.

Notifying authorities about a colleague's ethical misconduct can be a difficult matter in any context, and it can be especially so for students reporting misconduct among peers. Trainees may fear that whistle-blowing on a peer will lead to rejection from their group, retaliation from the person being identified, and unwarranted scrutiny or reprimand from their superiors. As a novice, the potential whistle-blower may doubt his or her own judgment about what is appropriate behavior. In this case, the intern writing the dissertation is clearly violating the ethical principles and practice of scientific research by altering her data. Saying nothing about the matter is to be tacitly complicit in the fraudulent activity. Writing an anonymous letter is one way of exposing this behavior, although the letter may not be taken seriously because of its anonymity. Calling the interns together to discuss this matter as a group is an unnecessary violation of the offending intern's privacy. Going to the supervisor or contacting the dissertation advisor may ultimately be required, but a reasonable and fair first step is to try to convince the colleague in a nonjudgmental way to discuss her disappointing results with her advisor or another supervisor. Should this fail, then the intern to whom the fraud was disclosed does have an obligation to notify the appropriate supervisor. (Pawlik 2009) *Answer 6.31: C*

6.32

For each of the following topics, indicate whether the topic is appropriate or inappropriate for an employer to raise with a job candidate at the time of an initial employment interview. Each answer option may be used once, more than once, or not at all.

A. Inappropriate.
B. Appropriate.

_____ Asking an applicant for a position as a child care worker whether the applicant has a child.

_____ Asking an applicant for a position as a fellow in a child and adolescent psychiatry fellowship program about the applicant's sexual orientation.

_____ Asking an applicant for a position as a nurse at a psychiatric hospital about the applicant's religious background.

_____ Asking an applicant for a position as a mental health worker at a psychiatric hospital about prior work experience.

_____ Asking an applicant for a position as a physician at a rural hospital about availability to work "on call" on evenings and weekends.

_____ Asking an applicant for a position as a psychologist about past experience working with youth with mental health issues.

_____ Asking an applicant for a position as a psychiatrist at a veteran's hospital how "she can be a doctor and look so young?"

_____ Asking an applicant for a position as a psychologist about her political party affiliation.

Federal law prohibits employment discrimination on the basis of "race, color, religion, sex (including pregnancy, gender identity, and sexual orientation), national origin, disability, age (40 or older), or genetic information" (U.S. Equal Employment Opportunity Commission 2020c). It is only appropriate for the employer to ask questions that are relevant to the position and the candidate's ability to fulfill the functions of the position. *Answers 6.32: A, A, A, B, B, B, A, A*

6.33

A 13-year-old girl is referred for therapy to help her adjust to her brother's diagnosis of terminal cancer. The girl and her family members have given permission for the therapist and the brother's oncologist to communicate with each other. During the course of therapy, the 13-year-old discloses that her father recently beat her because he thought she was being selfish and disrespectful to her brother. She has bruises on her shoulder and back. The therapist telephones the girl's parents and informs them of her legal obligation to report the abuse to the state child protective services agency. As the therapist is preparing to make the report, the brother's oncologist pages her and asks her not to make the notification. The oncologist says that the boy's death is imminent and that such a report would further destabilize the family. The oncologist believes that the father does not have a history of being abusive and acted out because of the overwhelming stress of the boy's impending death.

In addition to providing emotional support to the girl and, to whatever extent possible, to her family, which of the following options is the therapist's most appropriate course of action?

A. Warn the father that she will file the report if he abuses his daughter again.

B. Wait until the brother dies and then file a report.

C. Recommend that the oncologist file the report because he knows the family well.

D. Make the report to the child protective services agency but do not inform the oncologist of this action.

E. Make the report to the child protective services agency and explain to the oncologist the ethical and legal requirements for reporting child abuse.

Despite what may appear to be extenuating circumstances in this case of a family under extreme stress, the therapist still has an ethical responsibility, and in most localities a legal one, to report a case of suspected child abuse. It is not the duty of the therapist or the oncologist to determine the severity or chronicity of the abuse, which is more appropriately handled by the children's protective services agency. In addition to making the report, the therapist should also attempt to educate the oncologist about the requirements for reporting child abuse, because he may not be as knowledgeable about these matters as mental health professionals, primary care doctors, or emergency physicians. (Children's Bureau 2019; Johnson et al. 2019) *Answer 6.33: E*

6.34

For each of the following scenarios, indicate whether it is an example of ethically appropriate behavior between supervising psychiatrists and trainees. Each answer option may be used once, more than once, or not at all.

A. Ethically appropriate behavior.
B. Ethically inappropriate behavior.

_____ A psychiatry resident who believes her clinic supervisor is incompetent works harder to make up for the supervisor's shortcomings but does not report the situation to protect the supervisor's reputation.

_____ To spend more time taking care of patients, an overworked attending psychiatrist asks the medical student on her team to run a few personal errands for the attending psychiatrist and senior resident.

_____ A psychiatry intern asks a third-year medical student for a date during the medical student's psychiatry rotation.

_____ A psychiatry resident verbally objects to her supervisor's recommendation to discharge a patient from the hospital, because the resident believes discharge is not in the patient's medical best interest.

_____ Based on mutual attraction and affection, an attending psychiatrist and a resident begin a sexual relationship while the attending psychiatrist is supervising the resident's work.

Of all the scenarios listed, only the case of the resident voicing her disagreement with a supervisor over patient management is appropriate behavior in the supervisor-trainee relationship. The other situations describe supervisors exploiting their power over trainees, or, in the first case, a trainee who fails to report an incompetent supervisor. (Hoop 2004; Plaut and Baker 2011) *Answers 6.34: B, B, B, A, B*

6.35

For each of the following descriptions of applicants with health conditions, select the correct statement regarding obligations of employers associated with the Americans with Disabilities Act. Each answer option may be used once, more than once, or not at all.

   A.   The request for an accommodation during the hiring interview must be honored because the condition/situation is covered by the Americans with Disabilities Act.
   B.   The request for an accommodation during the hiring interview is not required because the condition/situation is not covered by the Americans with Disabilities Act.

   _____   A person who recently broke his wrist applies for a position as a chef in a very large, rapid-paced restaurant
   _____   A psychiatrist with psychotherapy expertise, with a visual impairment, applies for a position as an academic faculty member at a large university
   _____   An intellectually disabled individual with a co-occurring mental disorder applies for a position performing landscaping work on a corporate headquarters campus
   _____   An individual with a substance disorder applies for a job working at a family-owned corner store with three employees

Under Title I of the Americans with Disabilities Act, "private employers with 15 or more employees, State and local governments, employment agencies, and labor unions" are prohibited from discriminating against qualified individuals with disabilities (U.S. Department of Justice 2020a). A "qualified individual" is able to perform the essential functions of a position with or without reasonable accommodation (Americans with Disabilities Act of 1990, as amended, 2009, Sec. 12102). A disability is defined as "a physical or mental impairment that substantially limits one or more major life activities" (Americans with Disabilities Act of 1990, as amended, 2009, Sec. 12102). *Answers 6.35: B, A, A, B*

6.36

A large institution asks all employees to disclose symptoms, daily temperature, whether or not they are smokers, vaccine status, family health history, and all other personal health information, including mental health information, to their managers. The institution states that this information is to be used to assess workplace safety in the context of the COVID-19 pandemic. Which of the following is the most accurate statement?

A. Employees are never required to provide personal health information, including mental health information, to their employers.

B. Employees must always provide personal health information, including mental health information, to their employers.

C. Employers are obligated to obtain all personal health information, including mental health information, from their employees during a pandemic.

D. Employers may, in times of a national emergency, request that employees provide relevant health information voluntarily to address workplace health issues.

E. Employers may never request personal health information, including mental health information, of their employees.

The Americans with Disabilities Act "prohibits an employer from making disability-related inquiries and requiring medical examinations, except under limited circumstances" (U.S. Equal Employment Opportunity Commission 2020b). Asking employees about influenza-like symptoms is permitted. If federal and public officials deem a pandemic to be severe, and sufficient objective evidence exists that employees face a direct threat of substantial harm, employers may inquire regarding disabilities or require medical examinations (e.g., the taking of body temperature). Employers are required to keep any and all health information confidential, including voluntarily disclosures of disability. CDC guidance encourages in-person or virtual health checks and workplace-based testing as part of a workplace preparedness, response, and control plan for COVID-19. Employee health screenings should check for the presence of fever and symptoms of COVID-19 and should be conducted as privately as possible. (Americans with Disabilities Act of 1990, 42 USC § 12112, 2009; Centers for Disease Control and Prevention 2021; U.S. Equal Employment Opportunity Commission 2020b) *Answer 6.36: D*

PART III

SELF-ASSESSMENT AND FURTHER STUDY

CHAPTER 7

ETHICS AND PROFESSIONALISM QUESTIONS FOR REVIEW

7.1

A male medical student is rotating through an outpatient gynecology clinic. The student accompanies the attending physician while interviewing and examining some patients. As he is passing the registration table of the clinic, the student is surprised to see his girlfriend's chart. The student picks up the chart to see why his girlfriend is coming to the clinic.

Which one of the following ethical principles is most clearly violated by the medical student looking at his girlfriend's chart?

- A. Autonomy.
- B. Beneficence.
- C. Confidentiality.
- D. Justice.
- E. Nonmaleficence.

7.2

A woman presents to the emergency department with her husband after being in an automobile crash. She is bleeding, and the emergency physician determines that she requires a blood transfusion. The patient is a devout Jehovah's Witness and consequently refuses the transfusion. She is determined to have decision-making capability, and her husband confirms both the woman's stated religion and her refusal to receive blood products.

Which of the following is the emergency physician's most appropriate course of action?

A.   Contact the psychiatrist on call and ask for an urgent consult to determine whether the woman has an untreated mental illness.
B.   Explain to the woman that the physician cannot ethically treat her because the Hippocratic Oath forbids harming patients.
C.   Obtain legal guardianship over the patient.
D.   Sedate the patient and give her the potentially life-saving transfusion.
E.   Talk to the patient about an alternative treatment to blood transfusion, even though it is medically suboptimal.

7.3

Gifts from patients to psychiatrists can become ethically problematic in which of the following circumstances?

A.   When motivated by a wish for enhanced clinical care in the future.
B.   When motivated by the need to adhere to cultural expectations.
C.   When motivated by a desire to become friends with the psychiatrist.
D.   When motivated by the hope to be seen more positively by the psychiatrist.
E.   All of the above.

7.4

For each of the following definitions or descriptions, select the most appropriate term. Each answer option may be used once, more than once, or not at all.

A.   Accountability.
B.   Adherence.
C.   Good clinical practice.
D.   Good laboratory practices.
E.   Nonexploitation.
F.   Peer review.
G.   Transparency.

_____ Complying with laws, institutional policies, and ethical guidelines in professional duties

_____ Enacting rules and procedures for designing and performing experiments or tests

_____ Taking personal responsibility for one's actions and professional conduct

_____ Using experts within an academic discipline to evaluate quality of work performed by colleagues

_____ Seeking not to take unfair advantage of a person or situation

_____ Enacting rules and procedures for conducting clinical trials safely and rigorously

7.5

Many ethics dilemmas involve conflicting ethical principles, and they require that clinicians choose one principle over the other. Identify which of the following choices best applies to the clinical scenarios that follow. Each answer option may be used once, more than once, or not at all.

A. Choosing beneficence over confidentiality.
B. Choosing beneficence over veracity.
C. Choosing confidentiality over beneficence.
D. Choosing respect for autonomy over beneficence.
E. Choosing respect for autonomy over justice.

_____ A patient who has a history of violence slaps his 8-year-old daughter in front of the therapist just prior to a family therapy session. The daughter is clearly injured. The therapist verbally confronts the man and contacts the local child protective services agency.

_____ A patient gives informed consent to undergo a course of electroconvulsive therapy (ECT) for treatment of major depression. The patient dramatically improves. After the fourth session of ECT, the patient refuses further ECT treatments. Although the psychiatrist believes continued sessions will be helpful, she accepts the patient's wishes and discontinues the ECT.

_____ During a couple's therapy session, the wife leaves the room to use the restroom. While she is gone, her husband divulges to the therapist that he has been engaging in sexual behaviors with prostitutes and thinks he may have "caught something." The therapist informs the husband that the wife will need to be informed. When the wife returns, the husband drops the topic and never returns to it despite some subtle urging by the therapist. The therapist knows this couple is sexually active with each other, and before the end of the session informs the wife in front of the husband that she may be at risk for contracting a sexually transmitted infection.

_____ A patient with a remote history of substance abuse is very reluctant to take medications. She has end-stage metastatic ovarian cancer. The physician orders an analgesic medication without telling her it is potentially addictive.

_____ A psychologist working with an employee assistance program hears from a patient that the patient has been having elaborate fantasies about killing her boss. The patient has a plan but promises not to act on it. The psychologist chooses not to inform the boss at this time.

7.6

A psychiatrist receives a phone call from a close friend one evening. The friend lost a parent 6 months ago and has been having difficulties concentrating at work and is having problems sleeping. The sleep problems have been particularly bad of late, and the friend tearfully asks if the psychiatrist would provide some medication to help with the insomnia and depression.

In addition to offering emotional support, which of the following is the psychiatrist's best response?

A. Advise the friend to take over-the-counter medications.

B. Agree to accept the friend as a patient for the usual fee and make an appointment during normal office hours.

C. Decline to comply with the request, explaining that the friend has committed an ethical boundary violation.

D. Phone in a prescription for an antidepressant and a sleep medication.

E. Refer the friend to a colleague who provides urgent care.

7.7

For each of the following descriptions, select the most appropriate ethical concept. Each answer option may be used once, more than once, or not at all.

A. Autonomy.
B. Beneficence.
C. Compassion.
D. Dignity.
E. Fidelity.
F. Justice.
G. Integrity.
H. Nonmaleficence.
I. Respect for persons.
J. Veracity.

____ Doing good
____ Self-governance
____ Truthfulness
____ "Do no harm"
____ Equitable distribution of benefits and burdens

7.8

A psychiatrist is caring for a professional football player admitted with a concussion. During the hospitalization, the patient develops signs and symptoms highly suggestive of alcohol withdrawal. The psychiatrist provides care according to the standard alcohol withdrawal protocol and the syndrome resolves. As the hospitalization progresses, the psychiatrist finds various staff people looking at the patient's hospital chart. Not all of these individuals are directly involved in his care.

Which of the following is the psychiatrist's best option to protect this patient's privacy?

A. Ask the nursing supervisor to lock up the chart in the nursing station so that no one can get to it without showing proper identification.
B. Confront any staff member found inappropriately looking through the chart, and notify hospital authorities of the violations of patient confidentiality.
C. Go through the chart and black out any references to alcohol use, withdrawal syndrome, or other potentially embarrassing or stigmatizing matters.
D. Inform the patient that because of his VIP status, it will be impossible to ensure confidentiality of his medical record.
E. Place a large sticker on the outside of the chart that reads, "VIP Patient: Highly Confidential."

7.9

A deaf teenage boy is brought to a hospital emergency department by his mother after a suicide attempt. The patient is stabilized and transferred to the psychiatry ward, where the boy's mother tells the psychiatrist that he communicates best through sign language. He does not write well or lip-read. The mother offers to interpret for the psychiatrist, but the boy vehemently shakes his head no. Medical translators who are proficient in sign language are available at the hospital.

What is the psychiatrist's best method of conducting the patient interview?

- A. Ask a medical translator who is proficient in sign language to interpret so that the patient can communicate in his preferred language.
- B. Ask the mother to interpret and encourage the son to explore his feelings about his mother being in this role.
- C. Ask the mother to interpret and use her presence as an opportunity to learn about the mother-son relationship.
- D. Begin the interview by using gestures and writing to interview the patient, and plan to stop and obtain a translator if the patient complains or becomes frustrated.
- E. Use gestures and writing to interview the patient to the best extent possible, to avoid the need for a third person in the room.

7.10

Which of the following statements most closely describes ethical analysis based on utilitarian approaches to moral philosophy?

- A. Emphasizes consequences: "The ends justify the means."
- B. Emphasizes the character of the moral agent.
- C. Emphasizes the role of adherence to duty.
- D. Emphasizes the particulars of a situation.

7.11

The chairman of the department of surgery at a medical school develops renal failure. He is maintained on hemodialysis and placed on the list of those seeking a renal transplant from an unrelated donor. A good match for the patient is found in a young trauma patient who dies at the medical school's hospital. According to the normal kidney allocation scheme, the kidney will go to a sicker, well-matched woman in another state who is higher on the transplant list. However, the medical school's renal transplant surgeon wishes to use the kidney for her department chairman.

Which one of the following is the bioethical principle that is most important in determining who receives the kidney?

A. Autonomy.
B. Beneficence.
C. Justice.
D. Nonmaleficence.
E. Respect for persons.

7.12

Decisional capacity is an essential feature of the informed consent process. It is a measurement of a person's global and specific cognitive abilities within a particular context and for a particular decision.

Which of the following is *not* an element of decisional capacity?

A. Advocacy.
B. Appreciation.
C. Communication.
D. Reasoning.
E. Understanding.

7.13

The obligation of a physician providing an expert opinion in a competency hearing is based on which of the following duties?

A. Duty of care.
B. Duty to report.
C. Duty to serve.
D. Duty to be truthful.
E. Duty to warn.

7.14

A 17-year-old girl reports to her therapist that she is having sexual relations with a 26-year-old man. She has a diagnosis of bipolar disorder and a history of impulsive behavior; however, she says that this is a meaningful relationship. She does not want her mother to know about it for fear of her disapproval and anger. The state allows a 17-year-old to consent to sexual relations with an older person and allows health care providers to maintain a 17-year-old's confidentiality on issues of sexuality and reproduction. The therapist determines that the girl has decision-making capability.

What is the therapist's most appropriate course of action regarding the patient's disclosure of the sexual relationship?

    A.   Contact her mother because the girl has a mental illness.
    B.   Contact her mother because the girl is legally a minor.
    C.   Contact the local law enforcement agency because this behavior is immoral.
    D.   Contact the local law enforcement agency because this behavior is statutory rape.
    E.   Do not contact her mother, any law enforcement, or other state agency.

7.15

Which of the following terms commonly denotes the situation in which a professional has a financial, personal, political, or other concern which is likely to bias her judgment or decision-making in performing her professional duties?

    A.   Conflict of concern.
    B.   Conflict of conduct.
    C.   Conflict of interest.
    D.   Conflict of practice.
    E.   Conflict of professionalism.

7.16

Which of the following terms refers to the behavior in which a person knowingly misrepresents the truth or conceals a key fact, often for personal gain, to induce or cause someone else to make a decision against his or her best interests?

A. Bias.
B. Conflict.
C. Cruelty.
D. Fraud.
E. Manipulation.

7.17

For each of the following descriptions, select the most accurate risk assessment according to U.S. human subjects regulations. Each answer option may be used once, more than once, or not at all.

A. Greater than minimal risk.
B. Minimal risk.

_____ Having one's blood pressure taken
_____ Undergoing routine psychological tests
_____ Having one's medical history taken

7.18

A psychiatry resident rotating on a pediatrics service has just completed a history and physical on a 16-year-old girl, whose primary complaint is of a sore throat and of "lumps" in the neck. The resident is concerned that the adenopathy may represent malignancy. The resident's differential diagnosis also includes mononucleosis, and he decides that a number of blood tests are indicated to screen for Epstein-Barr virus and for malignancy. The resident is not sure whether he should tell the mother and his patient his reason for ordering all the blood tests. It seems that they have the right to know the truth about why he is ordering the tests, but he doesn't want to unnecessarily alarm them about the possibility of malignancy.

The resident's dilemma is based primarily on which of the following ethical principles?

A. Beneficence, privacy, veracity.
B. Competence, justice, nonmaleficence.
C. Competence, privacy, respect for autonomy.

D.   Confidentiality, justice, veracity.
E.   Nonmaleficence, respect for autonomy, veracity.

7.19

A patient with chronic pain comes to a psychiatrist's office for a disability evaluation. After a careful review, the psychiatrist finds that the patient clearly meets disability criteria, and he completes the required report. A short time later, the patient brings him a check written for twice his usual fee because she is so grateful for the disability finding. When he refuses to accept any payment above his normal fee, she urges him to donate the excess to his favorite charity.

What is the clinician's best response?

A.   Accept the money and donate it to the charity in the psychiatrist's name.
B.   Accept the money and use it to subsidize a disability evaluation for a patient who cannot pay.
C.   Ask a trusted colleague to talk to the patient and evaluate whether it is appropriate to accept the extra money from her.
D.   Decline the offer politely and explain professional duties and boundaries in this situation.
E.   Tell the patient the name of the psychiatrist's favorite charity and suggest that the patient make the donation herself in her own name.

7.20

For each of the following descriptions, select the most appropriate concept. Each answer option may be used once, more than once, or not at all.

A.   Discrimination.
B.   Implicit bias.
C.   Neither discrimination nor implicit bias.

_____   Intentional unjust treatment of people on the basis of race, age, or gender
_____   Unintentional unjust treatment of people on the basis of race, age, or gender

_____ An employer not hiring a physician with an uncontrolled seizure disorder for a position as an attending surgeon

_____ An employer not hiring a physician for a position as an attending surgeon because of the physician's having a family history of depression

7.21

Select the most salient ethical principle for each scenario. Each answer option may be used once, more than once, or not at all.

A. Justice.
B. Nonmaleficence.
C. Privacy.
D. Respect for autonomy.
E. Veracity.

_____ A psychiatrist has a patient who commits suicide. Panicking about a potential lawsuit, he alters his treatment notes to hide the fact that the patient had previously reported suicidal ideation.

_____ A psychiatrist gives talks for a pharmaceutical company. He also lectures about psychopharmacology in a psychiatry residency training program. The psychiatrist informs the residents of his relationship with the pharmaceutical company prior to beginning his first lecture.

_____ A psychiatrist encourages an internal medicine attending physician to follow a decisionally capable patient's wish to stop tube feedings.

7.22

A 15-year-old is being treated for depression. Both the adolescent and her mother consented to psychotherapy from a child psychiatrist. After a trial of cognitive-behavioral therapy, the depression has not remitted and the psychiatrist recommends a trial of an antidepressant medication. The mother refuses to consent, citing her history of substance abuse and her subsequent opposition to all drugs. The 15-year-old wants to try the medication, understands the risks and benefits, and asks if she can consent for herself. The psychiatrist is unclear about state law as it relates to parental consent to treatment.

What is the psychiatrist's initial course of action?

A. Consult a colleague or legal counsel to determine if, and at what age, a minor can consent to receiving psychotropic medications without parental consent in the state.
B. Prescribe the medication because the adolescent is a mature minor, and inform the parent of the decision.
C. Prescribe the medication because the adolescent is a mature minor, but do not inform the parent of the decision.
D. Refer the patient to a forensic psychiatrist for an evaluation to determine if the patient is legally capable of consent.
E. Refuse to prescribe the medication because parental consent is always required when treating a minor.

7.23

A psychiatrist sees a new patient for a pharmacotherapy evaluation. Throughout the evaluation, the patient makes condescending remarks about the psychiatrist's appearance, the professionalism of his staff, and the décor of his office. The psychiatrist feels annoyed but says nothing to the patient. Afterward, he entertains his office staff with a humorous description of his encounter with the patient.

Which of the following ethical pitfalls has the psychiatrist committed?

A. Failure to provide informed consent.
B. Failure to respect patient autonomy.
C. Failure to respect patient confidentiality.
D. Patient abandonment.
E. Practicing outside one's scope of competence.

7.24

A patient experiencing a mixed mood episode of bipolar disorder presents to the emergency room with extreme abdominal pain. The treatment team believes that the patient has an "acute belly" because of a rapidly progressing and life-threatening volvulus. The patient vacillates between consenting to and refusing the life-saving surgery.

Which of the following is the most ethical course of action?

A. Administer a Mini-Mental State Examination.
B. Bring in a consulting psychiatrist for a second opinion on the patient's mental state.

C. Call the hospital attorney.
D. Perform the surgery.
E. Wait until an alternative decision-maker can be found.

7.25

Match the unethical human experiment with the appropriate definition or description.

A. Guatemala experiments.
B. Operation Midnight Climax.
C. The Milgram experiment.
D. Tearoom trade study.
E. Tuskegee experiment.
F. Willowbrook experiments.

_____ Intentionally observing without consent the sexual activities occurring in public restrooms

_____ Intentionally infecting vulnerable individuals with syphilis and withholding appropriate treatment to observe the natural history of the infection

_____ Intentionally infecting intellectually disabled children and adults with hepatitis to observe the natural history of the infection

_____ Intentionally deceiving and withholding appropriate treatment from vulnerable people with syphilis

_____ Intentionally observing effects of LSD administered without knowledge or consent of adults by sex workers paid by the CIA

_____ Intentionally observing volunteers administering an electric shock to punish other volunteers in a psychological experiment

7.26

A research volunteer expresses his understanding of the double-blind, placebo-controlled study he is entering. His description of the study is factually accurate. In talking with his personal physician, however, the volunteer says he feels certain he will receive some kind of medication from the study; otherwise, his doctor would never have suggested it.

What kind of thinking is the volunteer demonstrating?

A.   Appreciation of benefits.
B.   Clinical reasoning.
C.   Delusional thinking.
D.   Therapeutic misconception.
E.   Trust in one's physician.

7.27

A woman who is 32-weeks pregnant is hospitalized on a psychiatric unit. She is psychotic, refusing medication, and stating that she has a devil inside her that must be destroyed. As a result of her untreated psychosis, she is unable to understand or discuss the risks and benefits associated with antipsychotic medication. The attending psychiatrist is concerned that the patient may harm herself or the fetus and is considering treating her against her will.

Which of the following pairs of ethical principles represent the primary ethical conflict in this situation?

A.   Beneficence vs. respect for autonomy.
B.   Confidentiality vs. justice.
C.   Confidentiality vs. respect for autonomy.
D.   Justice vs. nonmaleficence.
E.   Respect for autonomy vs. veracity.

7.28

While visiting a patient on a medical inpatient unit, a consultation-liaison psychiatrist discovers that her faculty colleague has been also hospitalized. She is concerned about her colleague and would like to provide a gesture of support.

Which of the following is the best course of action for this psychiatrist?

A.   Approach the colleague-patient directly to find out what the problem is and to offer assistance.
B.   Do not acknowledge the hospitalization in any way.
C.   Look at the chart to see what the medical issue is before approaching the colleague-patient, but if it is a potentially embarrassing matter, do not approach the colleague-patient.

D.   Send a card or flowers to the colleague-patient, but do not look at the chart or speak with the colleague-patient directly.

E.   Send a card or flowers to the colleague-patient anonymously, but do not look at the chart or speak with the colleague-patient directly.

7.29

For each of the following scenarios, select the most appropriate phrase. Each answer option may be used once, more than once, or not at all.

A.   Assisted suicide.
B.   Active euthanasia.
C.   Both assisted suicide and active euthanasia.
D.   Neither assisted suicide nor active euthanasia.

_____   A nurse administers a lethal dose of medication
_____   A decisionally capable individual voluntarily requests to be provided with the means (e.g., medication) to commit suicide
_____   A patient accumulates over several months his prescribed medication without others knowing and then uses these medications to commit suicide
_____   A physician administers a lethal dose of medication

7.30

For each of the following descriptions, indicate the most appropriate ethical concept that applies. Each answer option may be used once, more than once, or not at all.

A.   Confidentiality.
B.   Fidelity.
C.   Justice.
D.   Nonmaleficence.
E.   Respect for autonomy.

_____   Providing emergency treatment to patients without regard for race, creed, culture, nationality, or ability to pay
_____   Agreeing to the request of a decisionally capable patient to leave the hospital prior to completion of recommended treatment

7.31

Medicine is a rapidly changing and dynamic scientific endeavor. Various governmental licensing bodies, institutions, and professional organizations monitor the individual practitioner's efforts to stay informed of medical advances.

Which of the following are ways in which organizations monitor practitioners' continued learning and professional development?

A. Certification examinations.
B. Documentation of continuing medical education activities.
C. Peer review and references.
D. Verification of status with the National Practitioner Data Bank.
E. All of the above.

7.32

State legal standards for involuntary commitment of individuals with mental disorders typically include which of the following?

A. Dangerousness toward self or others.
B. Definite or provisional diagnosis of mental disorder directly linked to need for intervention.
C. Inability to provide adequate self-care.
D. Proposed intervention is less restrictive than other alternatives.
E. All of the above.

7.33

A psychiatrist who specializes in the treatment of acutely ill patients with schizophrenia is invited to lead a clinical trial of a new antipsychotic medication. Earlier trials have suggested that in some patients the medication is more effective and has fewer side effects than existing drug treatments. The psychiatrist believes that society will benefit if the U.S. Food and Drug Administration (FDA) approves this medication, and he therefore decides to try to enroll all of his schizophrenia patients without exception into the trial.

What is the major ethical problem with this decision?

A. Acutely psychotic inpatients are incapable of giving informed consent and so cannot participate in such clinical trials.

B. By making global decisions about his patients based on the good of society, the psychiatrist is failing to fulfill his responsibility of beneficence to his individual patients.

C. If the clinical trial does not lead to FDA approval, his patients will have been participants in a purposeless clinical trial.

D. Newer medications are almost always more costly, so the psychiatrist may be subjecting patients to a more expensive medication.

E. Some of his inpatients may be involuntarily hospitalized and are therefore unable to give consent for research participation.

7.34

For each of the following definitions, select the most appropriate term. Each answer option may be used once, more than once, or not at all.

A. Compassion.
B. Courage.
C. Integrity.
D. Self-sacrifice.
E. Veracity.

_____ The habit of never saying anything false to the patient, saying only what is true, never misleading the patient, and pacing disclosure to the patient effectively

_____ The habit of practicing medicine consistently with the highest intellectual and moral standards, both professionally and individually

_____ The habit of recognizing when the patient is in pain, suffering, or distressed and of acting to prevent and relieve pain, suffering, and distress

_____ The habit of distinguishing between what one ought to fear and what one ought not to fear, of ignoring what one ought not to fear, and of not being excessively swayed by what one ought to fear

_____ The habit of taking reasonable risks to one's self-interest (in time, convenience, health, and even life) to protect and promote the interests of patients

7.35

In the past physicians knowingly endorsed use of certain tobacco products in print advertisements despite adequate safety data. Which of the following pairs of ethical principles are in jeopardy in this situation?

A. Autonomy and justice.
B. Compassion and respect for persons.
C. Fidelity and beneficence.
D. Nonmaleficence and veracity.
E. Respect for persons and beneficence.

7.36

A medical student notices an error in the electronic database that contains her grades. The error gives the student an A when in fact she earned a B. She appears to be the only student affected, and the error will never be noticed if it is not pointed out. The student decides to report the grade error.

Which of the following virtues is most clearly demonstrated by the medical student's actions?

A. Charity.
B. Compassion.
C. Fidelity.
D. Respect for autonomy.
E. Veracity.

7.37

After a motor vehicle crash, a 70-year-old man is ticketed for inattentive driving. His primary care physician conducts a work-up, which reveals an early dementia. His wife requests that the diagnosis be withheld from him.

Which of the following is the physician's most appropriate option?

A. Ask the wife to undergo psychotherapy to explore her desire to protect the patient.
B. Conduct an interview with the patient focused on whether he wishes to be informed about his diagnosis and whether he has capacity to understand it.
C. Tell the patient his diagnosis without further discussion or evaluation.
D. Withhold the diagnosis because all demented patients lack the capacity to understand such information.
E. Withhold the diagnosis because of the wife's request.

7.38

A psychologist working for a large company performing prospective employee evaluations is scheduled to assess a woman who is applying for a job delivering packages. The day before the evaluation, the woman leaves a message on his telephone voice mail saying that she is very nervous about the interview because "there's a lot of bad stuff" in her past. She says she hopes that the psychologist will not "make a big deal out of it" and prevent her from getting the job.

Which of the following is the psychologist's most appropriate response?

    A.   Inform her at the beginning of the assessment that because she is now his patient, he cannot mention anything she tells him to her prospective employer unless she gives written permission.

    B.   Inform her at the beginning of the assessment that because she is now his patient, he cannot mention anything she tells him to her prospective employer, but he also cannot deny anything if the employer asks outright.

    C.   At the beginning of the assessment, explain the limits of confidentiality in this setting and the nature of the dual role.

    D.   At the end of the assessment, explain the limits of confidentiality in this setting and the nature of the dual role.

    E.   Ask the patient to explain what she meant by "a lot of bad stuff" in her past and then explain the limits of confidentiality in this setting and the nature of the dual role.

7.39

A policy statement from the Chief of Staff of United States Southern Command, dated August 5, 2002, instructed health care providers at the Guantanamo Bay detention facility that communications from "enemy persons under U.S. control…are not confidential and are not subject to the assertion of privileges" by detainees, and instructed medical personnel to "convey any information concerning…the accomplishment of a military or national security mission…obtained from detainees in the course of treatment to nonmedical military or other United States personnel who have an apparent need to know the information."

Which one of the following most accurately describes the internationally accepted bioethical position on such a policy?

A. The policy is acceptable because of general limitations to the confidentiality of medical information of prisoners.

B. The policy is acceptable because of an exception to the confidentiality of medical information pertaining to national security.

C. The policy is acceptable because the ultimate legal authority at the Guantanamo Bay detention facility belongs to the U.S. military.

D. The policy is unacceptable because it violates the right of detainees to confidentiality of personal medical information.

E. The policy is unacceptable because it violates the right of detainees to legal representation.

7.40

A psychiatrist receives a telephone call from the husband of a patient with a history of multiple suicide attempts. The husband states that his wife has been acting strangely but refuses to talk to him about her emotional state. He begs the psychiatrist to inform him if his wife is contemplating suicide again so that he can be more watchful. When the psychiatrist sees the patient later that day, the patient states that she is having thoughts of suicide but that she has no intention to act on them and that she does not want her husband to be informed.

Which ethical issues or principles are clearly involved in this situation?

A. Confidentiality, justice.

B. Confidentiality, respect for autonomy.

C. Decisional capacity, fidelity.

D. Decisional capacity, justice.

E. Decisional capacity, voluntarism.

7.41

A patient on an inpatient psychiatry ward develops an acute dystonic reaction to a psychiatric medication. He pleads, "Help me! Help me, Doc!" to his psychiatrist, who quickly gives a verbal order for an appropriate injection. But when the nurse rushes toward the patient with a needle and syringe, the patient declares, "No shots! No shots!"

Which of the following best describes the conflicting ethical duties embodied by the patient's conflicting requests?

A. Beneficence vs. paternalism.
B. Beneficence vs. respect for autonomy.
C. Integrity vs. respect for autonomy.
D. Justice vs. fidelity.
E. Justice vs. veracity.

7.42

A young man sustained a C-6 spinal cord injury in a diving accident and is quadriplegic. One month after the accident, he cries often, is unable to sleep, and has decided that life is not worth living. He has very little appetite and will not make an effort to eat. He has requested that all medical treatment be stopped and that he be allowed to die.

Which of the following represents the best immediate course of action?

A. Consult with a legal expert to avoid malpractice litigation in the likely event that the patient or a family member will sue the treating physician.
B. Evaluate the patient for the presence of a treatable psychiatric condition such as depression, which may impair his ability to think rationally about the future.
C. Honor the patient's request because a C-6 spinal cord injury is not a condition that would deprive him of decision-making capacity.
D. Proceed with treatment despite the patient's request because he very likely does not have decision-making capacity.
E. Seek an alternative decision-maker for the patient.

7.43

For each of the following professional activities, select the most appropriate term. Each answer option may be used once, more than once, or not at all.

A. Advocacy.
B. Autonomy.
C. Charity.
D. Confidentiality.
E. Veracity.

_____ Documenting professional activities and accomplishments accurately on a curriculum vitae

_____ Keeping detailed psychotherapy notes separate from the main medical chart

_____ Seeking changes in laws or policies that stigmatize individuals with mental illness

7.44

The *Belmont Report* is important for which of the following reasons?

A. The *Belmont Report* emerged from the Nazi war crimes trials and required informed consent in experimentation.

B. The *Belmont Report* established that respect for persons, beneficence, and justice are the cardinal principles in research ethics.

C. The *Belmont Report* is also known as the "Common Rule" and is the set of regulations governing research in the United States.

D. The *Belmont Report* was produced by the World Medical Association as a statement of ethics in research.

E. The *Belmont Report* uncovered the Tuskegee experiments.

7.45

A psychiatrist is in the midst of a busy clinic day when she receives a call from the medical intensive care unit of a local hospital. One of the psychiatrist's long-term patients, who has schizoaffective disorder, has been admitted emergently with diabetic ketoacidosis. The patient has been psychiatrically stable for years on an atypical antipsychotic, which has been associated in the medical literature with weight gain and metabolic syndrome. When the psychiatrist sees the patient in the hospital, the patient asks if the antipsychotic medicine caused his diabetes.

The psychiatrist's best response would be which of the following?

A. Acknowledge that the atypical antipsychotic may have contributed to the development of diabetes.

B. Acknowledge that there is a relationship between glucose intolerance and some atypical antipsychotic medications, but imply that this doesn't pertain to the medication the patient has been taking.

C. Deny any relationship between the drug and his diabetes and explain that diabetes is primarily caused by eating too much and exercising too little.

D. Explain that scientists are unsure exactly what causes diabetes.

E. Offer to discuss the topic when the patient is less acutely ill.

7.46

Match the professional behavior in each of the following scenarios with the associated ethical principle. Each answer option may be used once, more than once, or not at all.

A. Beneficence.
B. Confidentiality.
C. Justice.
D. Nonmaleficence.
E. Veracity.

_____ A psychiatrist arranges for a pseudonym in the electronic medical record for a celebrity patient seen in the outpatient clinic.

_____ A psychology intern providing psychotherapy explains her status as a trainee to patients seeking care in the low-fee community clinic.

_____ A psychiatrist provides information regarding potentially serious cross-reactions with certain foods and medications to a patient who is prescribed an antidepressant medication.

_____ A psychiatrist offers cognitive-behavioral therapy to a patient who is diagnosed with depression.

_____ A psychiatrist verifies in the electronic health record the number of prescriptions for opioids written by other physicians in the health system for a patient with pain.

_____ A nurse speaks with family members about not using their cell phones to take pictures while visiting a patient on an inpatient unit.

_____ A psychologist informs the police of a serious, imminent threat toward a specific neighbor made by a patient with a known history of violent behavior and access to a firearm.

_____ A psychiatrist restricts his clinical practice to the patient population that best matches his expertise.

7.47

For each of the following descriptions, select the most closely aligned ethical concept.

    A.   Altruism.
    B.   Autonomy.
    C.   Beneficence.
    D.   Compassion.
    E.   Dignity.
    F.   Fidelity.
    G.   Justice.
    H.   Integrity.
    I.   Nonmaleficence.
    J.   Professionalism.
    K.   Respect for persons.
    L.   Veracity.

    ____   Being honest
    ____   Maximizing good outcomes
    ____   Minimizing negative outcomes
    ____   Keeping promises
    ____   Deciding for one's self
    ____   Sharing resources equitably
    ____   Sacrificing for the sake of others

7.48

Which of the following is an accurate statement of the position of the American Psychiatric Association and of the American Psychological Association regarding sexual relationships between psychotherapists and their clients or patients?

    A.   Sexual activity is ethically acceptable if it is consensual.
    B.   Sexual activity is ethically acceptable if it is consensual and occurs at least 2 months after the therapeutic relationship is terminated.
    C.   Sexual activity is ethically acceptable if it is consensual and occurs at least 2 years after the therapeutic relationship is terminated.
    D.   Sexual activity is ethically acceptable if it is consensual and occurs at least 2 years after the therapeutic relationship is terminated and if the client initiated the relationship.
    E.   Sexual activity is not ethically acceptable.

7.49

For each of the following descriptions, select the most relevant term in institutional review board oversight of human research protocols.

    A.   Adverse event.
    B.   Amendment.
    C.   Audit.
    D.   Assent.
    E.   Consent.
    F.   Serious adverse event.

    _____   Seeking advance approval for a revision in a protocol.
    _____   Taking a study participant who experiences extreme claustrophobia and has a panic attack while undergoing an imaging test as part of a research protocol.
    _____   Reviewing good clinical practice documentation to verify completeness and accuracy in research records.

7.50

A psychology fellow is riding a crowded staff elevator with a psychiatry intern and a medical student. The intern is quietly discussing an urgent case with the student. He mentions the patient's name, probable diagnosis, and the work-up and treatment that must be started immediately. Later, the fellow approaches the intern and cautions him not to discuss patient information on elevators because it is a violation of privacy. The intern replies that what he did was not a breach of confidentiality.

Which of the following best explains why this was or was not a breach of doctor-patient confidentiality?

    A.   It was a breach because information could be overheard by those not directly involved in the patient's case.
    B.   It was a breach because the psychology fellow's opinion carries more weight than the intern's.
    C.   It was not a breach because the information discussed was of an urgent nature.
    D.   It was not a breach because the intern's intention was not to cause harm.
    E.   It was not a breach because staff elevators are designed to be a confidential setting.

7.51

A 16-year-old girl is brought to treatment by her parents because they perceive her as distant and indifferent. She tells her therapist that she wants to obtain oral contraceptives, and then she requests that the therapist not tell her parents. She says she is afraid that her parents will become angry and send her to live with relatives in Mexico.

Which of the following describes the therapist's best course of action?

A. Do not inform the parents because if the patient is sent to Mexico, the therapy will be disrupted.
B. Do not inform the parents because it is unethical to violate a patient's confidentiality.
C. Inform the parents because the patient is a minor and has no independent right to confidentiality.
D. Inform the parents because the therapist must show respect for the traditional cultural values of the patient's family.
E. Refer to the state's statute on the legal age for a minor to make her own decisions regarding reproductive health and adhere to the legal guidelines.

7.52

For each of the following descriptions, select the most closely aligned term related to scientific misconduct.

A. Fabrication.
B. Falsification.
C. Plagiarism.

_____ Creating or making up data to deceive
_____ Manipulating data or analyses to deceive
_____ Omitting data to deceive
_____ Misrepresenting someone else's work as one's own to deceive

7.53

For each of the following scenarios, select the bioethical principle most clearly illustrated in the scenario. Each answer option may be used once, more than once, or not at all.

A. Charity.
B. Confidentiality.
C. Nonmaleficence.
D. Respect for autonomy.
E. Respect for persons.

_____ An 83-year-old man who has been maintained for many years on hemodialysis while he cared for his wife, who had Alzheimer's disease, decides to forgo further hemodialysis 11 months after her death. After much discussion and evaluation, the physician agrees to the request.

_____ A 25-year-old man with schizophrenia who requests bilateral orchiectomy (removal of both testicles) to cure him of his "sexual addiction" is turned down for surgery by the urological consultant.

_____ A newborn baby girl with Down syndrome and esophageal atresia is given the same evaluation for possible corrective surgery as is received by a child with esophageal atresia without Down syndrome.

7.54

A psychiatrist is asked to perform a consultation on a 45-year-old man hospitalized for diagnostic testing on a medicine ward. Tests indicate that the man has advanced lung cancer, but his family has asked the internist not to tell him the diagnosis. According to the family, doctors in their culture do not inform patients who have terminal cancer because doing so is thought to take away the will to live. The psychiatrist interviews the man and finds that he is alert, oriented, and capable of making his own health care decisions.

What should the psychiatrist advise the internist?

A. Contact the medical-legal office of the hospital because the risk of legal action by this family is high.

B. Do not inform the patient of his diagnosis because a caring and involved family should be trusted to make sound decisions on a patient's behalf.

C. Immediately inform the patient of his diagnosis because physicians are obligated to follow the ethical norms for the society in which they practice.

D. Meet privately with the patient, ask if he wants to be informed of his diagnosis—and, if so, under what circumstances—and then follow his wishes to whatever extent possible.

E.   Transfer the patient to someone who is more capable of providing care that will be acceptable to this family.

7.55

A person diagnosed with schizophrenia understands the risks, benefits,
and alternatives to an antipsychotic regimen that his psychiatrist offers.
He says, "That sounds great for the other patients here, but I don't have
schizophrenia."

This patient fails to demonstrate which element of decisional capacity?

A.   Appreciating the situation.
B.   Communicating a choice.
C.   Demonstrating the ability to reason.
D.   Making a reasonable decision.
E.   Understanding risks, benefits, and alternatives to the proposed
treatment.

7.56

A spry 86-year-old woman who has decision-making capacity is diagnosed with metastatic breast cancer. Radiation and chemotherapy are
suggested by the consulting oncologist. She declines, stating that she is
"just too old" for the treatments. Her primary care physician has been
treating the woman for many years, is fond of her, and is deeply disap-
pointed in her decision to decline treatment.

Which of the following is the physician's most appropriate response?

A.   Attempt to persuade the patient to change her mind by gently
suggesting he might have to transfer her care to another doctor
if she does not comply with treatment recommendations.
B.   Override her decision by activating her health care power of attorney or seeking guardianship.
C.   Sever the professional relationship to avoid risk of malpractice
action by her family.
D.   Talk with her about her decision, and if her decision is uncoerced
and voluntary, arrange for appropriate palliative treatment and
follow up with her.
E.   Transfer her care to another primary care physician who does
not have an emotional involvement with the patient.

7.57

For each of the following scenarios, indicate whether the action would be identified as a therapeutic boundary violation according to accepted ethics principles in psychiatry. Each answer option may be used once, more than once, or not at all.

A. A therapeutic boundary violation.
B. Not a therapeutic boundary violation.

_____ A psychiatrist bakes two loaves of bread for a bake sale at a local NAMI office. The psychiatrist sees several of his patients at the bake sale and one of them buys a loaf of bread.

_____ A psychiatrist bakes two loaves of bread for a neighbor who has been in a car crash. The neighbor has a mental illness but is not a patient of the psychiatrist.

_____ A psychiatrist bakes two loaves of bread for a patient who has been in long-term psychotherapy for 4 years; the patient's father owned a bakery shop.

_____ A psychiatrist bakes two loaves of bread for her office, where a wide variety of patients are seen. The platter of sliced bread is placed on a table in the waiting room. A typed sign invites patients, family members, and office staff to take a slice, and there is no indication which of the staff members has made the bread.

7.58

An emergency physician pages a psychiatrist after the psychiatrist's patient overdoses. The patient is unresponsive. The patient's records are unavailable and the emergency physician needs to know the patient's medication regimen.

The psychiatrist should give the information under which exception to the informed consent doctrine?

A. Best interest exception.
B. Emergency exception.
C. Incapacitation exemption.
D. Substituted judgment exception.
E. Therapeutic waiver exception.

7.59

Which of the following statements most closely describes ethical analysis based on virtue-based approaches to moral philosophy?

    A.   Emphasizes consequences: "The ends justify the means."
    B.   Emphasizes the character of the moral agent.
    C.   Emphasizes the role of adherence to duty.
    D.   Emphasizes the particulars of a situation.

7.60

One month after the suicide of his 30-year-old daughter, a father makes an appointment with his daughter's psychiatrist. During the appointment, the father asks the psychiatrist to tell him why his daughter killed herself and whether she blamed her parents for her unhappiness. Before her death, the patient had not consented to the release of confidential information to any family member.

According to national ethics standards, in addition to offering emotional support, what is the psychiatrist's most appropriate response?

    A.   Share with the father everything the psychiatrist knows about the patient's motivation for suicide and her feelings about her parents, because confidentiality need not be protected after a patient's death.
    B.   Explain to the father that psychiatrists cannot ethically reveal confidential information until 3 years after the death of a patient.
    C.   Divulge only information the psychiatrist sincerely believes the patient would not have minded being disclosed.
    D.   Decline to reveal any information and offer to personally provide pharmacologic or psychotherapeutic treatment for the father's grief.
    E.   Explain to the father that psychiatrists are ethically bound to maintain confidentiality of patients even after death.

7.61

For each of the following scenarios, indicate whether the activity meets criteria for human subjects research in the U.S. Department of Health and Human Services regulations. Each answer option may be used once, more than once, or not at all.

A. Does not meet criteria for human subjects research.
B. Meets criteria for human subjects research.

_____ Systematic examination of websites for information regarding suicides in the United States

_____ Systematic examination of pathology reports in the university hospital morgue for documented cause of death in suspected suicides

_____ Systematic examination of clinical charts of hospitalized patients after attempted suicide to serve as the basis of a peer-reviewed publication on suicidality

_____ Systematic examination of clinical charts of hospitalized patients after accidental ingestions to serve as the basis of a peer-reviewed publication on suicidality

7.62

A patient confides to his psychiatrist his plan to kill a named intimate partner. The psychiatrist is unable to dissuade his patient from this plan.

Which of the following is the psychiatrist's most appropriate next step?

A. Do not warn the intended victim because all psychotherapeutic communication is confidential.
B. Do not warn the intended victim because psychiatric predictions of violence are notoriously fallible.
C. Do not warn the intended victim because the psychiatrist has no legal or ethical duty to a third party.
D. Notify the police of the situation, because this falls within their domain.
E. Warn and reasonably protect the intended victim.

7.63

For each of the following scenarios, indicate whether the psychiatrist's action is acceptable based on current ethical guidelines for the treatment of prisoners. Each answer option may be used once, more than once, or not at all.

A. Acceptable.
B. Not acceptable.

_____ A psychiatrist administers a lethal injection in the legal execution of a person who was convicted of murder.

_____ A psychiatrist administers a lethal injection in the legal execution of a person who was convicted of murder, was decisionally capable, and expressed a clear wish to be executed rather than spend life in prison.

_____ A psychiatrist diagnoses and treats anxiety, depression, post-traumatic stress disorder, and other psychiatric disorders among inmates at a federal prison.

7.64

A young man who recently tested positive on a predictive genetic test for Huntington's disease seeks psychiatric treatment for anxiety and depression. Over the course of several months of psychotherapy, the man's symptoms improve markedly. He tells his psychiatrist that he has decided to marry and start a family and that he does not plan to tell his new fiancée that he carries the disease-causing mutation. It is virtually certain that the patient will develop Huntington's disease and that each of his children will have a 50% risk of inheriting the disorder.

Which of the following is the psychiatrist's most appropriate next step, based on the ethical principles of confidentiality and beneficence?

A. Accept the patient's decision without comment and do not discuss it further because genetics is a uniquely private matter.
B. Encourage the patient to fully consider the implications of not telling his fiancée.
C. Inform the patient that the psychiatrist has a duty to warn the fiancée about his genetic status and telephone her immediately.
D. Place an anonymous phone call to warn the fiancée.
E. Refuse to continue to treat the patient unless he tells the fiancée.

7.65

A physician needs to determine whether a particular treatment in the care of his patient will be futile or very unlikely to have a medical benefit. The first step in making a decision about medical futility is to consider which of the following?

A. The physician's personal intuition.
B. The policies of the hospital.
C. The preferences of the family.
D. The preferences of the patient.
E. The scientific evidence.

7.66

An elderly woman with mild dementia and major depression dies from what appears to be an intentional medication overdose. The woman's family is convinced that she was not aware of the consequences of her actions and wants the coroner to record the death as an accident rather than a suicide. The family asks the woman's psychiatrist to testify to this effect if the case goes to court. Given the facts of the case, the psychiatrist is not sure whether the death was accidental or not.

From an ethical standpoint, what is the psychiatrist's best response to the family's request?

A. Demonstrate awareness of scope of practice issues by refusing to testify unless board-certified in forensic psychiatry.
B. Demonstrate compassion for the patient's family by agreeing to testify that the death was accidental.
C. Demonstrate courage by refusing to testify because the psychiatrist is unsure about the cause of death.
D. Demonstrate justice by making a blanket decision never to testify on behalf of any patient or family.
E. Demonstrate veracity by agreeing to testify truthfully about the woman's condition so that the court may decide whether the death was accidental or suicide.

7.67

Cruzan vs. Director, Missouri Department of Public Health stands for which one of the following legal propositions?

A. All patients can refuse medical care.
B. All patients have the right to have life support withdrawn.
C. Competent patients can refuse medical care.
D. Conscious patients have the right to have life support withdrawn.
E. Patients can refuse medical care if the medical team concurs with the decision.

7.68

For each of the following scenarios, indicate whether the action is an ethically appropriate response to cultural differences between psychiatrists and patients. Each answer option may be used once, more than once, or not at all.

    A. Appropriate.
    B. Not appropriate.

_____ A psychiatrist who practices what he refers to as Christian psychotherapy fully informs new patients of his beliefs and approach to treatment and readily offers referrals to clinicians with a secular orientation.

_____ A therapist tells a patient that women who participate in arranged marriages are childlike and lack self-esteem.

_____ A white psychoanalyst encourages a Black psychotherapy patient to fully articulate her feelings about having a therapist of a different race.

_____ To demonstrate that she is truly "color blind" and that she does not judge patients by their ethnic background, a white therapist gently dismisses any attempt by her Black patients to point out their ethnic or cultural differences.

7.69

A small dose of a sedative-hypnotic is ordered for a hospitalized patient. A nurse dispenses it to the wrong patient. The patient who received the medicine became sleepy but no significant harm was done. The nurse involved has a history of previous errors and feels she is at risk for losing her job if the hospital administration finds out. The physician who wrote the order has known the nurse for years and believes her to be a good person. The nurse is a single mother who is struggling financially. The physician chooses not to report the error.

Which of the following ethics principles is most compromised by this decision?

    A. Beneficence.
    B. Integrity.
    C. Justice.
    D. Respect for persons.
    E. Scope of practice.

7.70

For each of the following vignettes, select the best manuscript authorship designation. Each answer option may be used once, more than once, or not at all.

A. First author.
B. Second or subsequent author.
C. Acknowledged.
D. Not acknowledged.

_____ A data entry employee from a temporary agency is hired to spend a month entering psychiatric research data into a spreadsheet. Two years later, after the data are analyzed, a manuscript is generated. The employee's role is _____.

_____ After obtaining all the necessary approvals, a psychiatrist creates a novel rating method to see if it predicts residents' performance a year after graduation. Unable to analyze the data himself, the psychiatrist asks the department statistician to do the computations. The psychiatrist writes the first draft of a paper describing the results. The statistician reads the draft and makes minor corrections. The psychiatrist's role is

_____ .

7.71

A man seeks personal health care from a psychiatrist who works in the occupational health office at his place of work. The psychiatrist determines that the man is not in acute distress, and she then explains that her principal role is to perform "fitness for duty" evaluations for the employer. She says that because of her role, she may be obligated to inform the employer of certain kinds of issues if they arise. The psychiatrist then offers names of colleagues who have private offices in the area.

The occupational health psychiatrist's disclosure of her dual role and the limits of confidentiality most clearly demonstrates which ethical ideal?

A. Charity.
B. Compassion.
C. Fidelity.
D. Justice.
E. Veracity.

7.72

The daughter of an elderly man with delusional disorder asks to meet with the patient's psychiatrist. The patient agrees to let the daughter talk privately to the psychiatrist about her concerns and to speak generally about his illness, but he does not give permission for the psychiatrist to divulge any specific information about him. During the daughter's meeting with the psychiatrist, she criticizes the psychiatrist for failing to improve her father's condition. She demands to be told details about the father's case or she will file a malpractice suit. The psychiatrist allows the daughter to express herself and provides education about the general treatment and course of delusional disorder.

Which ethical principle or concept is most clearly embodied by the psychiatrist's action?

A. Confidentiality.
B. Fidelity.
C. Informed consent.
D. Justice.
E. Scope of practice.

7.73

Which of the following is an example of research misconduct?

A. Demonstrating that a hypothesis is not correct.
B. Falsifying data.
C. Not demonstrating that a hypothesis is correct.
D. Performing post hoc statistical tests to consider secondary hypotheses.
E. Using standard techniques for imputing data that are missing.

7.74

A college student athlete with severe bipolar disorder and a history of multiple suicide attempts sees a psychiatrist at the university's student health center. The student complains that his medication regimen is adversely affecting his abilities on the football field and in the classroom. He asks the physician to taper off all his medications because he is worried about losing his starting position and becoming academically ineligible. He says he understands that stopping the medications may lead to a manic or depressive episode and perhaps another suicide attempt, but he says he is willing to take the risk.

Which ethics principles are most pertinent to this scenario?

A. Beneficence and nonmaleficence.
B. Confidentiality and respect for persons.
C. Justice and respect for autonomy.
D. Justice and veracity.
E. Nonmaleficence and respect for autonomy.

7.75

For each of the following scenarios, indicate whether the clinician involved appears to be impaired and, if so, whether a colleague has a professional duty to intervene in some fashion. Each answer option may be used once, more than once, or not at all.

A. The clinician does not appear to be impaired.
B. The clinician may be impaired but no intervention is warranted at this time.
C. The clinician may be impaired and a colleague should intervene.

_____ A therapist feels sexually attracted to a patient. She neither acts on the feelings nor discloses them to the patient. She seeks supervision from a senior colleague to better understand the significance of her feelings.

_____ A social worker drinks heavily at night but never during the day or at work. During morning appointments, she is sometimes irritable because of hangover symptoms.

_____ A psychiatrist is diagnosed with early dementia but does not perceive any detriment in his ability to practice medicine.

_____ A psychologist who has the flu asks clinic coordinators to reschedule her appointments for 3 days and asks a colleague to cover her pager.

_____ An intern has to be reprimanded because of poor grooming. On several occasions, colleagues observe the intern crying in the call room.

_____ A psychologist with stage 4 breast cancer needs increasing doses of opiates to relieve her bone pain. One of her patients complains to the clinic coordinator that the psychologist fell asleep during a therapy session.

7.76

E-cigarette use has been ethically controversial. Evaluate the following statements regarding their ethical relevance for e-cigarette use, against e-cigarette use, or neutral to e-cigarette use.

- A. For.
- B. Against.
- C. Neutral.

_____ E-cigarettes have been marketed with fruit flavorings intended to appeal to children, adolescents, and young adults.

_____ E-cigarettes have significant health risks that are as yet unknown.

_____ Use of e-cigarettes may reduce use of tobacco and tobacco-related health problems.

_____ Use of e-cigarettes may be associated with second-hand or "passive" vaping.

_____ E-cigarette packaging is harmful to the environment.

ANSWERS AND REFERENCES

7.1: **C** (see Chapters 3 and 4; Appelbaum 2002; Junkerman and Schiedermayer 1998; Lo 2020b)

7.2: **E** (see Chapter 4; Jonsen et al. 2002; Muramoto 2001)

7.3: **E** (see Chapter 4; Roberts 2006)

7.4: **B, D, A, F, E, C** (see Chapter 5)

7.5: **A, D, A, B, C** (see Chapters 3 and 4; Roberts 2016; Spellecy and Roberts 2006)

7.6: **E** (see Chapters 3 and 4; Roberts 2016)

7.7: **B, A, J, H, F** (see Chapters 2 and 3)

7.8: **B** (see Chapters 3, 4, and 6; Post 2004)

7.9: **A** (see Chapters 3 and 4; Tseng and Streltzer 2004)

7.10: **A** (see Chapters 1 and 3)

7.11: **C** (see Chapters 3 and 4; Junkerman and Schiedermayer 1998; Lo 2020b)

7.12: **A** (see Chapters 3, 4, and 5; Grisso and Appelbaum 1998; Roberts 2016)

7.13: **D** (see Chapter 4)

7.14: **E** (see Chapter 4; American Psychiatric Association 2010; Boonstra and Nash 2000; Koocher and Keith-Spiegel 1990)

7.15: **C** (see Chapters 2 and 3)

7.16: **D** (see Chapter 3)

7.17: **B, B, B** (see Chapter 5; Roberts 2016)

7.18: **E** (see Chapter 4; American Psychiatric Association 2001a; Sugarman 2000)

7.19: **D** (see Chapters 3 and 4; Epstein 1994)

7.20: **A, B, C, A** (see Chapters 3 and 6; Chapman et al. 2013; U.S. Department of Justice 2020a; Americans with Disabilities Act of 1990, as amended, 2009, Sec. 12102)

7.21: **E, E, D** (see Chapters 3 and 4; Beauchamp and Childress 2001; Roberts 2016; Spellecy and Roberts 2006)

7.22: **A** (see Chapters 3 and 4; Boonstra and Nash 2000; Roberts 2016)

7.23: **C** (see Chapters 3 and 4; American Psychiatric Association 2010; Roberts 2016)

7.24: **D** (see Chapters 3 and 4; Jonsen et al. 2002; Lo 2020b; Roberts 2016)

7.25: **D, A, F, E, B, C** (see Chapter 3; Beecher 1966; Fletcher et al. 1997)

7.26: **D** (see Chapter 5; Grisso and Appelbaum 1998)

7.27: **A** (see Chapters 3 and 4; Roberts 2016)

7.28: **B** (see Chapters 3 and 4; Roberts 2016)

7.29: **B, A, D, B** (see Chapters 2 and 3; Materstvedt et al. 2003; Meisel 2020; Roberts 2016)

7.30: **C, E** (see Chapters 3 and 4; Beauchamp and Childress 2001; Boyd et al. 1997)

7.31: **E** (see Chapter 3; Roberts 2016)

7.32: **E** (see Chapters 2 and 3; Byatt et al. 2007; Menninger 2001)

7.33: **B** (see Chapter 5; Roberts 2002a, 2002b; World Medical Association 1964)

7.34: **E, C, A, B, D** (see Chapters 3 and 4; Beauchamp and Childress 2001)

7.35: **D** (see Chapter 2)

7.36: **E** (see Chapters 3 and 5; Beauchamp and Childress 2001; Roberts 2016)

7.37: **B** (see Chapters 3 and 4; Appelbaum and Grisso 1988; Lo 2020b; President's Commission for the Study of Ethical Problems in Medicine and Biomedical and Behavioral Research 1982)

7.38: **C** (see Chapters 3 and 4; Malley and Reilly 1999)

7.39: **D** (see Chapters 3 and 4; Bloche and Marks 2005a, 2005b; Rubenstein et al. 2005)

7.40: **B** (see Chapters 3 and 4; American Psychiatric Association 2010)

7.41: **B** (see Chapters 3 and 4; Roberts 2016)

7.42: **B** (see Chapter 4; Lo 2020b; Sullivan and Youngner 1994)

7.43: **E, D, A** (see Chapters 3 and 4; Beauchamp and Childress 2001; Boyd et al. 1997)

7.44: **B** (see Chapter 5; National Commission for the Protection of Human Subjects of Biomedical and Behavioral Research 1979; Pincus et al. 1999; Roberts 2016)

7.45: **A** (see Chapter 4; Hérbert et al. 2001; Lo 2020b)

7.46: **B, E, D, A, D, B, D, D**

7.47: **L, C, I, F, B, G, A** (see Chapters 2 and 3)

7.48: **E** (see Chapter 4; American Psychiatric Association 2010; Dewald and Clark 2001; Roberts 2016)

7.49: **B, F, C** (see Chapter 5; ICH 2016; Office for Human Research Protections 2016)

7.50: **A** (see Chapter 4; American Psychiatric Association 2010; Ubel et al. 1995)

7.51: **E** (see Chapter 4; American Psychological Association 2003; Boonstra and Nash 2000)

7.52: **A, B, B, C** (see Chapter 5; Caplan and Redman 2018)

7.53: **D, C, E** (see Chapters 3 and 4; Beauchamp and Childress 2001; Jonsen et al. 2002; Junkerman and Schiedermayer 1998; Lo 2020b)

7.54: **D** (see Chapter 4; Jonsen et al. 2002; Okasha et al. 2000)

7.55: **A** (see Chapters 4 and 5; Grisso and Appelbaum 1998)

7.56: **D** (see Chapter 4; Lo 2020b)

7.57: **B, B, A, B** (see Chapters 3 and 4; Dewald and Clark 2001; Gutheil and Gabbard 1998; Roberts 2016)

7.58: **B** (see Chapter 4; Berg et al. 2001; Roberts 2016)

7.59: **B** (see Chapters 2 and 3)

7.60: **E** (see Chapters 3 and 4; Roberts 2005)

7.61: **A, A, B, B** (see Chapter 5; Roberts 2016; U.S. Department of Health and Human Services 2018)

7.62: **E** (see Chapter 4; Appelbaum 1985; Lo 2020b)

7.63: **B, B, A** (see Chapters 3 and 4; American Psychiatric Association 2010; World Medical Association 2003)

7.64: **B** (see Chapter 4; Farmer and McGuffin 1999; Group for the Advancement of Psychiatry 1990)

7.65: **E** (see Chapter 4; Jonsen et al. 2002; Marco and Larkin 2000)

7.66: **E** (see Chapters 3 and 4; Beauchamp and Childress 2001; Gutheil and Appelbaum 2019)

7.67: **C** (see Chapter 4; Roberts 2005)

7.68: **A, B, A, B** (see Chapter 4; American Psychiatric Association 2001a; Okasha et al. 2000)

7.69: **B** (see Chapters 3 and 4; Roberts 2016; Spellecy and Roberts 2006)

7.70: **D, A** (see Chapters 5 and 6; Fine and Kurdek 1993; International Committee of Medical Journal Editors 2006)

7.71: **E** (see Chapters 3 and 4; Malley and Reilly 1999)

7.72: **A** (see Chapters 3 and 4; Bloch et al. 1999)

7.73: **B** (see Chapter 5; Caplan and Redman 2018; Office of Science and Technology Policy 2000)

7.74: **E** (see Chapters 3 and 4; Beauchamp and Childress 2001)

7.75: **A, C, C, A, C, C** (see Chapter 6; American Psychiatric Association 2001a; Group for the Advancement of Psychiatry 1990)

7.76: **B, B, A, B, B** (see Chapter 3; Franck et al. 2016)

REFERENCES

Abeles N: Ethics and the interrogation of prisoners: an update. Ethics Behav 20:243–249, 2010

Abràmoff MD, Lavin PT, Birch M, et al: Pivotal trial of an autonomous AI-based diagnostic system for detection of diabetic retinopathy in primary care offices. NPJ Digit Med August 28, 1:39, 2018

Accreditation Council for Graduate Medical Education (ACGME): Common Program Requirements (Residency). June 10, 2018. Available at: www.acgme.org/Portals/0/PFAssets/ProgramRequirements/CPRResidency2019.pdf. Accessed March 10, 2020.

Accreditation Council for Graduate Medical Education: Psychiatry Milestones. Second Revision. March 2020. Available at: www.acgme.org/Portals/0/PDFs/Milestones/Psychiatry Milestones2.0.pdf?ver=2020-03-10-152105-537. Accessed May 24, 2020.

Addington v. Texas, 441 U.S. 418 (1979)

Alexander L, Moore M: Deontological ethics. Stanford Encyclopedia of Philosophy. Revised October 17, 2016. Available at: https://plato.stanford.edu/entries/ethics-deontological. Accessed August 5, 2020.

Amdur RJ, Bankert EA: Institutional Review Board Management and Function. Boston, MA, Jones & Bartlett Publishers, 2002

American Academy of Psychiatry and the Law: Ethics Guidelines for the Practice of Forensic Psychiatry. May 2005. Available at: www.aapl.org/ethics.htm. Accessed August 10, 2020.

American Board of Internal Medicine: Project Professionalism. Philadelphia, PA, American Board of Internal Medicine Communications, 1999

American Board of Internal Medicine Foundation, American College of Physicians–American Society of Internal Medicine, European Federation of Internal Medicine: Medical professionalism in the new millennium: a physician charter. Ann Intern Med 136(3):243–246, 2002

American Board of Psychiatry and Neurology: Continuing Certification/MOC Program. August 2020. Available at: www.abpn.com/wp-content/uploads/2015/05/ABPN_MOC_Booklet-1.pdf. Accessed August 6, 2020.

American Hospital Association: Management Advisory: Ethics Committee. Chicago, IL, American Hospital Association, 1990

American Medical Association: Principles of Medical Ethics—1957. JAMA 164(13):1482, 1957

American Medical Association: Sexual harassment in the practice of medicine. 2016. Available at: www.ama-assn.org/delivering-care/ethics/sexual-harassment-practice-medicine. Accessed July 24, 2020.

American Medical Association: Expansion of AMA Policy on Female Genital Mutilation H-525.980. 2017. Available at: https://policysearch.ama-assn.org/policyfinder/detail/female%20genital%20mutilation?uri=%2FAMADoc%2FHOD.xml-0-4716.xml. Accessed August 5, 2020.

American Medical Association: Physician-assisted suicide. Available at: www.ama-assn.org/delivering-care/ethics/physician-assisted-suicide. Accessed February 10, 2020.

American Medical Association, Council on Ethical and Judicial Affairs: Medical futility in end-of-life care. JAMA 281:937–941, 1999

American Medical Association, Council on Ethical and Judicial Affairs: Code of Medical Ethics, Current Opinions with Annotations. Chicago, IL, American Medical Association, 2002

American Medical Association, Council on Ethical and Judicial Affairs: Code of Medical Ethics Current Opinions with Annotations. Chicago, IL, American Medical Association, 2005

American Medical Association, Council on Ethical and Judicial Affairs: Code of Medical Ethics, Current Opinions with Annotations. Chicago, IL, American Medical Association, 2006

American Medical Association, Council on Ethical and Judicial Affairs: CEJA Report 2—A-16 Modernized Code of Medical Ethics. Proceedings of the House of Delegates, 165th Annual Meeting. Chicago, IL: American Medical Association, 2016a

American Medical Association, Council on Ethical and Judicial Affairs: Preface to the AMA Code of Medical Ethics. 2016b. Available at: www.ama-assn.org/sites/ama-assn.org/files/corp/media-browser/preface-and-preamble-to-opinions.pdf. Accessed February 24, 2020.

American Nurses Association, Center for Ethics and Human Rights: Code of Ethics for Nurses: With Interpretive Statements, 2nd Edition. Silver Spring, MD, American Nurses Association, 2015

American Psychiatric Association: Principles of informed consent in psychiatry. APA Document Reference No. 960001. Approved by the Board of Trustees, June 1996

American Psychiatric Association: Ethics Primer of the American Psychiatric Association. Washington, DC, American Psychiatric Association, 2001a

American Psychiatric Association: Opinions of the Ethics Committee on the Principles of Medical Ethics With Annotations Especially Applicable to Psychiatry, 2001 Edition. Washington, DC, American Psychiatric Association, 2001b

American Psychiatric Association: Resource Document on Psychotherapy Notes Provision of the Health Insurance Portability and Accountability Act Privacy Rule. March 2002. Available at: www.psychiatry.org/File%20Library/Psychiatrists/Directories/Library-and-Archive/resource_documents/rd2002_PsychotherapyNotesHIPAA.pdf. Accessed August 4, 2020.

American Psychiatric Association: Position Statement on Psychiatric Participation in Interrogation of Detainees. Arlington, VA, American Psychiatric Association, 2006

American Psychiatric Association: The Principles of Medical Ethics With Annotations Especially Applicable to Psychiatry, 2013 Edition. Arlington, VA, American Psychiatric Association, 2010. Available at: www.psychiatry.org/File%20Library/Psychiatrists/Practice/Ethics/principles-medical-ethics.pdf. Accessed April 13, 2021.

American Psychiatric Association: APA Commentary on Ethics in Practice. December 2015. Available at: www.psychiatry.org/File%20Library/Psychiatrists/Practice/Ethics/APA-Commentary-on-Ethics-in-Practice.pdf. Accessed April 13, 2021.

American Psychiatric Association: Position Statement on Medical Euthanasia. December 2016. Available at: www.psychiatry.org/File%20Library/About-APA/Organization-Documents-Policies/Policies/Position-2016-Medical-Euthanasia.pdf. Accessed April 13, 2021.

American Psychiatric Association: APA reiterates strong opposition to conversion therapy. November 15, 2018. Available at: www.psychiatry.org/newsroom/news-releases/apa-reiterates-strong-opposition-to-conversion-therapy. Accessed March 18, 2021.

American Psychiatric Association: Opinions of the Ethics Committee on The Principles of Medical Ethics, With Annotations Especially Applicable to Psychiatry. Washington, DC, American Psychiatric Association, 2020. Available at: www.psychiatry.org/File%20Library/Psychiatrists/Practice/Ethics/Opinions-of-the-Ethics-Committee.pdf. Accessed April 13, 2021.

American Psychiatric Association, Task Force on Research Ethics: Ethical principles and practices for research involving human participants with mental illness. Psychiatric Serv 57:552–557, 2006

American Psychoanalytic Association: Ethics Casebook of the American Psychoanalytic Association, 2nd Edition. Edited by Dewald PA, Clark RW. New York, American Psychoanalytic Association, 2008

American Psychological Association: Guidelines for Providers of Psychological Services to Ethnic, Linguistic, and Culturally Diverse Populations. Washington, DC, American Psychological Association, 1990

American Psychological Association: Guidelines on Multicultural Education, Training, Research, Practice, and Organizational Change for Psychologists. Am Psychol 58(5):377–402, 2003

American Psychological Association: Ethical Principles of Psychologists and Code of Conduct, Including 2010 and 2016 Amendments. January 1, 2017. Available at: www.apa.org/ethics/code. Accessed August 6, 2020.

American Psychological Association, Advisory Committee on Colleague Assistance: Advancing Colleague Assistance in Professional Psychology. Washington, DC, American Psychological Association, 2006

American Psychological Association, Committee on Animal Research and Ethics: Guidelines for Ethical Conduct in the Care and Use of Nonhuman Animals in Research. February 4, 2012. Available at: www.apa.org/science/leadership/care/guidelines. Accessed October 13, 2020.

Americans with Disabilities Act of 1990, as amended. June 15, 2009. Available at: www.ada.gov/pubs/adastatute08.htm#12102. Accessed July 27, 2020.

Andrews LB, Burruss JW: Core Competencies for Psychiatric Education: Defining, Teaching, and Assessing Resident Competence. Washington, DC, American Psychiatric Publishing, 2004

Anfang SA, Appelbaum PS: Twenty years after Tarasoff: reviewing the duty to protect. Harv Rev Psychiatry 4:67–76, 1996

Annas GJ, Grodin MA (eds): The Nazi Doctors and the Nuremberg Code: Human Rights in Human Experimentation. New York, Oxford University Press, 1992

Appelbaum PS: Tarasoff and the clinician: problems in fulfilling the duty to protect. Am J Psychiatry 142:425–429, 1985

Appelbaum PS: Privacy in psychiatric treatment: threats and responses. Am J Psychiatry 159:1809–1818, 2002

Appelbaum PS: Ethical issues in psychiatric genetics. J Psychiatr Pract 10:343–351, 2004

Appelbaum PS: Decisional capacity of patients with schizophrenia to consent to research: taking stock. Schizophr Bull 32:22–25, 2006

Appelbaum PS, Gold A: Psychiatrists' relationships with industry: the principal-agent problem. Harv Rev Psychiatry 18(5):255–265, 2010

Appelbaum PS, Grisso T: Assessing patients' capacities to consent to treatment. N Engl J Med 319:1635–1638, 1988; erratum: N Engl J Med 320:748, 1989

Appelbaum PS, Grisso T: The MacArthur Competence Study, I: mental illness and competence to consent to treatment. Law Hum Behav 19:105–126, 1995

Appelbaum PS, Gutheil T: Legal issues in emergency psychiatry and involuntary commitment, in Clinical Handbook of Psychiatry and the Law, 5th Edition. Philadelphia, PA, Wolters Kluwer Baltimore, MD, Williams & Wilkins, 2020, pp 36–71

Appelbaum PS, Roth LH: Competency to consent to research: a psychiatric overview. Arch Gen Psychiatry 39:951–958, 1982

Arnold L, Stern DT: What is medical professionalism? in Measuring Medical Professionalism. Edited by Stern DT. New York, Oxford University Press, 2006, pp 15–38

Arnold LE, Stoff DM, Cook E, et al: Ethical issues in biological psychiatric research with children and adolescents. J Am Acad Child Adolesc Psychiatry 34:929–939, 1995

Arras J: Theory and bioethics. Stanford Encyclopedia of Philosophy. May 18, 2010. Available at: https://plato.stanford.edu/entries/theory-bioethics. Accessed August 5, 2020.

Association of American Medical Colleges: Guidelines for maintaining active and permanent individual student records in the registrar's office. November 10, 2015. Available at: www.aamc.org/system/files/c/2/448950-guidelinesformaintainingactiveandpermanent.pdf. Accessed July 24, 2020.

Association of American Medical Colleges: Medical School Graduation Questionnaire: 2019 All School Summary Report. July 2019. Available at: www.aamc.org/data-reports/students-residents/report/graduation-questionnaire-gq. Accessed March 8, 2020.

Austin W, Rankel M, Kagan L, et al: To stay or to go, to speak or stay silent, to act or not to act: moral distress as experienced by psychologists. Ethics Behav 15:197–212, 2005

Babaria P, Abedin S, Nunez-Smith M: The effect of gender on the clinical clerkship experiences of female medical students: results from a qualitative study. Acad Med 84(7):859–866, 2009

Backlar P, Cutler DL (eds): Ethics in Community Mental Health Care: Commonplace Concerns. New York, Kluwer Academic/Plenum, 2002

Barak-Corren Y, Castro VM, Javitt S, et al: Predicting suicidal behavior from longitudinal electronic health records. Am J Psychiatry 174(2):154–162, 2017

Barrangou R, Doudna JA: Applications of CRISPR technologies in research and beyond. Nat Biotechnol 34(9):933–941, 2016

Barocas S, Selbst A: Big data's disparate impact. 104 Calif L Rev 671 (2016)

Bartlett P: The test of compulsion in mental health law: capacity, therapeutic benefit and dangerousness as possible criteria. Med Law Rev 11:326–352, 2003

Batha E: US toughens ban on "abhorrent" female genital mutilation. Reuters. January 7, 2021. Available at: www.reuters.com/article/us-usa-law-fgm-idUSKBN29C2OF. Accessed March 11, 2021.

Beauchamp TL: The philosophical basis of psychiatric ethics, in Psychiatric Ethics, 3rd Edition. Edited by Bloch S, Chodoff P, Green SA. New York, Oxford University Press, 1999, pp 25–48

Beauchamp TL, Childress JF: Principles of Biomedical Ethics, 5th Edition. New York, Oxford University Press, 2001

Beeber LS: Disentangling mental illness and violence. J Am Psychiatr Nurses Assoc 24(4):360–362, 2018

Beecher H: Ethics and clinical research. N Engl J Med 274:1354–1360, 1966

Behrendt A, Moritz S: Posttraumatic stress disorder and memory problems after female genital mutilation. Am J Psychiatry 162(5):1000–1002, 2005

Belitz J: How to intervene with unethical and unprofessional colleagues, in Roberts Academic Medicine Handbook: A Guide to Achievement and Fulfillment for Academic Faculty, 2nd Edition. Edited by Roberts LW. Cham, Switzerland, Springer, 2020, pp 183–189

Berg JW, Appelbaum PS, Lidz CW, Parker LS: Informed Consent: Legal Theory and Clinical Practice, 2nd Edition. New York, Oxford University Press, 2001

Berkman ND, Wynia MK, Churchill LR: Gaps, conflicts, and consensus in the ethics statements of professional associations, medical groups, and health plans. J Med Ethics 30:395–401, 2004

Biesecker BB, Peay HL: Ethical issues in psychiatric genetics research: points to consider. Psychopharmacology (Berl) 171:27–35, 2003

Blackett T: Trademarks. Cham, Switzerland, Springer, 2016

Bloch S, Reddaway P: Soviet Psychiatric Abuse: The Shadow Over World Psychiatry. London, Routledge, 2019

Bloch S, Chodoff P, Green SA (eds): Psychiatric Ethics, 3rd Edition. New York, Oxford University Press, 1999

Bloche MG, Marks JH: Doctors and interrogators at Guantanamo Bay. N Engl J Med 353:6–8, 2005a

Bloche MG, Marks JH: When doctors go to war. N Engl J Med 352:3–6, 2005b

Bolukbasi T, Chang KW, Zou J, et al: Man is to computer programmer as woman is to homemaker? Debiasing word embeddings. Advances in Neural Information Processing Systems June 2016

Boonstra H, Nash E: Minors and the right to consent to health care. Issues Brief (Alan Guttmacher Inst) September; (2):1–6, 2000

Boroughs MS, Andres Bedoya C, O'Cleirigh C, Safren SA: Toward defining, measuring, and evaluating LGBT cultural competence for psychologists. Clin Psychol (New York) 22(2):151–171, 2015

Bourgeois JA, Cohen MA, Geppert CM: The role of psychosomatic-medicine psychiatrists in bioethics: a survey study of members of the Academy of Psychosomatic Medicine. Psychosomatics 47:520–526, 2006

Boyd KM, Higgs R, Pinching AJ: The New Dictionary of Medical Ethics. London, BMJ Publishing, 1997

Brandeis LD: Business: A Profession. Boston, MA, Hole, Cushman & Flint, 1993

Braun UK: Surrogate decision-making and advance care planning, in Ethical Considerations and Challenges in Geriatrics. Edited by Catic AG. Cham, Switzerland, Springer, 2017, pp 23–34

Brody BA: The Ethics of Biomedical Research: An International Perspective. New York, Oxford University Press, 1998

Brody H, Doukas D: Professionalism: a framework to guide medical education. Med Educ 48(10):980–987, 2014

Bugental JFT: The Search for Authenticity: An Existential-Analytic Approach to Psychotherapy. New York, Holt, Rinehart & Winston, 1965

Buolamwini J, Gebru T: Gender shades: intersectional accuracy disparities in commercial gender classification. Proceedings of Machine Learning Research 81:1–15, 2018

Burke W, Pinsky LE, Press NA: Categorizing genetic tests to identify their ethical, legal, and social implications. Am J Med Genet 106:233–240, 2001

Burnham JC: A clinical alternative to the public health approach to mental illness: a forgotten social experiment. Perspect Biol Med 49:220–237, 2006

Byatt N, Pinals D, Arikan R: Involuntary hospitalization of medical patients who lack decisional capacity: an unresolved issue. Focus 5(4):438-443, 2007

Candilis P, Foti ME, Holzer J: End-of-life care and mental illness: a model for community psychiatry and beyond. Community Ment Health J 40:3–16, 2004

Caplan AL, Redman BK: Research misconduct, in Getting to Good: Research Integrity in the Biomedical Sciences. Cham, Switzerland, Springer, 2018, pp 385–433

Carman D, Britten N: Confidentiality of medical records: the patient's perspective. Br J Gen Pract 45(398):485–488, 1995

Carpenter WT Jr, Gold JM, Lahti AC, et al: Decisional capacity for informed consent in schizophrenia research. Arch Gen Psychiatry 57:533–538, 2000

Cavaliere G: Background Paper: The Ethics of Human Genome Editing. World Health Organization Expert Advisory Committee on Developing Global Standards for Governance and Oversight of Human Genome Editing. March 18–19, 2019. Available at: www.who.int/ethics/topics/human-genome-editing/WHO-Commissioned-Ethics-paper-March19.pdf. Accessed August 6, 2020.

Centers for Disease Control and Prevention: Firearm violence prevention. May 22, 2020. Available at: https://www.cdc.gov/violenceprevention/firearms/fastfact.html. Accessed July 29, 2020.

Centers for Disease Control and Prevention: Guidance for Businesses and Employers Responding to Coronavirus Disease 2019 (COVID-19). March 8, 2021. Available at: www.cdc.gov/coronavirus/2019-ncov/community/guidance-business-response.html. Accessed April 20, 2021.

Chapman EN, Kaatz A, Carnes M: Physicians and implicit bias: how doctors may unwittingly perpetuate health care disparities. J Gen Intern Med 28(11):1504–1510, 2013

Char DS, Shah NH, Magnus D: Implementing machine learning in health care—addressing ethical challenges. N Engl J Med 378(11):981–983, 2018

Children's Bureau: Mandatory reporters of child abuse and neglect. Child Welfare Information Gateway. 2019. Available at: www.childwelfare. gov/pubPDFs/manda.pdf. Accessed August 5, 2020.

Chiles JA, Strosahl KD, Roberts LW: Clinical Manual for the Assessment and Treatment of Suicidal Patients, 2nd Edition. Washington, DC, American Psychiatric Association Publishing, 2019

Chisolm MS, Peters ME, Burkhart K, Wright SM: Clinical excellence in psychiatry: a review of the psychiatric literature. Prim Care Companion CNS Disord 14(2), 2012

Chouldechova A: Fair prediction with disparate impact: a study of bias in recidivism prediction instruments. October 24, 2016 [cited January 21, 2020]. Available at: http://arxiv.org/abs/1610.07524. Accessed January 21, 2020.

Christakis DA, Feudtner C: Ethics in a short white coat: the ethical dilemmas that medical students confront. Acad Med 68:249–254, 1993

Chu J, Leino A, Pflum S, Sue S: A model for the theoretical basis of cultural competency to guide psychotherapy. Professional Psychology: Research and Practice 47(1):18–29, 2016

Clement S, Schauman O, Graham T, et al: What is the impact of mental health-related stigma on help-seeking? A systematic review of quantitative and qualitative studies. Psychol Med 45:11–27, 2015

Coburn WJ: The vision in supervision: transference-countertransference dynamics and disclosure in the supervision relationship. Bull Menninger Clin 61:481–494, 1997

Cohen JJ: Viewpoint: Linking professionalism to humanism: what it means, why it matters. Acad Med 82:1029–1032, 2007

Colliver JA, Markwell SJ, Verhulst SJ, Robbs RS: The prognostic value of documented unprofessional behavior in medical school records for predicting and preventing subsequent medical board disciplinary action: the Papadakis studies revisited. Teach Learn Med 19(3):213–215, 2007

Committee on Publication Ethics: COPE ethical guidelines for peer reviewers. September 2017. Available at: https://publicationethics.org/files/Ethical_Guidelines_For_Peer_Reviewers_2.pdf. Accessed August 6, 2020.

Committee on Publication Ethics: Discussion document: authorship. 2019. Available at: https://publicationethics.org/files/COPE_DD_A4_Authorship_SEPT19_SCREEN_AW.pdf. Accessed July 24, 2020.

Committee on the Science of Changing Behavioral Health Social Norms; Board on Behavioral, Cognitive, and Sensory Sciences; Division of Behavioral and Social Sciences and Education; National Academies of Sciences, Engineering, and Medicine: Ending Discrimination Against People with Mental and Substance Use Disorders. Washington, DC, National Academies Press, 2016

Compton MT, Shim RS: The social determinants of mental health. Focus 13(4):419–425, 2015

Conner KO, Copeland VC, Grote NK, et al: Mental health treatment seeking among older adults with depression: the impact of stigma and race. Am J Geriatr Psychiatry 18(6):531–543, 2010

Corbett-Davies S, Pierson E, Feller A, et al: Algorithmic decision making and the cost of fairness. Proceedings of ACM SIGKDD International Conference on Knowledge Discovery and Data Mining, July 2017

Council for International Organizations of Medical Sciences: International Ethical Guidelines for Biomedical Research Involving Human Subjects, Fourth Revision. Geneva, Council for International Organizations of Medical Sciences, 2016

Counts NZ, Wrenn G, Muhlestein D: Accountable care organizations' performance in depression: lessons for value-based payment and behavioral health. J Gen Intern Med 34(12):2898–2900, 2019

Coverdale J, Roberts L, Louie A, et al: Writing the methods. Acad Psychiatry 30:361–364, 2006

Coverdale JH, Balon R, Roberts LW: Cultivating the professional virtues in medical training and practice. Acad Psychiatry 35(3):155–159, 2011

Coverdale JH, Gordon MR, Nguyen PT (eds): Human Trafficking: A Treatment Guide for Mental Health Professionals. Washington, DC, American Psychiatric Association Publishing, 2020

Creative Commons: About the licenses. Available at: https://creativecommons.org/licenses. Accessed August 5, 2020.

Cripps SN, Swartz MS: Update on assisted outpatient treatment. Curr Psychiatry Rep 20(12):112, 2018

Crowden A, Gildersleeve M: Place, virtue ethics and physician-researcher dual-role consent in clinical research. Am J Bioeth 19(4):37–39, 2019

Cruzan v. Director, Missouri Department of Public Health, 497 U.S. 261 (1990)

de Araujo Reinert C, Kowacs C: Patient-targeted "googling": when therapists search for information about their patients online. Psychodyn Psychiatry 47(1):27–38, 2019

DeGrazia D, Beauchamp TL: Philosophical foundations and philosophical methods, in Methods in Medical Ethics. Edited by Sugarman J, Sulmasy DP. Washington, DC, Georgetown University Press, 2001, pp 31–46

Dehon E, Weiss N, Jones J, et al: A systematic review of the impact of physician implicit racial bias on clinical decision making. Acad Emerg Med 24(8):895–904, 2017

Dermatis H, Lesko LM: Psychological distress in parents consenting to child's bone marrow transplantation. Bone Marrow Transplant 6:411–417, 1990

DesRoches CM, Rao SR, Fromson JA, et al: Physicians' perceptions, preparedness for reporting, and experiences related to impaired and incompetent colleagues. JAMA 304(2):187–193, 2010

Dewald PA, Clark RW (eds): Ethics Case Book of the American Psychoanalytic Association. New York, American Psychoanalytic Association, 2001

Dilday JC, Miller EA, Schmitt K, et al: Professionalism: a core competency, but what does it mean? A survey of surgery residents. J Surg Educ 75:601–605, 2018

Dingle AD, Kolli V: Ethics in child and adolescent psychiatry training: what and how are we teaching? Acad Psychiatry 44:168–178, 2020

Dinwiddie SH, Hoop J, Gershon ES: Ethical issues in the use of genetic information. Int Rev Psychiatry 16:320–328, 2004

Drane J: Competency to give an informed consent: a model for making clinical assessments. JAMA 252:925–927, 1984

Drescher J, Roberts LW, Termuehlen G: Lesbian, gay, bisexual, and transgender patients, in The American Psychiatric Association Publishing Textbook of Psychiatry, 7th Edition. Edited by Roberts LW. Washington, DC, American Psychiatric Association Publishing, 2019, pp 1185–1212

Dressel J, Farid H: The accuracy, fairness, and limits of predicting recidivism. Science Advances American Association for the Advancement of Science January 17; 4(1):eaao5580, 2018. Available at: http://advances.sciencemag.org/lookup/doi/10.1126/sciadv.aao5580. Accessed April 13, 2021.

Druss BG, Bradford DW, Rosenheck RA, et al: Mental disorders and use of cardiovascular procedures after myocardial infarction. JAMA 283(4):506–511, 2000

Dubbai H, Adelstein B-A, Taylor S, Shulruf B: Definition of professionalism and tools for assessing professionalism in pharmacy practice: a systematic review. J Educ Eval Health Prof 16:22, 2019

DuBois JM, Walsh HA, Chibnall JT, et al: Sexual violations of patients by physicians: a mixed-methods, exploratory analysis of 101 cases. Sex Abuse 31(5):503–523, 2019

Dubois M, Gilbert H, Rich B, et al: Ethics forum: Quality of care, teaching responsibilities, and patients' preference. Pain Med 5:206–211, 2004

Dudley R, Taylor P, Wickham S, Hutton P: Psychosis, delusions and the "jumping to conclusions" reasoning bias: a systematic review and meta-analysis. Schizophr Bull 42(3):652–665, 2016

Dumais A, Lesage AD, Alda M, et al: Risk factors for suicide completion in major depression: a case-control study of impulsive and aggressive behaviors in men. Am J Psychiatry 162(11):2116–2124, 2005

Dunn LB, Gordon NE: Improving informed consent and enhancing recruitment for research by understanding economic behavior. JAMA 293:609–612, 2005

Dunn LB, Jeste DV: Enhancing informed consent for research and treatment. Neuropsychopharmacology 24:595–607, 2001

Dunn LB, Roberts LW: Emerging findings in ethics of schizophrenia research. Curr Opin Psychiatry 18:111–119, 2005

Dunn LB, Roberts LW: Psychiatric research, in Psychiatric Ethics, 5th Edition. Edited by Bloch S, Green SA. New York, Oxford University Press, 2021

Dunn LB, Candilis PJ, Roberts LW: Emerging empirical evidence on the ethics of schizophrenia research. Schizophr Bull 32:47–68, 2006a

Dunn LB, Nowrangi MA, Palmer BW, et al: Assessing decisional capacity for clinical research or treatment: a review of instruments. Am J Psychiatry 163(8):1323–1334, 2006b

Dunn LB, Palmer BW, Karlawish JH: Frontal dysfunction and capacity to consent to treatment or research: conceptual considerations and empirical evidence, in The Human Frontal Lobes: Functions and Disorders, 2nd Edition. Edited by Miller BL, Cummings JL. New York, Guilford, 2007, pp 335–344

Edelstein L: The Hippocratic Oath. Baltimore, MD, Johns Hopkins Press, 1943

Edelstein L: The Idea of Progress in Classical Antiquity. Baltimore, MD, Johns Hopkins University Press, 1967

Edelstein A, Alici Y, Breitbart W, Chochinov HM: Palliative care, in The American Psychiatric Publishing Textbook of Psychosomatic Medicine. Edited by Levenson JL. Washington, DC, American Psychiatric Association Publishing, 2019, pp 1297–1334

Educational Commission for Foreign Medical Graduates: ACGME Core Competencies. July 5, 2012. Available at: www.ecfmg.org/echo/acgme-core-competencies.html. Accessed May 24, 2020.

Emanuel EJ, Wendler D, Grady C: What makes clinical research ethical? JAMA 283:2701–2711, 2000

Epstein RS: Monetary compensation in psychotherapy: balancing the therapist's financial needs against those of the patient, in Keeping Boundaries: Maintaining Safety and Integrity in the Psychotherapeutic Process. Washington, DC, American Psychiatric Press, 1994, pp 159–179

Epstein RS, Simon RI: The exploitation index: an early warning indicator of boundary violations in psychotherapy. Bull Menninger Clin 54:450–465, 1990

Esteva A, Kuprel B, Novoa RA, et al: Dermatologist-level classification of skin cancer with deep neural networks. Nature 542(7639):115–118, 2017

Faden RR, Beauchamp TL: Decision-making and informed consent: a study of the impact of disclosed information. Soc Indic Res 7:313–336, 1980

Faden RR, Beauchamp TL, King N: A History and Theory of Informed Consent. New York, Oxford University Press, 1986

Fadus MC, Ginsburg KR, Sobowale K, et al: Unconscious bias and the diagnosis of disruptive behavior disorders and ADHD in African American and Hispanic youth. Acad Psychiatry 44(1):95–102, 2020

Fan R, Tao J: Consent to medical treatment: the complex interplay of patients, families, and physicians. J Med Philos 29:139–148, 2004

Fann JR, Hunt DD, Schaad D: A sociological calendar of transitional stages during psychiatry residency training. Acad Psychiatry 27:31–38, 2003

Fargen KM, Drolet BC, Philibert I: Unprofessional behaviors among tomorrow's physicians: review of the literature with a focus on risk factors, temporal trends, and future directions. Acad Med 91(6):858–864, 2016

Farmer A, McGuffin P: Ethics and psychiatric genetics, in Psychiatric Ethics, 3rd Edition. Edited by Bloch S, Chodoff P, Green SA. New York, Oxford University Press, 1999, pp 479–493

Field MJ, Lo B (eds): Conflict of Interest in Medical Research, Education, and Practice. Washington, DC, National Academies Press, 2009

Fine MA, Kurdek LA: Reflections on determining authorship credit and authorship order on faculty-student collaborations. Am Psychol 48:1141–1147, 1993

Fisher CD: Ethical issues in therapy: therapist self-disclosure of sexual feelings. Ethics Behav 14:105–121, 2004

FitzGerald C, Hurst S: Implicit bias in healthcare professionals: a systematic review. BMC Med Ethics 18(1):19, 2017

Flecknell P: Replacement, reduction, and refinement. ALTEX 19(2):73–78, 2002

Fletcher JC, Lombardo PA, Marshall MF, et al (eds): Introduction to Clinical Ethics, 2nd Edition. Hagerstown, MD, University Publishing Group, 1997

Flores AW, Bechtel K, Lowenkamp CT: False positives, false negatives, and false analyses: a rejoinder to "machine bias": There's software used across the country to predict future criminals. And it's biased against blacks. Federal Probation Journal 80(2), September 2016

Flory J, Emanuel E: Interventions to improve research participants' understanding in informed consent for research: a systematic review. JAMA 292:1593–1601, 2004

Fortney JC, Pyne JM, Turner EE, et al: Telepsychiatry integration of mental health services into rural primary care settings. Int Rev Psychiatry 27(6):525–539, 2015

Fox AB, Smith BN, Vogt D: How and when does mental illness stigma impact treatment seeking? Longitudinal examination of relationships between anticipated and internalized stigma, symptom severity, and mental health service use. Psychiatry Res 268:15–20, 2018

Franck C, Filion KB, Kimmelman J, et al: Ethical considerations of e-cigarette use for tobacco harm reduction. Respir Res 17(1):53, 2016

Freedman B: Equipoise and the ethics of clinical research. N Engl J Med 317:141–145, 1987

Freidson E: Profession of Medicine: A Study of the Sociology of Applied Knowledge. New York, Dodd Mead, 1970

Friedman PJ: Mistakes and fraud in medical research. Law Med Health Care 20:17–25, 1992

Frye V, Camacho-Rivera M, Salas-Ramirez K, et al: Professionalism: the wrong tool to solve the right problem? Acad Med 95:860–863, 2020

Gabbard GO (ed): Sexual Exploitation in Professional Relationships. Washington, DC, American Psychiatric Press, 1989

Gabbard GO: Boundary violations, in Psychiatric Ethics, 3rd Edition. Edited by Bloch S, Chodoff P, Green SA. New York, Oxford University Press, 1999, pp 141–160

Gabbard GO: Post-termination sexual boundary violations. Psychiatr Clin North Am 25:593–603, 2002

Gabbard GO, Lester EP: The early history of boundary violations in psychoanalysis, in Boundaries and Boundary Violations in Psychoanalysis. New York, Basic Books, 1995, pp 68–86

Gabbard GO, Nadelson C: Professional boundaries in the physician-patient relationship. JAMA 273:1445–1449, 1995

Gabbard GO, Kassaw KA, Perez-Garcia G: Professional boundaries in the era of the internet. Acad Psychiatry 35(3):168–174, 2011

Gallegos AM, Trabold N, Cerulli C, Pigeon WR: Sleep and interpersonal violence: a systemic review. Trauma Violence Abuse May 26; 1524838019852633, 2019

Garg N, Schiebinger L, Jurafsky D, Zou J: Word embeddings quantify 100 years of gender and ethnic stereotypes. 2017. Available at: https://arxiv.org/pdf/1711.08412.pdf. Accessed April 13, 2021.

Gengoux G, Zack SE, Derenne JL, et al: Professional Well-Being: Enhancing Wellness Among Psychiatrists, Psychologists, and Mental Health Clinicians. Washington, DC, American Psychiatric Association Publishing, 2020

Geppert CM: Voluntarism in consultation psychiatry: the forgotten capacity. Am J Psychiatry 164:409–413, 2007

Germline gene-editing research needs rules. Nature 567(7747):145, 2019

Ghaemi SN: The Concepts of Psychiatry: A Pluralistic Approach to the Mind and Mental Illness. Baltimore, MD, Johns Hopkins University Press, 2003

Gilligan C: Moral orientation and moral development, in Women and Moral Theory. Edited by Kittay E, Meyers D. Totowa, NJ, Rowman & Littlefield, 1987, pp 19-33

Glannon W: Phase I oncology trials: why the therapeutic misconception will not go away. J Med Ethics 32:252–255, 2006

Gostin LO: Public Health Law and Ethics: A Reader. Berkeley, University of California Press, 2002

Gottesman II, Bertelsen A: Legacy of German psychiatric genetics: hindsight is always 20/20. Am J Med Genet 67:317–322, 1996

Grady C: Money for research participation: does it jeopardize informed consent? Am J Bioeth 1:40-4, 2001

Grady C: Payment of clinical research subjects. J Clin Invest 115:1681–1687, 2005

Green AR, Carney DR, Pallin DJ, et al: Implicit bias among physicians and its prediction of thrombolysis decisions for black and white patients. J Gen Intern Med 22(9):1231–1238, 2007

Grisso T, Appelbaum PS: The MacArthur Competence Study, III: abilities of patients to consent to psychiatric and medical treatments. Law Hum Behav 19:149–174, 1995

Grisso T, Appelbaum PS: Assessing Competence to Consent to Treatment: A Guide for Physicians and Other Health Professionals. New York, Oxford University Press, 1998

Grisso T, Appelbaum PS, Mulvey EP, et al: The MacArthur Competence Study, II: measures of abilities related to competence to consent to treatment. Law Hum Behav 19:127–148, 1995

Grootens-Wiegers P, Hein IM, van den Broek JM, de Vries MC: Medical decision-making in children and adolescents: developmental and neuroscientific aspects. BMC Pediatr 17(1):120, 2017

Grosch WN, Olsen DC: When Helping Starts to Hurt: A New Look at Burnout Among Psychotherapists. New York, WW Norton, 1994

Group for the Advancement of Psychiatry: A Casebook in Psychiatric Ethics. New York, Brunner/Mazel, 1990

Gulshan V, Rajan RP, Widner K, et al: Performance of a deep-learning algorithm vs manual grading for detecting diabetic retinopathy in India. JAMA Ophthalmol 137(9):987–993, 2019

Gupta M, Forlini C, Lenton K, et al: The hidden ethics curriculum in two Canadian psychiatry residency programs: a qualitative study. Acad Psychiatry 40(4):592–599, 2016

Gutheil TG, Appelbaum PS: Clinical Handbook of Psychiatry and the Law, 5th Edition. Philadelphia, PA, Lippincott Williams & Wilkins, 2019

Gutheil TH, Gabbard GO: Misuses and misunderstandings of boundary theory in clinical and regulatory settings. Am J Psychiatry 155:409–414, 1998

Hantoot MS: Lying in psychotherapy supervision: why residents say one thing and do another. Acad Psychiatry 24:179–187, 2000

Health Information Privacy: Guidance regarding methods for de-identification of protected health information in accordance with the Health Insurance Portability and Accountability Act (HIPAA) privacy rule. November 6, 2015. Available at: www.hhs.gov/hipaa/for-professionals/privacy/special-topics/de-identification/index.html. Accessed August 6, 2020.

Hellinger FJ: The impact of financial incentives on physician behavior in managed care plans: a review of the evidence. Med Care Res Rev 53(3):294–314, 1996

Hendelman W, Byszewski A: Formation of medical student professional identity: categorizing lapses of professionalism, and the learning environment. BMC Med Educ 14:139, 2014

Hérbert PC, Levin AV, Robertson G: Bioethics for clinicians: 23. Disclosure of medical error. CMAJ 164(4):509–513, 2001

Herlihy B, Corey G: Boundary Issues in Counseling: Multiple roles and Responsibilities. 3rd Edition. New York, Wiley, 2014

Herx L, Cottle M, Scott J: The "normalization" of euthanasia in Canada: the cautionary tale continues. World Med J 66:28–39, 2020

Hester DM: The anatomy of bioethical consultations. Am J Bioeth 1(4):57–58, 2001

Hickman SE, Nelson CA, Moss A, et al: Use of the Physician Orders for Life-Sustaining Treatment (POLST) Paradigm Program in the hospice setting. J Palliat Med 12:133–141, 2009

Hilty DM, Leamon MH, Roberts LW: Approaching research, evaluation, and continuous quality improvement projects, in Handbook of Career Development in Academic Psychiatry and Behavioral Sciences. Edited by Roberts LW, Hilty DM. Washington, DC, American Psychiatric Publishing, 2006, pp 273–282

HIV.gov: U.S. statistics. June 30, 2020. Available at: hwww.hiv.gov/hiv-basics/overview/data-and-trends/statistics. Accessed August 5, 2020.

Hoge SK, Appelbaum PS: Ethics and neuropsychiatric genetics: a review of major issues. Int J Neuropsychopharmacol 15(10):1547–1557, 2012

Holder SM, Warren C, Rogers K, et al: Involuntary processes: knowledge base of health care professionals in a tertiary medical center in upstate South Carolina. Community Ment Health J 54(2):149–157, 2018

Hoonpongsimanont W, Sahota PK, Chen Y, et al: Physician professionalism: definition from a generation perspective. Int J Med Educ 9:246–252, 2018

Hoop JG: Hidden ethical dilemmas in psychiatric residency training: the psychiatry resident as dual agent. Acad Psychiatry 28:183–189, 2004

Hoop JG, Di Pasquale T, Hernandez JM, et al: Ethics and culture in mental health care. Ethics and Behavior 18(4):353–372, 2008

Howe EG: Medical ethics—are they different for the military physician? Mil Med 146:837–841, 1981

Hurley JC, Underwood MK: Children's understanding of their research rights before and after debriefing: informed assent, confidentiality, and stopping participation. Child Dev 73:132–143, 2002

ICH (International Council for Harmonisation of Technical Requirements for Registration of Pharmaceuticals for Human Use): International Council for Harmonisation (ICH) Harmonized Guideline: Integrated Addendum to ICH E6(R1): Guideline for Good Clinical Practice E6(R2). November 9, 2016. Available at: https://database.ich.org/sites/default/files/E6_R2_Addendum.pdf. Accessed August 6, 2020.

Illes J (ed): Neuroethics: Anticipating the Future. Oxford, UK, Oxford University Press, 2017

Institute of Medicine, Committee on Quality of Health Care in America: Crossing the Quality Chasm: A New Health System for the 21st Century. Washington DC, National Academies Press, 2001

Institute of Medicine: Committee on Identifying and Preventing Medication Errors: Preventing Medication Errors: Quality Chasm Series. Washington, DC, National Academies Press, July 20, 2006

International Committee of Medical Journal Editors: Recommendations for the Conduct, Reporting, Editing, and Publication of Scholarly Work. December 2019. Available at: www.icmje.org/icmje-recommendations.pdf. Accessed April 13, 2021.

Jackson L, Kuhlman C, Jackson F, Fox PK: Including vulnerable populations in the assessment of data from vulnerable populations. Frontiers in Big Data [cited 2019 Nov 26] 2:19, June 28, 2019. Available at: https://doi.org/10.3389/fdata.2019.00019. Accessed April 13, 2021.

Jaffee v. Redmond, 518 U.S. 1, 116 S.Ct. 1923, 135 L.Ed.2d 337 (1996)

Jain S: Understanding Physician-Pharmaceutical Industry Interactions: A Concise Guide. Cambridge, UK, Cambridge University Press, 2007

Jain S: Aspects of physician and pharmaceutical industry relationships for trainees. Acad Psychiatry 34(2):98–101, 2010

Jain S, Dunn LB, Warner CH, Roberts LW: Results of a multisite survey of U.S. psychiatry residents on education in professionalism and ethics. Acad Psychiatry 35(3):175–183, 2011a

Jain S, Lapid MI, Dunn LB, Roberts LW: Psychiatric residents' needs for education about informed consent, principles of ethics and professionalism, and caring for vulnerable populations: results of a multisite survey. Acad Psychiatry 35(3):184–190, 2011b

James SE, Herman JL, Rankin S, et al: The Report of the 2015 US Transgender Survey. Washington, DC, National Center for Transgender Equality, 2016

Jansen LA, Mahadevan D, Appelbaum PS, et al: Dispositional optimism and therapeutic expectations in early-phase oncology trials. Cancer 122:1238–1246, 2016

Jha V, Bekker HL, Duffy SR, et al: Perceptions of professionalism in medicine: a qualitative study. Med Educ 40:1027–1036, 2006

Jiang H, Nachum O: Identifying and correcting label bias in machine learning. arXiv.org January 15, 2019 [cited January 13, 2020]. Available at: http://arxiv.org/abs/1901.04966. Accessed January 13, 2020.

Johnson MR, Hatzis NM, Jutla A: Children and adolescents, in The American Psychiatric Association Publishing Textbook of Psychiatry, 7th Edition. Edited by Roberts LW. Washington, DC, American Psychiatric Association Publishing, 2019, pp 1147–1183

Jonsen AR, Toulmin S: The Abuse of Casuistry: A History of Moral Reasoning. Berkeley, University of California Press, 1988

Jonsen AR, Siegler M, Winslade WJ: Clinical Ethics: A Practical Approach to Ethical Decisions in Clinical Medicine, 5th Edition. New York, McGraw-Hill, Medical Publishing Division, 2002

Joyce C, Ochoa TT, Carroll MW, et al: Copyright Law. Durham, NC, Carolina Academic Press, 2016

Junkerman C, Schiedermayer D: Practical Ethics for Students, Interns and Residents: A Short Reference Manual, 2nd Edition. Frederick, MD, University Publishing Group, 1998

Kaminsky A, Roberts LW, Brody JL: Influences upon willingness to participate in schizophrenia research: an analysis of narrative data from 63 people with schizophrenia. Ethics Behav 13:279–302, 2003

Karlawish JH, Lantos J: Community equipoise and the architecture of clinical research. Camb Q Healthc Ethics 6:385–396, 1997

Kass LR: Professing ethically. On the place of ethics in defining medicine. JAMA 249:1305–1310, 1983

Katz J: Experimentation With Human Beings: The Authority of the Investigator, Subject, Professions, and State in the Human Experimentation Process. New York, Russell Sage Foundation, 1972

Kelly E, Nisker J: Increasing bioethics education in preclinical medical curricula: what ethical dilemmas do clinical clerks experience? Acad Med 84(4):498–504, 2009

Kim SY, Caine ED, Currier GW, et al: Assessing the competence of persons with Alzheimer's disease in providing informed consent for participation in research. Am J Psychiatry 158:712–717, 2001

Kim SYH, De Vries RG, Peteet JR: Euthanasia and assisted suicide of patients with psychiatric disorders in the Netherlands 2011 to 2014. JAMA Psychiatry 73:362–368, 2016

Klein EJ, Jackson JC, Kratz L, et al: Teaching professionalism to residents. Acad Med 78:26–34, 2003

Knoll JL IV: Ethics in forensic psychiatry, in The American Psychiatric Association Publishing Textbook of Forensic Psychiatry, 3rd Edition. Edited by Gold LH, Frierson RL. Washington, DC, American Psychiatric Association Publishing, 2018, pp 27–40

Koch T: Professionalism: an archaeology. HEC Forum 31:219–232, 2019

Kong D, Whitaker R: Doing harm: research on the mentally ill: Testing takes human toll. The Boston Globe, November 15, 1998a. Available at: http://web.archive.org/web/19991008230951/boston.com/globe/nation/packages/doing_harm/day1.htm. Accessed September 28, 2007.

Kong D, Whitaker R: Doing harm: research on the mentally ill: Debatable forms of consent. The Boston Globe, November 16, 1998b. Available at: http://web.archive.org/web/20000916151238/boston.com/globe/nation/packages/doing_harm/day2.htm. Accessed September 28, 2007.

Kong D, Whitaker R: Doing harm: research on the mentally ill: Lures of riches fuels testing. The Boston Globe, November 17, 1998c. Available at: http://web.archive.org/web/20000916151306/boston.com/globe/nation/packages/doing_harm/day3.htm. Accessed September 28, 2007.

Kong D, Whitaker R: Doing harm: research on the mentally ill: Still no solution in the struggle on safeguards. The Boston Globe, November 18, 1998d. Available at: http://web.archive.org/web/20010613014648/boston.com/globe/nation/packages/doing_harm. Accessed September 28, 2007.

Koocher GP, Keith-Spiegel PC: Children, Ethics, and the Law. Lincoln, University of Nebraska Press, 1990

Kovnick JA, Appelbaum PS, Hoge SK, et al: Competence to consent to research among long-stay inpatients with chronic schizophrenia. Psychiatr Serv 54:1247–1252, 2003

Krill Williston S, Martinez JH, Abdullah T: Mental health stigma among people of color: an examination of the impact of racial discrimination. Int J Soc Psychiatry 65(6):458–467, 2019

Krupat E, Dienstag JL, Padrino SL, et al: Do professionalism lapses in medical school predict problems in residency and clinical practice? Acad Med 95(6):888–895, 2020

LaCombe MA: On professionalism. Am J Med 94(3):329, 1993

Lafollette MC: Stealing Into Print: Fraud, Plagiarism, and Misconduct in Scientific Publishing. Berkeley, University of California Press, 1992

Lake v. Cameron, 364 F.2d 657 (DC Cir 1966)

Lane LW, Lane G, Schiedermayer DL, et al: Caring for medical students as patients. Arch Intern Med 150:2249–2253, 1990

Lane-McKinley K: Creating a culture of belonging, respect, and support on campus, in Student Mental Health: A Guide for Psychiatrists, Psychologists, and Leaders Serving in Higher Education. Edited by Roberts LW. Washington DC, American Psychiatric Association Publishing, 2018, pp 17–32

Lapid MI, Rummans TA, Poole KL, et al: Decisional capacity of severely depressed patients requiring electroconvulsive therapy. J ECT 19:67–72, 2003

Lapid M, Moutier C, Dunn L, et al: Professionalism and ethics education on relationships and boundaries: psychiatric residents' training preferences. Acad Psychiatry 33(6):461–469, 2009

Lawrence RE, Appelbaum PS: Genetic testing in psychiatry: a review of attitudes and beliefs. Psychiatry 74(4):315–331, 2011

Layde JB, Roberts LW: How to write effective letters of recommendation, in Roberts Academic Medicine Handbook, 2nd Edition. Edited by Roberts LW. Cham, Switzerland, Springer, 2020, pp 135–136

Lazarus JA: Ethics in split treatment. Psychiatr Ann 31:611–614, 2001

Levenson JL: Psychiatric commitment and involuntary hospitalization: an ethical perspective. Psychiatr Q 58:106–112, 1986–1987

Levine C, Faden R, Grady C, et al: The limitations of "vulnerability" as a protection for human research participants. Am J Bioeth 4:44–49, 2004

Lidz CW, Appelbaum PS, Grisso T, et al: Therapeutic misconception and the appreciation of risks in clinical trials. Soc Sci Med 58:1689–1697, 2004

Link BG, Phelan JC: Stigma and its public health implications. Lancet 367:528–529, 2006

Link BG, Struening EL, Rahav M, et al: On stigma and its consequences: evidence from a longitudinal study of men with dual diagnoses of mental illness and substance abuse. J Health Soc Behav 38:177–190, 1997

Link BG, Struening EL, Neese-Todd S, et al: Stigma as a barrier to recovery: the consequences of stigma for the self-esteem of people with mental illnesses. Psychiatr Serv 52:1621–1626, 2001

Lo B: Answers and questions about ethics consultations. JAMA 290:1208–1210, 2003

Lo B: Informed consent, in Resolving Ethical Dilemmas: A Guide for Clinicians. Philadelphia, PA, Wolters Kluwer Health, 2020a, pp 18–30

Lo B: Resolving Ethical Dilemmas: A Guide for Clinicians, 4th Edition. Philadelphia, PA, Lippincott Williams & Wilkins, 2020b

Lopez F: Confidentiality of Patient Records for Alcohol and Other Drug Treatment. Technical Assistance Publication (TAP) Series 13. DHHS Publ No (SMA) 95-3018. Rockville, MD, Substance Abuse and Mental Health Services Administration, 1994

Luciano A, Bond GR, Drake RE: Does employment alter the course and outcome of schizophrenia and other severe mental illnesses? A systematic review of longitudinal research. Schizophr Res 159:312–321, 2014

Macapagal K, Bhatia R, Greene GJ: Differences in healthcare access, use, and experiences within a community sample of racially diverse lesbian, gay, bisexual, transgender, and questioning emerging adults. LGBT Health 3(6):434–442, 2016

Macklin R: Ethical relativism in a multicultural society. Kennedy Inst Ethics J 8(1):1–22, 1998

Malley PB, Reilly EP: Legal and Ethical Dimensions for Mental Health Professionals. Philadelphia, PA, Accelerated Development, 1999

Mandal J, Parija SC: Ethics of involving animals in research. Trop Parasitol 3(1):4–6, 2013

Mangino DR, Nicolini ME, De Vries RG, Kim SYH: Euthanasia and assisted suicide of persons with dementia in the Netherlands. Am J Geriatr Psychiatry 28(4):466–477, 2020

Marcello PW: Working with industry: what is the conflict? Clin Colon Rectal Surg 26:12–16, 2010

Marco CA, Larkin GL: Ethics seminars: case studies in "futility"—challenges for academic emergency medicine. Acad Emerg Med 7:1147–1151, 2000

Marks M: Artificial intelligence for suicide prediction. November 6, 2018. Available at: https://blog.petrieflom.law.harvard.edu/2018/11/06/artificial-intelligence-for-suicide-prediction. Accessed May 23, 2020.

Martinez-Martin N, Dunn LB, Roberts LW: Is it ethical to use prognostic estimates from machine learning to treat psychosis? AMA J Ethics 20(9):E804–E811, 2018

Maslach C, Jackson SE: The measurement of experienced burnout. Journal of Organizational Behavior 2(2):99–113, 1981

Maslach C, Leiter MP: Understanding the burnout experience: recent research and its implications for psychiatry. World Psychiatry 15(2):103–111, 2016

Materstvedt LJ, Clark D, Ellershaw J, et al: Euthanasia and physician-assisted suicide: a view from an EAPC Ethics Task Force. Palliat Med 17(2):97–101, 2003

McCarty T, Roberts LW: The difficult patient, in Medicine: A Primary Care Approach. Edited by Rubin RH, Voss C, Derksen DJ, et al. Philadelphia, PA, WB Saunders, 1996, pp 395–399

McCullough LB, Coverdale J, Chervenak FA: Teaching professional formation in response to the COVID-19 pandemic. Acad Med 95(10):1488–1491, 2020

McGirr A, Renaud J, Bureau A, et al: Impulsive-aggressive behaviours and completed suicide across the life cycle: a predisposition for younger age of suicide. Psychol Med 38(3):407–417, 2008

McHugh PR: Psychotherapy awry. Am Scholar 63:17–30, 1994

McHugh PR: Hippocrates à la mode. Nat Med 2:507–509, 1996

McHugh PR, Slavney PR: The Perspectives of Psychiatry, 2nd Edition. Baltimore, MD, Johns Hopkins University Press, 1998

McKinney SM, Sieniek M, Godbole V, et al: International evaluation of an AI system for breast cancer screening. Nature 577(7788):89–94, 2020

Meisel A: A history of the law of assisted dying in the United States. 73 SMU Law Review 119, 2020

Menninger JA: Involuntary treatment: hospitalization and medications, in Psychiatric Secrets, 2nd Edition. Edited by Jacobson JL, Jacobson AM. Philadelphia, PA, Hanley & Belfus, 2001, pp 477–484

Michels R: Are research ethics bad for our mental health? N Engl J Med 340:1427–1430, 1999

Michels R: Research on persons with impaired decision making and the public trust. Am J Psychiatry 161:777–779, 2004

Mischoulon D: An approach to the patient seeking psychiatric disability benefits. Acad Psychiatry 23:128–136, 1999

Morrison J, Wickersham P: Physicians disciplined by a state medical board. JAMA 279:1889–1893, 1998

Moser DJ, Schultz SK, Arndt S, et al: Capacity to provide informed consent for participation in schizophrenia and HIV research. Am J Psychiatry 159:1201–1207, 2002

Moser DJ, Reese RL, Hey CT, et al: Using a brief intervention to improve decisional capacity in schizophrenia research. Schizophr Bull 32:116–120, 2006

Mostaghimi A, Crotty BH: Professionalism in the digital age. Ann Intern Med 154(8):560–562, 2011

Muramoto O: Bioethical aspects of the recent changes in the policy of refusal of blood by Jehovah's witnesses. BMJ 322:37–39, 2001

Murden RA, Way DP, Hudson A, Westman JA: Professionalism deficiencies in a first-quarter doctor-patient relationship course predict poor clinical performance in medical school. Acad Med 79(10 suppl):S46–S48, 2004

Murray H, Wortzel HS: Psychiatric advance directives: origins, benefits, challenges, and future directions. J Psychiatr Pract 25(4):303–307, 2019

Nachum O, Jiang H: Group-based fair learning leads to counter-intuitive predictions. October 4, 2019 [cited January 13, 2020]. Available at: http://arxiv.org/abs/1910.02097. Accessed January 13, 2020.

National Association of Social Workers: NASW Revised Code of Ethics. 2017. Available at: www.socialworkers.org/About/Ethics/Code-of-Ethics/Code-of-Ethics-English. Accessed February 25, 2020.

National Bioethics Advisory Commission: Research Involving Persons with Mental Disorders That May Affect Decisionmaking Capacity. Rockville, MD, National Bioethics Advisory Commission, 1998

National Board for Certified Counselors: Code of ethics. October 7, 2016. Available at: www.nbcc.org/Assets/Ethics/NBCCCodeofEthics.pdf. Accessed February 25, 2020.

National Commission for the Protection of Human Subjects of Biomedical and Behavioral Research: The Belmont Report: Ethical Principles and Guidelines for the Protection of Human Subjects of Research. Washington, DC, U.S. Government Printing Office, April 18, 1979. Available at: www.hhs.gov/ohrp/regulations-and-policy/belmont-report/read-the-belmont-report/index.html. Accessed October 14, 2007.

National Institutes of Health: Genetic discrimination. 2008. Available at: www.genome.gov/about-genomics/policy-issues/Genetic-Discrimination. Accessed March 5, 2020.

Nemani K, Li C, Olfson M, et al: Association of psychiatric disorders with mortality among patients with COVID-19. JAMA Psychiatry 78(4):380–386, 2021

New Freedom Commission on Mental Health: Achieving the Promise: Transforming Mental Health Care in America. Executive Summary. Rockville, MD, Department of Health and Human Services, 2003

New York State Office of Mental Health: Kendra's Law: final report on the status of assisted outpatient treatment. New York, Office of Mental Health, 2005

Norris DM, Gutheil TG, Strasburger LH: This couldn't happen to me: boundary problems and sexual misconduct in the psychotherapy relationship. Psychiatr Serv 54:517–522, 2003

Notredame CE, Morgiève M, Morel F, et al: Distress, suicidality, and affective disorders at the time of social networks. Curr Psychiatry Rep 21:98, 2019

Nurcombe B: Malpractice, in Child and Adolescent Psychiatry: A Comprehensive Textbook, 3rd Edition. Edited by Lewis M. Philadelphia, PA, Lippincott Williams & Wilkins, 2002

O'Connor v. Donaldson, 422 U.S. 563 (1975)

Office for Civil Rights: Summary of the HIPAA Privacy Rule. U.S. Department of Health and Human Services. July 26, 2013. Available at: www.hhs.gov/hipaa/for-professionals/privacy/laws-regulations/index.html. Accessed April 8, 2021.

Office for Civil Rights: Guidance Regarding Methods for De-identification of Protected Health Information in Accordance with the Health Insurance Portability and Accountability Act (HIPAA) Privacy Rule. U.S. Department of Health And Human Services. November 6, 2015. Available at: www.hhs.gov/hipaa/for-professionals/privacy/special-topics/de-identification/index.html. Accessed April 13, 2021.

Office for Human Research Protections: Special protections for children as research subjects. 2005. Available at: www.hhs.gov/ohrp/regulations-and-policy/guidance/special-protections-for-children/index.html. Accessed February 2, 2007.

Office for Human Research Protections: Unanticipated problems involving risks & adverse events guidance. 2016. Available at: www.hhs.gov/ohrp/regulations-and-policy/guidance/reviewing-unanticipated-problems/index.html. Accessed April 24, 2021.

Office for Human Research Protections: Revised common rule Q&As. July 30, 2018. Available at: www.hhs.gov/ohrp/education-and-outreach/revised-common-rule/revised-common-rule-q-and-a/index.html. Accessed July 28, 2020.

Office of Science and Technology Policy: Federal research misconduct policy. Federal Register Dec 6; 65(235):76260–76264, 2000

Ojeda VD, McGuire TG: Gender and racial/ethnic differences in use of outpatient mental health and substance use services by depressed adults. Psychiatr Q 77:211–222, 2006

Okasha A, Arboleda-Florez J, Sartorius N (eds): Ethics, Culture, and Psychiatry: International Perspectives. Washington, DC, American Psychiatric Press, 2000

Oldham JM, Haimowitz S, Delano SJ: Protection of persons with mental disorders from research risk: a response to the report of the National Bioethics Advisory Commission. Arch Gen Psychiatry 56:688–693, 1999

Ostman M, Kjellin L: Stigma by association: psychological factors in relatives of people with mental illness. Br J Psychiatry 181:494–498, 2002

Overstreet MM: Duty to report colleagues who engage in fraud or deception, in Ethics Primer of the American Psychiatric Association. Washington, DC, American Psychiatric Association, 2001, pp 51–56

Ozdemir S, Jafar TH, Choong LHL, Finkelstein EA: Family dynamics in a multi-ethnic Asian society: comparison of elderly CKD patients and their family caregivers experience with medical decision making for managing end stage kidney disease. BMC Nephrol 20(1):73, 2019

Palmer BW, Dunn LB, Appelbaum PS, et al: Assessment of capacity to consent to research among older persons with schizophrenia, Alzheimer disease, or diabetes mellitus: comparison of a 3-item questionnaire with a comprehensive standardized capacity instrument. Arch Gen Psychiatry 62:726–733, 2005

Palmer BW, Dunn LB, Depp CA, et al: Decisional capacity to consent to research among patients with bipolar disorder: comparison with schizophrenia patients and healthy subjects. J Clin Psychiatry 68(5):689–696, 2007

Papadakis MA, Hodgson CS, Teherani A, Kohatsu ND: Unprofessional behavior in medical school is associated with subsequent disciplinary action by a state medical board. Acad Med 79(3):244–249, 2004

Papadakis MA, Teherani A, Banach MA, et al: Disciplinary action by medical boards and prior behavior in medical school. N Engl J Med 353(25):2673–2682, 2005

Pawlik TM: Suspected ethical misconduct in research. Virtual Mentor 11(4):287–290, 2009

Pellegrino ED, Hart RJ Jr, Henderson SR, et al: Relevance and utility of courses in medical ethics. A survey of physicians' perceptions. JAMA 253:49–53, 1985

Percival T: Medical Ethics; or, A Code of Institutes and Precepts, Adapted to the Professional Conduct of Physicians and Surgeons...to Which is Added an Appendix Containing a Discourse on Hospital Duties. Manchester, UK, Russell, 1803

Peris TS, Teachman BA, Nosek BA: Implicit and explicit stigma of mental illness: links to clinical care. J Nerv Ment Dis 196(10):752–760, 2008

Phelan JC, Bromet EJ, Link BG: Psychiatric illness and family stigma. Schizophr Bull 24:115–126, 1998

Pincus HA, Lieberman JA, Ferris S (eds): Ethics in Psychiatric Research: A Resource Manual for Human Subjects Protection. Washington, DC, American Psychiatric Association, 1999

Plaut SM, Baker D: Teacher-student relationships in medical education: Boundary considerations. Med Teach 33(10):828–833, 2011

Post SG (ed): Encyclopedia of Bioethics, 3rd Edition. New York, MacMillan Reference USA, 2004

Post SG, Whitehouse PJ, Binstock RH, et al: The clinical introduction of genetic testing for Alzheimer disease: an ethical perspective. JAMA 277:832–836, 1997

President's Commission for the Study of Ethical Problems in Medicine and Biomedical and Behavioral Research: Making Health Care Decisions: A Report on the Ethical and Legal Implications of Informed Consent in the Patient-Practitioner Relationship, Vol 1: Report—President's Commission for the Study of Ethics Problems in Medicine and Biomedical and Behavioral Research, Washington, DC, U.S. Government Printing Office, 1982

Quill T: Dutch practice of euthanasia and assisted suicide: a glimpse at the edges of the practice, J Med Ethics 44:297–298, 2018

Racy J: Professionalism: sane and insane. J Clin Psychiatry 51:138–140, 1990

Raymont V, Bingley W, Buchanan A, et al: Prevalence of mental incapacity in medical inpatients and associated risk factors: cross-sectional study. Lancet 364:1421–1427, 2004

Reynolds CF 3rd, Frank E: US Preventive Services Task Force Recommendation Statement on Screening for Depression in Adults: not good enough. JAMA Psychiatry 73(3):189–190, 2016

Reynolds PP: Reaffirming professionalism through the education community. Ann Intern Med 120:609–614, 1994

Roberts LW: Ethical dimensions of psychiatric research. A constructive criterion-based approach to protocol preparation: the Research Protocol Ethics Assessment Tool (RePEAT). Biol Psychiatry 46:1106–1119, 1999

Roberts LW: Ethics and mental illness research. Psychiatr Clin North Am 25:525–545, 2002a

Roberts LW: Informed consent and the capacity for voluntarism. Am J Psychiatry 159:705–712, 2002b

Roberts LW: Ethics in psychiatry, in Kaplan & Sadock's Comprehensive Textbook of Psychiatry, 8th Edition. Edited by Sadock BJ, Sadock VA. Philadelphia, PA, Lippincott Williams & Wilkins, 2005, pp 4441–4448.

Roberts LW: Ethical philanthropy in academic psychiatry. Am J Psychiatry 163:772–778, 2006

Roberts LW: A Clinical Guide to Psychiatric Ethics. Arlington, VA, American Psychiatric Association Publishing, 2016

Roberts LW: Addressing authorship issues prospectively: a heuristic approach. Acad Med 92(2):143–146, 2017

Roberts LW: High road, low road: professionalism, trust, and medical education. Acad Med 95(6):817–818, 2020

Roberts LW, Dunn LB: Ethical considerations in psychiatry, in The American Psychiatric Association Publishing Textbook of Psychiatry. Edited by Roberts LW. Washington DC, American Psychiatric Association Publishing, 2019, pp 177–200

Roberts LW, Dyer A: Concise Guide to Ethics in Mental Health Care. Washington, DC, American Psychiatric Publishing, 2004

Roberts LW, Heinrich T: Walking a tightrope: ethics and neuropsychiatric research. Psychiatric Times 22:24–26, 2005

Roberts LW, Kim JP: Giving voice to study volunteers: comparing views of mentally ill, physically ill, and healthy protocol participants on ethical aspects of clinical research. J Psychiatr Res 56:90–97, 2014

Roberts LW, Roberts B: Psychiatric research ethics: an overview of evolving guidelines and current ethical dilemmas in the study of mental illness. Biol Psychiatry 46:1025–1038, 1999

Roberts JS, Uhlmann WR: Genetic susceptibility testing for neurodegenerative diseases: ethical and practice issues. Prog Neurobiol 110:89–101, 2013

Roberts LW, Hardee JT, Franchini G, et al: Medical students as patients: a pilot study of their health care needs, practices, and concerns. Acad Med 71:1225–1232, 1996a

Roberts LW, McCarty T, Roberts BB, et al: Clinical ethics teaching in psychiatric supervision. Acad Psychiatry 20:176–188, 1996b

Roberts LW, Battaglia J, Smithpeter M, et al: An office on Main Street. Health care dilemmas in small communities. Hastings Cent Rep 29:28–37, 1999

Roberts LW, Warner TD, Carter D, et al: Caring for medical students as patients: access to services and care-seeking practices of 1,027 students at nine medical schools. Collaborative Research Group on Medical Student Healthcare. Acad Med 75:272–277, 2000a

Roberts LW, Warner TD, Brody JL: Perspectives of patients with schizophrenia and psychiatrists regarding ethically important aspects of research participation. Am J Psychiatry 157:67–74, 2000b

Roberts LW, Geppert CM, Brody JL: A framework for considering the ethical aspects of psychiatric research protocols. Compr Psychiatry 42:351–363, 2001a

Roberts LW, Warner TD, Lyketsos C, et al: Perceptions of academic vulnerability associated with personal illness: a study of 1,027 students at nine medical schools. Collaborative Research Group on Medical Student Healthcare. Compr Psychiatry 42:1–15, 2001b

Roberts LW, Geppert CM, Bailey R: Ethics in psychiatric practice: essential ethics skills, informed consent, the therapeutic relationship, and confidentiality. J Psychiatr Pract 8:290–305, 2002a

Roberts LW, Warner TD, Brody JL, et al: Patient and psychiatrist ratings of hypothetical schizophrenia research protocols: assessment of harm potential and factors influencing participation decisions. Am J Psychiatry 159:573–584, 2002b

Roberts LW, Geppert C, McCarty T, et al: Evaluating medical students' skills in obtaining informed consent for HIV testing. J Gen Intern Med 18:112–119, 2003

Roberts LW, Green Hammond KA, Geppert CM, et al: The positive role of professionalism and ethics training in medical education: a comparison of medical student and resident perspectives. Acad Psychiatry 28:170–182, 2004a

Roberts LW, Hammond KA, Warner TD, et al: Influence of ethical safeguards on research participation: comparison of perspectives of people with schizophrenia and psychiatrists. Am J Psychiatry 161:2309–2311, 2004b

Roberts LW, Warner TD, Anderson CT, et al: Schizophrenia research participants' responses to protocol safeguards: recruitment, consent, and debriefing. Schizophr Res 67:283–291, 2004c

Roberts LW, Warner TD, Green Hammond KA, et al: Becoming a good doctor: perceived need for ethics training focused on practical and professional development topics. Acad Psychiatry 29:301–309, 2005

Roberts LW, Hammond KG, Hoop J: An inverse relationship between perceived harm and participation willingness in schizophrenia research protocols. Am J Psychiatry 163:2002–2004, 2006

Roberts LW, Warner TD, Dunn L, et al: Shaping medical students' attitudes toward ethically important aspects of clinical research: results of a randomized, controlled educational intervention. Ethics Behav 17:19–50, 2007

Roberts LW, Warner TD, Moutier C, et al: Original Research Reports: Are doctors who have been ill more compassionate? Attitudes of resident physicians regarding personal health issues and the expression of compassion in clinical care. Psychosomatics 52(4):367–374, 2011

Rosato J: The ethics of clinical trials: a child's view. J Law Med Ethics 28:362–378, 2000

Rosenman S: Psychiatrists and compulsion: a map of ethics. Aust N Z J Psychiatry 32:785–793, 1998

Ross LF, Moon MR: Ethical issues in genetic testing of children. Arch Pediatr Adolesc Med 154:873–879, 2000

Ross LF, Loup A, Nelson RM, et al: Nine key functions for a human subjects protection program for community-engaged research: points to consider. J Empir Res Hum Res Ethics 5:33–47, 2010

Rossant J: Gene editing in human development: ethical concerns and practical applications. Development 145(16):dev150888, 2018

Rubenstein L, Pross C, Davidoff F, et al: Coercive US interrogation policies: a challenge to medical ethics. JAMA 294:1544–1549, 2005

Sabin JE, Harland JC: Professional ethics for digital age psychiatry: boundaries, privacy, and communication. Curr Psychiatry Rep 19(9):55, 2017

Sabin JE, Nosek BA, Greenwald A, Rivara FP: Physicians' implicit and explicit attitudes about race by MD race, ethnicity, and gender. J Health Care Poor Underserved 20(3):896–913, 2009

Sachs GA, Stocking CB, Stern R, et al: Ethical aspects of dementia research: informed consent and proxy consent. Clin Res 42:403–412, 1994

Sah S, Fugh-Berman A: Physicians under the influence: social psychology and industry marketing strategies. J Law Med Ethics 41(3):665–672, 2013

Saigle V, Racine E: Ethical challenges faced by healthcare professionals who care for suicidal patients: a scoping review. Monash Bioeth Rev 35(1–4):50–79, 2018

Sallam M, Debabseh D, Eid H, et al: High rates of COVID-19 vaccine hesitancy and its association with conspiracy beliefs: a study in Jordan and Kuwait among other Arab countries. Vaccines 9(1):42, 2021

Samartzis L, Talias MA: Assessing and improving the quality in mental health services. Int J Environ Res Public Health 17(1):249, 2019

Sansone RA, Sansone LA: Crossing the line: sexual boundary violations by physicians. Psychiatry 6:45–48, 2009

Santen SA, Hemphill RR, McDonald MF, et al: Patients' willingness to allow residents to learn to practice medical procedures. Acad Med 79:144–147, 2004

Santen SA, Hemphill RR, Spanier CM, et al: "Sorry, it's my first time!" Will patients consent to medical students learning procedures? Med Educ 39:365–369, 2005

Saposnik G, Redelmeier D, Ruff CC, Tobler PN: Cognitive biases associated with medical decisions: a systematic review. BMC Med Inform Decis Mak 16(1):138, 2016

Saxena A: Ethical understanding among students about bioethical issues, in Ethics in Science: Pedagogic Issues and Concerns. Cham, Switzerland, Springer, 2019, pp 209–230

Schneider BJ, Bradley JC: Ethical considerations of the practice of psychiatry in the military, in Military and Veteran Mental Health. Edited by Roberts LW, Warner CH. New York, Springer, 2018, pp 73–93

Schneider JA, Arora V, Kasza K, et al: Residents' perceptions over time of pharmaceutical industry interactions and gifts and the effect of an educational intervention. Acad Med 81:595–602, 2006

Schraufnagel TJ, Wagner AW, Miranda J, et al: Treating minority patients with depression and anxiety: what does the evidence tell us? Gen Hosp Psychiatry 28:27–36, 2006

Schwartz LM, Woloshin S: Medical marketing in the United States, 1997–2016. JAMA 321(1):80–96, 2019

Shen SC, Dubey V: Addressing vaccine hesitancy: clinical guidance for primary care physicians working with parents. Can Fam Physician 65(3):175–181, 2019

Shenoy A, Appel JM: Safeguarding confidentiality in electronic health records. Camb Q Healthc Ethics 26(2):337–341, 2017

Shim R, Vinson S (eds): Social (In)Justice and Mental Health. Washington, DC, American Psychiatric Association Publishing, 2021

Siegler M: Sounding boards. Confidentiality in medicine—a decrepit concept. N Engl J Med 307:1518–1522, 1982

Siegler M: Training doctors for professionalism: some lessons from teaching clinical medical ethics. Mt Sinai J Med 69:404–409, 2002

Siegler M: Clinical medical ethics, in Clinical Medical Ethics: Landmark Works of Mark Siegler. Edited by Roberts LW, Siegler M. Cham, Switzerland, Springer, 2017, pp 9–16

Simon RI: Clinical Psychiatry and the Law, 2nd Edition. Washington, DC, American Psychiatric Press, 1992

Simon RI, Williams IC: Maintaining treatment boundaries in small communities and rural areas. Psychiatr Serv 50:1440–1446, 1999

Siu AL, US Preventive Services Task Force (USPSTF), Bibbins-Domingo K, et al: Screening for Depression in Adults: US Preventive Services Task Force Recommendation Statement. JAMA 315(4):380–387, 2016

Sjöstrand M, Karlsson P, Sandman L, et al: Conceptions of decision-making capacity in psychiatry: interviews with Swedish psychiatrists. BMC Med Ethics May 21; 16:34, 2015

Slavney PR, McHugh PR: The life-story method in psychotherapy and psychiatric education: the development of confidence. Am J Psychother 39:57–67, 1985

Slavney PR, McHugh PR: Psychiatric Polarities: Methodology and Practice. Baltimore, MD, Johns Hopkins University Press, 1987

Smith E, Master Z: Best practice to order authors in multi-interdisciplinary health sciences research publications. Accountability in Research 24(4):243–267, 2017

Smith RC: Teaching interviewing skills to medical students: the issue of "countertransference." J Med Educ 59:582–588, 1984

Snyder Sulmasy L, Bledsoe TA, for the ACP Ethics, Professionalism and Human Rights Committee: American College of Physicians Ethics Manual: Seventh Edition. Ann Intern Med 170:S1–S32, 2019

Spellecy R, Roberts LW: Developing your ethics skills, in Handbook of Career Development in Academic Psychiatry and Behavioral Sciences. Edited by Roberts LW, Hilty DM. Washington, DC, American Psychiatric Publishing, 2006, pp 133–144

Springmann RR: Reflections on the role of the supervisor. Br J Med Psychol 62:217–228, 1989

Srebnik D, Appelbaum PS, Russo J: Assessing competence to complete psychiatric advance directives with the competence assessment tool for psychiatric advance directives. Compr Psychiatry 45:239–245, 2004

Srebnik DS, Rutherford LT, Peto T, et al: The content and clinical utility of psychiatric advance directives. Psychiatr Serv 56:592–598, 2005

Stern DT, Frohna AZ, Gruppen LD: The prediction of professional behaviour. Med Educ 39(1):75–82, 2005

Stern TA, Freudenreich O, Smith FA, et al (eds): Massachusetts General Hospital Handbook of General Hospital Psychiatry, 7th Edition. Edinburgh, Scotland, Elsevier, 2018

Stobo JD, Blank LL: American Board of Internal Medicine's Project Professionalism: staying ahead of the wave. Am J Med 97:1–3, 1994

Stockman AF: Dual relationships in rural mental health practice: an ethical dilemma. Journal of Rural Community Psychology 11:31–45, 1990

Stoudemire A, Rhoads JM: When the doctor needs a doctor: special considerations for the physician-patient. Ann Intern Med 98:654–659, 1983

Strasburger LH, Gutheil TG, Brodsky A: On wearing two hats: role conflict in serving as both psychotherapist and expert witness. Am J Psychiatry 154:448–456, 1997

Stroup S, Appelbaum P, Swartz M, et al: Decision-making capacity for research participation among individuals in the CATIE schizophrenia trial. Schizophr Res 80(1):1–8, 2005

Studdert DM, Mello MM, Brennan TA: Financial conflicts of interest in physicians' relationships with the pharmaceutical industry—self-regulation in the shadow of federal prosecution. N Engl J Med 351:1891–1900, 2004

Sue DW, Capodilupo CM, Torino GC, et al: Racial microaggressions in everyday life: implications for clinical practice. Am Psychol 62(4):271–286, 2007

Sugarman J: Twenty Common Problems: Ethics in Primary Care. New York, McGraw-Hill Professional, 2000

Sullivan MD, Youngner SJ: Depression, competence, and the right to refuse lifesaving medical treatment. Am J Psychiatry 151:971–978, 1994

Swanson JW, Swartz MS: Why the evidence for outpatient commitment is good enough. Psychiatr Serv 65(6):808–811, 2014

Swanson JW, McGinty EE, Fazel S, Mays VM: Mental illness and reduction of gun violence and suicide: bringing epidemiologic research to policy. Ann Epidemiol 25(5):366–376, 2015

Szasz TS: Involuntary psychiatry. University of Cincinnati Law Rev 45:347–365, 1976

Talbott JA, Mallott DB: Professionalism, medical humanism, and clinical bioethics: the new wave—does psychiatry have a role? J Psychiatr Pract 12:384–390, 2006

Tarasoff v. Regents of the University of California, 17 Cal.3d 425; 551 P.2d 334 (Cal. Rptr 14, 1976)

Testa M, West SG: Civil commitment in the United States. Psychiatry (Edgmont) 7(10):30–40, 2010

Thienpont L, Verhofstadt M, Van Loon T, et al: Euthanasia requests, procedures and outcomes for 100 Belgian patients suffering from psychiatric disorders: a retrospective, descriptive study. BMJ Open 5(7), 2015

Toomey J: On social suicide prevention. Don't let the perfect be the enemy of the good. February 20, 2019. Available at: https://blog.petrieflom.law.harvard.edu/2019/02/20/on-social-suicide-prevention-dont-let-the-perfect-be-the-enemy-of-the-good. Accessed May 23, 2020.

Torous J, Roberts LW: The ethical use of mobile health technology in clinical psychiatry. J Nerv Ment Dis 205(1):4–8, 2017

Trials of War Criminals Before the Nuremberg Military Tribunals Under Control Council Law No 10, Vol 1. Washington, DC, U. S. Government Printing Office, 1946–1949

Tseng W, Streltzer J: Introduction: culture and psychiatry, in Cultural Competence in Clinical Psychiatry. Edited by Tseng W, Streltzer J. Washington, DC, American Psychiatric Publishing, 2004, pp 1–20

Ubel PA, Zell MM, Miller DJ, et al: Elevator talk: observational study of inappropriate comments in a public space. Am J Med 99:190–194, 1995

United Nations: Principles of Medical Ethics Relevant to the Role of Health Personnel, Particularly Physicians, in the Protection of Prisoners and Detainees Against Torture and Other Cruel, Inhuman or Degrading Treatment or Punishment. Adopted by General Assembly resolution 37/194 of 18 December 1982

United Nations Office on Drugs, Crime, Division for Treaty Affairs Staff, United Nations Office on Drugs & Crime, Division for Treaty Affairs: Legislative Guides for the Implementation of the United Nations Convention Against Transnational Organized Crime and the Protocols Thereto. Geneva, United Nations, 2004

U.S. Advisory Committee on Human Radiation Experiments: Final Report of the President's Advisory Committee on Human Radiation Experiments. New York, Oxford University Press, 1996

U.S. Copyright Office: Copyright Law of the United States and Related Laws Contained in Title 17 of the United States Code. Circular 92. June 2020. Available at: www.copyright.gov/title17/title17.pdf. Accessed August 5, 2020

U.S. Department of Health and Human Services: The Health Insurance Portability and Accountability Act (HIPAA) of 1996. Available at: https://aspe.hhs.gov/report/health-insurance-portability-and-accountability-act-1996. Accessed April 24, 2021

U.S. Department of Health and Human Services: Mental Health: A Report of the Surgeon General—Executive Summary. Rockville, MD, U.S. Department of Health and Human Services, Substance Abuse and Mental Health Services Administration, Center for Mental Health Services, National Institutes of Health, National Institute of Mental Health, 1999

U.S. Department of Health and Human Services: Mental Health: Culture, Race, and Ethnicity—A Supplement to Mental Health: A Report of the Surgeon General. Rockville, MD, Department of Health and Human Services, Substance Abuse and Mental Health Services Administration, Center for Mental Health Services, 2001

U.S. Department of Health and Human Services: HIPAA Administrative Simplification. March 26, 2013. Available at: www.hhs.gov/sites/default/files/hipaa-simplification-201303.pdf. Accessed July 26, 2020.

U.S. Department of Health and Human Services: CFR: Title 45 Public Welfare Department of Health and Human Services Part 46 Protection of Human Subjects. 2018. Available at: www.ecfr.gov/cgi-bin/text-idx?SID=ebb7d1155f77df9745c0f2b93e906228&mc=true&tpl=/ecfrbrowse/Title45/45cfr46_main_02.tpl. Accessed July 30, 2020

U.S. Department of Justice: Fighting discrimination in employment under the ADA Information and Technical Assistance on the Americans with Disabilities Act. 2020a. Available at: www.ada.gov/employment.htm. Accessed July 27, 2020.

U.S. Department of Justice: Harvard University professor and two Chinese nationals charged in three separate China related cases. January 28, 2020b. Available at: www.justice.gov/opa/pr/harvard-university-professor-and-two-chinese-nationals-charged-three-separate-china-related. Accessed March 4, 2020.

U.S. Equal Employment Opportunity Commission: Harassment. 2020a. Available at: www.eeoc.gov/harassment. Accessed July 29, 2020.

U.S. Equal Employment Opportunity Commission: Pandemic Preparedness in the Workplace and the Americans with Disabilities Act. March 21, 2020b. Available at: www.eeoc.gov/laws/guidance/pandemic-preparedness-workplace-and-americans-disabilities-act. Accessed April 7, 2021.

U.S. Equal Employment Opportunity Commission: What is employment discrimination? 2020c. Available at: https://www.eeoc.gov/youth/what-employment-discrimination. Accessed July 27, 2020.

Van de Camp K, Vernooij-Dassen MJ, Grol RP, et al: How to conceptualize professionalism: a qualitative study. Med Teach 8:696–702, 2004

Vayena E, Blasimme A, Cohen IG: Machine learning in medicine: addressing ethical challenges. PLoS Med 15(11):e1002689, 2018

Walsh CG, Ribeiro JD, Franklin JC: Predicting risk of suicide attempts over time through machine learning. Clin Psychol Sci 5(3):457–469, 2017

Warner TD, Roberts LW: Scientific integrity, fidelity and conflicts of interest in research. Curr Opin Psychiatry 17:381–385, 2004

Wazana A: Physicians and the pharmaceutical industry: is a gift ever just a gift? JAMA 283:373–380, 2000

Wear D, Nixon LL: Literary inquiry and professional development in medicine: against abstractions. Perspect Biol Med 45(1):104–124, 2004

Werner RM, Alexander GC, Fagerlin A, et al: Lying to insurance companies: the desire to deceive among physicians and the public. Am J Bioeth 4:53–59, 2004

West J, Zarin DA, Hill T, et al: Industry and academia collaboration in psychiatric research, in Research Funding and Resource Manual: Mental Health and Addictive Disorders. Edited by Pincus HA. Washington, DC, American Psychiatric Association, 1995

Williams JH, Dawson A: Prioritising access to pandemic influenza vaccine: a review of the ethics literature. BMC Medical Ethics 21:40, 2020

Williams LM: Precision psychiatry: a neural circuit taxonomy for depression and anxiety. Lancet Psychiatry 3(5):472–480, 2016

Wilson N, Kariisa M, Seth P, et al: Drug and opioid-involved overdose deaths—United States, 2017–2018. MMWR Morb Mortal Wkly Rep 69(11):290–297, 2020

Wilson ST, Stanley B: Ethical concerns in schizophrenia research: looking back and moving forward. Schizophr Bull 32:30–36, 2006

Winsper C, Singh SP, Marwaha S, et al: Pathways to violent behavior during first-episode psychosis: a report from the UK National EDEN study. JAMA Psychiatry 70(12):1287–1293, 2013

Wofford JL, Ohl CA: Teaching appropriate interactions with pharmaceutical company representatives: the impact of an innovative workshop on student attitudes. BMC Med Educ 5:5, 2005

Woltmann E, Grogan-Kaylor A, Perron B, et al: Comparative effectiveness of collaborative chronic care models for mental health conditions across primary, specialty, and behavioral health care settings: systematic review and meta-analysis. Am J Psychiatry 169(8):790–804, 2012

World Health Organization: Care of Girls and Women Living With Female Genital Mutilation: A Clinical Handbook. Geneva, World Health Organization, 2018

World Medical Association: Declaration of Helsinki: ethical principles for medical research involving human subjects. World Medical Association, Ferney-Volatire, France, 1964. Available at: www.wma.net/policies-post/wma-declaration-of-helsinki-ethical-principles-for-medical-research-involving-human-subjects. Accessed August 3, 2020.

World Medical Association: Declaration of Tokyo—Guidelines for Physicians Concerning Torture and Other Cruel , Inhuman or Degrading Treatment or Punishment in Relation to Detention and Imprisonment. Adopted by the 29th World Medical Assembly, Tokyo, Japan, October 1975

World Medical Association: Resolution on the responsibility of physicians in the denunciation of acts of torture or cruel or inhuman or degrading treatment of which they are aware. Adopted by the World Medical Association in 2003.

Wynia MK: The role of professionalism and self-regulation in detecting impaired or incompetent physicians. JAMA 304(2):210–212, 2010

Wynia MK, Latham SR, Kao AC, et al: Medical professionalism in society. N Engl J Med 341(21):1612–1616, 1999

Yarbrough E: Transgender Mental Health. Washington, DC, American Psychiatric Association Publishing, 2018

Yarbrough E: Gender dysphoria, in The American Psychiatric Association Publishing Textbook of Psychiatry, 7th Edition. Edited by Roberts LW. Washington, DC, American Psychiatric Association Publishing, 2019, pp 597–611

Yellowlees P: Physician Suicide: Cases and Commentaries. Washington, DC, American Psychiatric Association Publishing, 2019

Yeung S, Downing NL, Fei-Fei L, Milstein A: Bedside computer vision—moving artificial intelligence from driver assistance to patient safety. N Engl J Med 378(14):1271–1273, 2018

Yeung S, Rinaldo F, Jopling J, et al: A computer vision system for deep learning-based detection of patient mobilization activities in the ICU. NPJ Digit Med March 1; 2:11, 2019

Young SD, Monin B, Owens D: Opt-out testing for stigmatized diseases: a social psychological approach to understanding the potential effect of recommendations for routine HIV testing. Health Psychol 28(6):675–681, 2009

Yu R, Geddes JR, Fazel S: Personality disorders, violence, and antisocial behavior: a systematic review and meta-regression analysis. J Pers Disord 26(5):775–792, 2012

Zilber C: Is it ethical to "google" patients? Psychiatric News 49:20, August 5, 2014. Available at: https://psychnews.psychiatryonline.org/doi/full/10.1176/appi.pn.2014.9a22. Accessed February 26, 2020.

Subject Index

Page numbers printed in **boldface** type refer to tables or figures.

Q&A Index

Principles of Medical Ethics With Anno-
tations Especially Applicable to
Psychiatry (American Psychiatric
Association), 6.5, 6.9
Prisoners
ethical guidelines for treatment
of, 7.63
as research subjects, 5.19
Privacy Rule, and data deidentifica-
tion, 5.35
Process-based approach, to end-of-
life treatment, 4.49
Professionalism. *See* Fidelity; Justice;
Veracity
Public health, 3.2, 4.12, 4.25
Psychiatric advance directives, 3.28,
4.32
Psychology, 6.14, 6.18, 6.22
Psychosis, 4.45, 5.10, 7.27
Pythagoras, 3.32

Quality of life, 3.20, 4.49

Referrals, 3.26, 4.47, 6.1, 7.6
Refusal of treatment, 4.39, 6.24, 7.2,
7.56, 7.67
Release-of-information forms, 4.31
Religion, 3.17, 3.19, 3.41, 6.24, 7.2
Reporting. *See* Child abuse
Research. *See also Belmont Report;*
Institutional review boards
adverse events and audit of, 5.30
animals and ethical conduct of,
5.8, 5.32
anonymous methods for data collection, 5.14
children and, 5.21, 5.22
conflicts of interest and, 5.11, 5.27
data safety and data use, 5.35
errors in, 5.24
examples of ethical violations,
3.21, 5.9, 7.25
human subjects and regulations,
3.15, 5.16, 5.19, 5.26, 5.34,
5.36, 7.17, 7.61

incentives for participation, 5.12
informed consent for, 3.11, 5.12,
5.21
justice as bioethics principle for,
5.6, 5.9
"minimal risk" benchmark for,
5.34
misconduct and, 5.2, 5.5, 5.24,
5.28, 7.52, 7.73
motivations for participation, 5.3
safeguards for patients with mental illness, 5.10, 5.19
scientific equipoise and, 5.15
scientific rigor and value of, 5.18
therapeutic misconceptions and,
3.11, 7.26
Residents. *See also* Education; Medical students; Trainees
depression and suicidality in, 6.15
pharmaceutical industry and conflicts of interest, 6.16
power and requests for personal
errands, 6.26
social relationships with faculty,
6.11
use of titles, 6.24
veracity of process notes, 6.19
veracity in letters of recommendation, 6.20
working relationships and behavior of, 6.8
Respect. *See also* Autonomy
definition of, 5.33
examples of, 7.53
group therapy and, 3.17
history of psychiatry and violations of, 3.34
human subjects research and, 5.1,
5.9
Risk assessment
human subjects research and,
7.17
suicide and, 4.55
Rural psychiatry, 3.14, 3.23
Rush, Benjamin, 3.27